The Homeopathic Journey

The Homeopathic Journey

A Guide for Learners, Teachers, and Leaders

by Todd Rowe, MD, MD(H), CCH, DHt

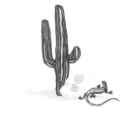

Desert Institute Publishing

Published by Desert Institute Publishing
Printed in the United States of America.

Editing and project management by Via Press, Phoenix, AZ
Cover and interior design by The Printed Page, Phoenix, AZ

Library of Congress Card Number: 2002108272
ISBN: 0-9720224-0-6

To my mother, Bonnie Rowe
who devoted her life to learning
and teaching

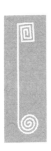

Acknowledgments

This book was a community effort. I received extensive input and advice from the homeopathic community.

In particular I wish to greatly thank Karla Olson of Via Press. In addition, my thanks go to Thelma Rowe, PsyD, and Sara Cota, MSW, for assistance in editing. Thanks to Lisa Liddy of the Printed Page for book design.

I am also greatly indebted to the following:
Loretta Bardewyck, RN
Iris Bell, MD, MD(H)
Mark Brody, MD
Ted Chapman, MD
Melanie Chimes, MD, MD(H)
Yolande Grill, CCH, HMA
Patrick Hesselmann
Greta Holmes
Cheryl Johnnson, HMA
Kathy Lukas
Bill Mann, LAc
Kirk Mann, LAc
Jose Mullen, MD, MD(H)
Marlena Mulvey
Eileen Nauman, EMT
Richard Plant, DC, CCH
Joie Rowles, PharmD, HMA
Louise Sanchione, ND, HMA
Dana Ulman, MPH
Julian Winston

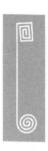

Foreword

Todd Rowe tackles a largely neglected topic—homeopathic education with thoroughness, creativity and great personal insight. He lays out a detailed road map for the homeopathic journey which many of us have been compelled to pursue, often with little formal preparation. Rowe acknowledges that being either a competent practitioner or an able teacher does not automatically ensure a successful homeopathic educator; one must be both.

Rowe's book provides in-depth guidance for all participants—be they students, teachers or administrators. His guide delineates what a perspective homeopathic student should look for and what an engaged homeopathic student can expect. Rowe's broad knowledge of current educational theory and practice provides the homeopathic teacher with a framework for defining their profession and ample means to assess their success. For homeopathic administrators, he skillfully explores the vital and complementary roles of leadership and management.

The Homeopathic Journey is a book which fills a definite need in today's homeopathic community—the need to know what we are about, and how to go about, teaching the "Great Subject" of homeopathy. The journey is finely described with clear and well-defined markers at every turn. This book will be a helpful companion for every homeopathic student, learner and leader.

—Eric Sommermann, Ph.D., RSHom,
Dean, Northwestern Academy of Homeopathy

Contents

We shall not cease from exploration
And the end to all our exploring
Will be to arrive where we started
And know the place for the first time.
—T. S. Eliot

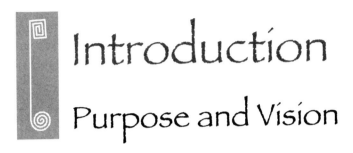

Introduction

Purpose and Vision

Education is not the filling of a pail,
but the lighting of a fire.
—William Butler Yeats

The Homeopathic Journey was written to help individuals take the next step in their homeopathic education, whether as student, teacher or administrator. It provides a basic road map and describes what can be expected on one's homeopathic educational journey.

The book is also an attempt to portray the heart of homeopathic education. The hope is that readers will find herein that which sustains, supports and motivates them through the vicissitudes of their own educational process. The wonder and majesty of homeopathic education are explored to help inspire the reader.

Homeopathic education is concerned with more than content. Most students are taught what to learn in homeopathy, but not how to learn it. Similarly most teachers and administrators are taught what to teach and administrate, but not how. This book focuses more on process than content. It describes the dynamics of transformation on the homeopathic journey.

I've been involved in homeopathic education for many years. Much of this work has been at the Desert Institute School of Classical Homeopathy in Phoenix, Arizona. I've also taught and learned at several other schools around the country, as well as being on the board of directors of the Council on Homeopathic Education. My work as the president of the National Center for Homeopathy and on the board of the Council for Homeopathic Certification has helped me explore homeopathic leadership.

This project began in response to the many students and faculty who have asked how they might become more effective learners and teachers. It also originated from their struggles with the process of homeopathic education and their desire for a road map to guide them on their journey. Lastly, it grew out of my own and my colleagues' struggles in administrating homeopathic schools and training programs.

This work represents a first step in articulating what it is to engage in the journey of homeopathic education. It is the outgrowth of a community project and reflects a shared vision of homeopathic education. As no one has examined many of these issues in homeopathy before, this book embarks on new ground.

Few issues engender more controversy than education. This book itself may appear controversial to some. Inevitably, there will be material with which the reader disagrees. Please note that I've focused more on inspiring wonder and stimulating readers' thinking, feelings and memories than on providing answers to the difficult questions mentioned herein.

For some, this book may seem complex and difficult. It holds forth the highest ideals of homeopathic education. The reader should not expect to encompass all the requisite qualities, knowledge and skills contained herein. This is a journey, and it is important to work on one piece at a time. For others, this material may appear too oversimplified and romanticized. Yet, homeopathy is both an art and a science. It offers learners both a well-laid out logic and a deep sense of mystery.

Who Should Read this Book?

Education is not a product:
mark, diploma, job, money-in that order;
it is a process, a never-ending one.
—Bel Kaufman

This book is designed for anyone with an interest in homeopathic education. In particular, it is for students, teachers, leaders and administrators. Homeopathic education is life-long process; there is always another step along the way. This work is a guide to that process.

Many students drop out of homeopathic training, lacking awareness of what to expect on the homeopathic journey. The book will help students of all levels identify the skills, attitudes and knowledge necessary to the effective study of homeopathy. It also will assist them in determining where they are on their educational journey and what their next steps will be.

For teachers, the book will help pinpoint the skills, attitudes and knowledge necessary for the effective teaching of homeopathy. It is designed as much for beginning lecturers as for veteran teachers, public speakers, and clinical educators.

Finally, this work provides material to aid homeopathic educational leaders and administrators in identifying the skills, attitudes and knowledge necessary to effective leadership in homeopathy. Further, it describes both the leadership and management qualities needed for good homeopathic administration.

On the Nature of Homeopathic Education

I have never let my school interfere with my education.
—Mark Twain

There is little written about homeopathic education. The majority of the greatest homeopaths remain silent on this subject, despite years of dedicated teaching. Most of today's writing about homeopathic education focuses on curriculum content and training standards. It is beyond the scope of this book to discuss these issues, although some of these standards are included in the appendices.

Much of the homeopathic education of the past has been allopathically focused. ("Allopathy" is another term for conventional medicine.) Even today, homeopathic educators typically borrow administrating, teaching and learning methods from allopathic medicine and apply them to homeopathy. Allopathic methods, inculcated into them in their own past, are the methods they know. Many are surprised when this approach fails. A goal of this book is to explore a method of educating that is homeopathically oriented. This is a challenge. It means leading, teaching and learning in ways that are new and may not be comfortable. This takes courage.

Homeopathic education is different from many other fields of education. At bottom, it is learning about all life. It is extraordinarily broad in its scope. Because of this, learning and teaching homeopathy is not easy. It necessitates change and requires growth on deep levels. The training is prolonged, individualized and emotionally charged. This book is an attempt to be honest about this, as well as to describe the great joys in the process.

Homeopathy as a Craft

Every time we teach a child something,
we keep him from inventing it himself.
—Jean Piaget

Homeopathy is a profession. A profession is defined as "an occupation that regulates itself through systematic required training and collegial discipline and that has a base in specialized knowledge and that has a service, rather than profit orientation in its code of conduct (Starr 1982).

There are three types of professional practice. These include technologies, arts and crafts (Oakeshott 1962). Technologies use and require definitely classifiable circumstances. They demand specialized technical knowledge. Arts utilize methods that are more idiosyncratic, relying on insight. Arts require predominantly practical knowledge. Crafts employ well established methods of practice. These methods are used in a wide range of circumstances and are aimed toward an indefinite, but desired result. Crafts require significant components of both technical and practical knowledge. Homeopathy is predominantly a craft. Homeopathic education must be targeted not only toward technical knowledge, but also toward practical knowledge.

Contemporary professional education is in trouble. Educational literature contains many studies that demonstrate a large gap between education and practice. The vast majority of professionals, regardless of discipline, feel that they have been poorly prepared for practice. Homeopathy is no exception. Most homeopathic training programs have neglected clinical training and skill development, while focusing on academic knowledge and allopathic models of teaching. Homeopathic and professional education must reform or become a target of an increasingly skeptical society.

The Educational Journey

It is in passionate leaps of faith that we propel the human spirit forward.
The safety of the known, which only leads to boredom, stifles
the experience of life. As with heroes everywhere, the course of
our lives may become a beacon to others who are on their own quests.
—Carl Hammerschlag

One description of the homeopathic educational journey is miasmatic. In homeopathy, miasms describe an underlying predisposition towards disease. They were initially described by Hahnemann as the source and "tinder to chronic diseases." He described three main miasms, psoric, sycotic and syphilitic. Later, others have added new miasms, including the acute miasm. Sankaran (1994) expanded the concept of miasms and described them as important in categorizing disease states, describing different types of reactions and embodying differing perceptions of reality.

Recently, the concept of miasms has been expanded to describe phases of human development and evolution (Van der Zee 2000). In this way, miasms can also be used to describe growth during the homeopathic educational journey. They become part of the process of becoming who we truly are.

The initial phase of the journey is the "acute miasm." This is the phase in which students respond to the calling and begin their odyssey. Here individuals make a break from their previous life and world. It is a departure from their usual state, from the known, and requires courage. It is their first contact with homeopathy. Often during this stage there is a shock, a feeling of freedom. This is coupled with excitement, enthusiasm, fear and insight. The mythologies that best describe this are the creation myths, where a movement is made out of the known into the unknown.

Next comes the "psoric miasm," the world of the student. This is the stage of establishing identity, curiosity, initiative, optimism, expectation, knowledge development, confidence, nostalgia and trying. Here the student learns the work and forms an identity as a homeopath in relationship to the world. The mythologies that best describe this phase are the hero myths. These myths typically involve a journey and confrontations of both inner and outer dragons. The hero ultimately sees things once invisible and does things once impossible.

This book describes the difficult transition from student to teacher. Most homeopathic teachers engage in teaching with much enthusiasm but little teaching experience. We expect, naively, to be able to move from being a good practitioner to becoming a good teacher with ease. Good practitioners do not necessarily make the best teachers. The skills required are quite different. The "sycotic miasm" is the world of the teacher and practitioner. This is the stage of exploring issues concerning endurance, empathy, tolerance and freedom from prejudice, exploring the shadow and the unconscious, forgiveness, honesty, self-appreciation and self-condemnation. In this phase of the journey, the teacher and practitioner encounter those hidden and unaccepted parts of themselves ("shadow work") which are brought to the surface to be examined. The mythologies that best describe this are the underworld myths. The underworld myths involve a movement into the darkness to better see the light.

Another difficult transition is that from teacher to administrator. An administrator is often described as a "teacher leader" or "teacher supervisor." Chapter Three attempts to explore how this process occurs and the challenges and pitfalls that accompany it.

Finally, the "syphilitic miasm" is the realm of the leader and administrator. This is the stage of issues concerning death and rebirth, creativity, courage, responsibility, performance, self-assertion, isolation, egotism, altruism and service. Here homeopaths find that they are not enough in themselves, and the need for community increasingly grows. Individuals learn to take responsibility for their actions and integrate their work with that of others. This is the alchemical phase of the journey where lead is transmuted into gold. The mythologies that best describe this are the transformation myths.

Ultimately, the homeopathic journey moves full circle as leaders become students once again. In the syphilitic miasm phase of the journey, leaders destroy their creations to make room for new learning and growth. The end of one quest becomes the beginning of another. Through this transformational process homeopaths realize themselves and their potential in the world.

Educating Homeopathically

> *It will now be clear that the science of homeopathic therapeutics makes exacting demands on the physician who prefers it to other forms of treatment. Homeopathy refuses to reveal its secrets to a casual inquirer. It caters essentially to the idealistic type of mind which craves of the satisfaction that comes from a job well done and which considers material gains as only incidental. It will suit the hard working conscientious physician with a philosophical bent of mind which takes readily to the study of emotional and intellectual sides of man.*
> —"Principles and Practice of Homeopathy"

Through incorporating homeopathic methodology into the teaching process, homeopathic students learn not only the content but also the process of homeopathy. What would it mean to find a "homeopathic" method for homeopathic education? The following is a summary of some key ideas expanded on throughout this book.

Law of Similars

Most important, educating homeopathically means finding a method of education that is "similar" to what is being learned. Likes are educated by likes. Good educators incorporate the material of what they teach into the process of education itself.

Individualization

The uniqueness of each learner, teacher and school must be sought and honored. This also means matching the uniqueness of the student with the uniqueness of the teacher, matching the uniqueness of each student with the uniqueness of a training program and matching the uniqueness of each faculty with that of educational administration. Good educators honor their own and their students' individuality.

Holistic View

Wholeness is an important goal of education. Homeopathic education is more than knowledge (often the focus of allopathic education). It also addresses the actions, heart and spirit. Homeopathic education flows from experience.

Homeopathy is in part a vocation. A set of skills and behaviors must be modeled by the homeopathic teacher and practiced by the homeopathic student. Similarly, this skill must be modeled by the homeopathic administrator and practiced by the homeopathic teacher.

The emotional side of homeopathic education is often neglected but critical to developing homeopaths. What attitudes and emotions are necessary to becoming a good homeopath? On this subject, homeopathic education parallels the education of psychotherapists, and much can be learned from this model.

Education also has a spiritual side that is seldom discussed. Most contemporary education takes the allopathic approach of separating the material from the spiritual. What does it mean to educate spiritually? Most schools abandon the inner world, yet by ignoring the spiritual side, wholeness is not achieved. True learning requires openness to the unknown and to mystery. It requires practicing basic respect and openness to the world, to our craft, to our faculty, to our students and to ourselves. Good educators live their craft.

Homeopathy as a Great Subject

There are three models to teaching: a teacher-centered model, a student-centered model and a subject-centered model. In the teacher-centered model, the teacher becomes the center of the classroom, pontificating from the lectern. This is the traditional method of teaching that encourages authoritarianism in the teacher and passive dependence in the students.

In the student-centered model, the students are the center of the classroom, while the teacher tends to function as a facilitator on the periphery. This is a newer model that is quite popular today. It encourages independence and self-learning in the student, yet in doing so often misses the heart and mystery of homeopathy. Lacking a clear sense of purpose, such classes can degenerate and wander.

In the subject-centered model, the "Great Subject" becomes the center of the classroom. Here the students, teachers and administrators keep coming back to the greatness of the source, which is homeopathy. The great subject rests on a firm, unchanging foundation that inspires its learners on all levels of their being. Unlike allopathic medicine, homeopathy represents a great subject:

> *Homeopathy while not perfect, is complete in all its essentials*
> *as a system. It is supreme within its legitimate sphere because*
> *it is the only method of therapeutic medication which is based*
> *on a fixed and definite law of nature. Medicine (allopathy) is*
> *a vast plain where a multitude of people pass back and forth;*
> *some carry bricks, others pebbles, others grains of sand, but no*
> *one dreams of the cement. The mass of such labors and facts is*
> *enormous, no reader can wade through them—but no one has*
> *any general doctrine except the homeopaths.*
> —Marchand de Calvi

Resonance

Resonance of energy occurs throughout the educational process. This resonance leads individuals forward on their homeopathic journey. Ancient wisdom says "when the student is ready, the teacher appears." Similarly, when the teacher is ready, the leader appears. Finally, when the leader is ready, the student appears. It is also the resonance between students, teachers and administrators that allows effective homeopathic education to occur.

Less Is More

By the Law of the Minimum Dose, less is more. Teaching and learning homeopathy means being comfortable with silence. Silence is seldom honored in the allopathic classroom. In an increasingly hurried world, the pace of education has dramatically increased, leaving little time for reflection and self-observation. Yet reflection and silence are that part of education where the greatest learning takes place. This involves developing the capacity to listen actively, perceive deeply and see the whole. It requires patience and comfort with waiting.

Freedom from Prejudice

In homeopathy, the concept of prejudice is central in the development of quality case taking and case analysis skills. Good homeopaths strive work to be free of any kind of prejudice of the mind to be effective in their work.

Homeopathic education also means developing freedom from prejudice. Prejudice prevents educators from being fully present in their work. To develop freedom from prejudice, one must first know oneself. This is a never-ending process. Education is a mirror that allows the individual to glimpse his own face. This self-awareness is vital to effective homeopathic practice, teaching and administration.

It is also necessary to develop the capacity for openness of the mind, heart and spirit. This means understanding the psyche and becoming comfortable with such concepts as transference, counter-transference and projection. It requires embracing all types of diversity.

Succussion, Dilution and Potency

The process of the preparation of homeopathic remedies requires both succussion (vigorous shaking) and dilution for potentization (maximum strength) to occur. Homeopathic education is a constant process of succussion, dilution and potentization. It is an ebb-and-flow, a movement forward here and backward there. Education is a chaotic and non-linear process. It can be very hard at times to see where the individual learner stands in this process. Yet with each repetition of the material, the student is brought deeper into the wonder and mystery of homeopathy. Each homeopathic class is a preparation of the remedy that is homeopathy.

Empiricism

Homeopathy reflects a system of healing based upon the therapeutic tradition of Empiricism, whereas allopathic medicine is based upon the tradition of Rationalism (Coulter 1973). These two forms of healing have been in conflict throughout the centuries. Education has much to learn from both the Rational and Empiric traditions.

Rationalistic education predominates in the world today. Rationalist education focuses on knowledge, rigid logic and pathologic theory. It seeks to put labels on phenomena and strongly separates students, teachers and leaders. The rationalistic educator needs to stay in command and become the ultimate judge of how education should occur.

What would it mean to find an empirical basis to teaching, learning and leading? Empirical education values experience and careful observation. It seeks to identify the manifest patterns of disease, health and education. It explores the commonalties of the educational process and the similarities between student, teacher and leader.

Dynamis

Homeopathy is a form of energy medicine. Hahnemann described it as a field that is concerned with "dynamis." This "dynamis" represents the vital force that is found within our clients, our remedies and ourselves. Homeopathic education must also be dynamic, energetic, movement-oriented and transformative. Homeopathic educators bring their dynamic vital force into their work through their energy and enthusiasm for homeopathy.

Obstacles

Effective treatment in homeopathy requires removing the "obstacles to cure" in the healing process (Hahnemann). These obstacles consist of behaviors within the client that prevent homeopathic treatment from moving forward. There are also "obstacles to learn" in homeopathy that must be overcome before the learning journey can begin. Learning cannot commence until these obstacles are removed. There are similar "obstacles to teach" and "obstacles to leadership" in homeopathy.

Structure of this Book

In seed time learn,
in harvest teach,
in winter enjoy.
—William Blake

The book is divided into three parts: learning, teaching and administrating. In designing a book on homeopathic education, it is impossible to talk about one without the others. Appendix A includes a diagram of the dynamic interplay between teaching, learning and administrating in homeopathic education.

Part One

The first part of this text focuses on learning homeopathy. It examines the qualities, skills and knowledge necessary for effective homeopathic learning, and describes the developmental stages of that process. The reasons for embarking on the study of homeopathy and the various levels of involvement in homeopathic learning are explored. A section on how to choose a homeopathic program will help students find a training program that best fits their needs. Obstacles that prevent each student from moving forward in the learning process are examined. Finally, there is a discussion of key issues in didactic and clinical training.

Teaching and learning represent two sides of the same coin and are inseparably bound together. In order to teach effectively, a teacher must remember both what it was like to be a student, and that a student aspires to give back to others what he has learned. Education at its best is an exchange of minds, hearts and spirits between teachers and students.

Part Two

The book's second part is dedicated to teaching. It explores the qualities of a good homeopathic teacher and outlines the skills and techniques necessary for homeopathic teaching. Although technical skills can be very helpful in the education process, it has been said that "technique is what you do until the teacher arrives."

Chapter Three investigates when and how a practitioner moves into teaching. It examines the importance of modeling, building trust and handling uncertainty. The developmental stages of growth as a teacher, diversity in teaching styles, and obstacles to teaching are also discussed. One of the most important sections focuses on adult learning. Although teaching children is the reference point of most beginning homeopathic teachers, teaching adult learners is very different from teaching children. Different skills and attitudes are required. The chapter concludes with a section on the importance of teacher renewal. Teachers must always seek new ways to recreate themselves in their work and to keep the dynamic spark that is homeopathy alive for their students.

Chapter Four explores didactic teaching. Lecture formats are often over-utilized in homeopathic education. Strategies such as problem-based learning, class exercises, role-playing and class discussions are effective alternatives. The importance of emotions and critical thinking in teaching and learning also are discussed. Teachers must model emotional connection to their students and cannot remain dispassionate observers. Critical thinking involves openness and questioning what one has been taught. Good teachers help students to think for themselves, to question and challenge.

A much-neglected issue in didactic teaching is failure. Students are often exposed to successful cases and develop a jaundiced view of the ease of the work, which prepares them poorly for eventual practice. It is important that teachers present a balanced view of both successes and failures. As the chapter continues, it describes the different challenges in teaching licensed versus non-licensed students. It goes on to review specific strategies focusing on the teaching of philosophy, materia medica, repertory, ethics, research, case-taking, case analysis, case management, history and medical competency.

Lastly, the concept of mentorship is explored. Mentorship provides a powerful method for students to see where they are on their respective homeopathic journeys and what their next steps need to be. Mentorship also helps students to balance their professional, student and personal lives.

Clinical training is the subject of Chapter Five. Clinical training has been given short shrift in homeopathic education. In this chapter, the difficulties in designing clinical training programs are explored, as well as their structure, importance and purpose. Specific core clinical skills and knowledge bases are discussed. The handling of emergencies and practical business issues are separate areas often overlooked in professional training.

Four specific clinical training models are proposed, representing varying degrees of autonomy for the student. These are observation, training clinics, supervision and consultation. Observation involves watching an experienced homeopath at work. Training clinics offer a collaborative approach where students work directly with a clinical teacher, creating opportunities for direct feedback. Supervision generally involves students working homeopathic cases independently and then presenting their work to their supervisors. Supervisors take responsibility for the clinical work of their supervisee. Consultation is more collegial and consultants do not take responsibility for the consultee's work.

Public speaking and introductory talks are the focus of Chapter Six. These are the most important means by which a homeopathic practitioner begins to move into teaching and establish a practice. Strategies for helping the teacher overcome performance anxiety are explored. Specific skills for designing, organizing, preparing and delivering presentations are outlined. The chapter concludes with a discussion of the importance of introductory talks and key elements to include in them.

Part Three

The last section of this book focuses on administration. Administration is a combination of leadership and management. This section explores the dynamic underpinnings of effective homeopathic administration, management and leadership.

Chapter Eight is concerned with homeopathic educational leadership. Quality homeopathic leadership is vital to the success and growth of homeopathy in the world today. Homeopathic leadership is contrasted with allopathic leadership. Homeopathic leadership is community-based and dispersed throughout an organization. Allopathic leadership uses the image of the isolated hero and is narcissistically power-based.

The chapter explores why homeopaths would wish to become leaders and the challenges they face in building a homeopathic organization. The predictable stages of leadership development are discussed. The remainder of the chapter focuses on the creation of a strong homeopathic community and the developmental stages of its growth. A strong homeopathic community is vital for the continued growth and development of homeopathy in the new millennium.

Chapter Nine focuses on homeopathic educational management or stewardship. An overview of schools in North America is provided, followed by a discussion of the importance of certification and licensure. Administrators must choose a central learning approach before embarking on curriculum development. Several learning approaches are presented, such as problem-based learning and liberal learning. Strategies for curriculum design and curriculum improvement are explored. It is important to create a curriculum that focuses not just on becoming a successful homeopathic prescriber, but also a successful homeopath.

The book concludes with a discussion of the skills, qualities and knowledge necessary for effective homeopathic administration (Chapter Ten). Teachers and students often attempt to minimize the role of administrators in the education process, but effective administration is vital to the success of any educational program, whether it is a study group or a more formal training program. The transition from practitioner or teacher to administrator is often difficult. The pitfalls that beset the new administrator are explored.

Quotations and Literary Tools

Learn from everyone, from everywhere, from every source, from every incident. Learn, apply and utilize. Life is a glorious opportunity. Utilize this opportunity to the maximum so that we can say at the end as Hahnemann said, "Non inutilis vixi." (I did not live in vain.)
—Dr. P. Sankaran

There are many quotations included in the text. This was important to me because I wanted to include the words of masters. We must respect the masters who have preceded us. We must be aware of our roots to see clearly where we are going. I wanted to demonstrate that we are not alone on this journey. Many great teachers, leaders and learners have gone before us. The quotations also help to lead the reader deeper and give pause to the material. They are intended to provide inspiration and should not be seen as a lofty standard to which the reader compares himself.

Although it includes an extensive bibliography, this work purposely avoids too many scholarly and technical references. That is because I wanted to focus on the heart of that which is homeopathic education. This writing does rely on the texts of many others. I am particularly indebted to the works of Palmer, Banner and Cunningham.

There is much repetition throughout this book. You will find that many basic ideas are repeated in each section (learning, teaching and administrating). This reflects the holistic and holographic nature of homeopathic education. Repetition is also central to learning and to the process of homeopathic education.

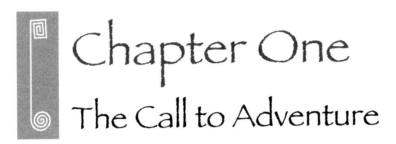

Chapter One
The Call to Adventure

Every age has a kind of universal genius,
which inclines those that live in it to some particular studies.
—John Dryden

Many who choose to study homeopathy are called. Often they can remember the exact circumstances in which they heard the call. They become impassioned about their learning and their voyage of discovery.

Others come kicking and screaming. They are hesitant and uncertain, often skeptical of what they are learning. Yet, with time and careful study, they prove homeopathy for themselves and become dedicated.

Hearing a call and not following it creates disease within each of us. Following the call permits students to express themselves at their deepest levels. Healing happens for the learner to the extent that they identify what they love and live that in their lives.

The learning of homeopathy is a life-long adventure. The adventure often begins with the feeling that something is lacking in a student's life. This inner sense of emptiness is coupled with a desire to know more and become more. To realize that desire, the student must be willing to move out of a place of safety and embark into the unknown.

True learning is learning that touches all aspects of who we are. It gets to the heart of what it is to be human. It gives us the capacity to recreate ourselves, to do what we never could do before and to change our relationship to the world. Homeopathic education changes the student, providing new ways of seeing and perceiving the world. There is a deep need inside each of us for this kind of learning.

The homeopathic journey is full of surprises, unexpected delights and excitement. There are perils along the way, monsters to be conquered and monsters to be avoided. There are islands of relative calm where some will be tempted to linger and go no farther. There are guides to lead the way, although ultimately one must make the last part of the journey alone. Finally, when students have accomplished their goal of becoming homeopaths, they must return to serve all of life, with the realization that the journey has just begun. This chapter and the next attempt to provide a road map for that journey.

Why Study Homeopathy?

Just sheer life cannot be said to have a purpose, because look at all the different purposes it has all over the place. But each incarnation, you might say, has a potentiality, and the mission of life is to live that potentiality. How do you do it? My answer is "follow your bliss." There is something inside you that knows when you're in the center, that knows when you're on the beam or off the beam.
—Joseph Campbell

The reasons to study homeopathy are as diverse as the individuals who study. However, some common themes emerge when students are asked about what brought them to homeopathic training.

Holistic View

A homeopathic practitioner treats individuals on all levels of their being. This includes the physical, emotional, mental and spiritual levels. In this way, homeopathy has the capacity to get to the root cause of illness.

Good homeopathic practitioners use all of themselves in their work. Homeopaths take the time to connect with their patients, and homeopathic clients respond by feeling deeply understood. Many practitioners are attracted to the slower pace of homeopathy and the opportunity it affords to spend more time with their patients.

Intrinsic Beauty

Homeopathy is a beautiful field of study. It is a complete healing system unto itself. It is a tremendously rich tapestry that captures the hearts of those who study it and touches them deeply. It explores the harmony and resonance that occurs between individuals and their world. Homeopathy ultimately involves the study and learning of all life.

Plus Factor

Many practitioners pursue a variety of forms of healing before learning homeopathy. With each field of study, they struggle until they can integrate it and then they move on. Yet when they come to homeopathy, they find it to be boundless. They are unable to fully encompass the field. This realization is accompanied by feelings of wonderment. In this way, homeopathy represents a "great thing." The poet Rilke once said that "community is held together by the power of the grace of great things" (Rilke 1986). It is this "great thing" around which students, teachers and administrators gather in their work.

Nurturing the Spirit

Many homeopaths find homeopathy deeply satisfying and fulfilling. It captivates the mind, fires the imagination, holds the heart and frees the spirit. Homeopaths feel part of a supportive and nurturing tradition that stems back for several hundred years.

Balancing Science with Art

Homeopathy is both an art and a science. A considerable and growing body of empirical medical evidence supports its efficacy (Gray 2000). The art of homeopathy is embodied in a series of qualities, skills and knowledge necessary for practice (see Chapter Three). Through this unique marriage of science and art, homeopathy becomes a craft that requires both technical and practical knowledge (see Introduction).

It Works

Homeopathy works. Many students come to homeopathy because they or a family member have been successfully treated homeopathically. Many allopaths have been converted to homeopathy after successful homeopathic treatment. This experience can turn a skeptic into a believer.

It Is in Demand

Homeopathy is thought to be the world's fastest-growing form of alternative medicine. Currently, the demand for homeopathic care far exceeds the supply of practicing homeopaths in most areas of the world. What attracts many is its affordability. Homeopathic treatment is generally much less expensive to patients than conventional medical care. With demand for their services already high and increasing, students of homeopathy can count on steady work and a healthy income. Most medically trained homeopaths find they can make a salary equivalent to that of conventional medical doctors in private practice.

Philosophy

Homeopathy is founded on clear laws and principles. This is not true of allopathic (conventional) medicine. Unlike traditional science, in which 50 percent of what is held true will eventually be proved untrue, homeopathy maintains a firm foundation while its practitioners continuously add to the field's existing body of knowledge.

A main philosophical principle that attracts students to homeopathy is "non-suppression." Homeopathy, unlike allopathic medicine, does not tend to suppress illness deeper into the organism. For example, when a young child with eczema is treated allopathically with steroid creams, this condition can resolve and be replaced by asthma. In homeopathic treatment of asthma, it is not uncommon when the asthma resolves, for the eczema to temporarily recur and then gradually resolve as the suppressed condition comes back to the surface. It is expected that many diseases of the 21st century (e.g. antibiotic-resistant organisms, multiple chemical sensitivity) will not respond well to allopathic treatment but will respond to the many forms of alternative medicine that are better suited to address these conditions. Another fundamental principle of homeopathy that attracts students is "individualization." Homeopathy does not treat patients as diseases but as individuals. Thus practitioners of classical homeopathy will prescribe for a patient only one medication at a time. The average American is commonly thought to be taking on taking on average eight allopathic medications at any given time (JAMA 2000).

Possibility of Cure

Much of conventional medicine is concerned with managing rather than curing disease. Homeopathy offers the possibility of cure. Many modern diseases are potentially curable utilizing homeopathic treatment. Homeopathy also offers treatment for chronic conditions that are not treatable by traditional methods such as multiple sclerosis, hepatitis, chronic fatigue syndrome and fibromyalgia.

Lack of Side Effects

Unlike conventional treatments, homeopathic medicines do not have toxic side effects. When prescribed correctly, homeopathic medicines are quite safe and well tolerated by patients.

Second Career

Some individuals fear that they are too old to learn a discipline such as homeopathy. Clinical evidence does not substantiate this concern. Many have embarked on the study of homeopathy as a second career and met with success. Growth is a never-ending process.

My personal journey into homeopathy began in my last year of medical school. I was interested in learning more about alternative medicine and spent one month studying with a homeopathic physician in Chicago. In his practice, I saw rapid and highly beneficial responses to his treatments for acute illnesses. I also saw remarkable cures of patients with chronic illnesses, many of which were considered untreatable by conventional medicine. The experience transformed my view of health and healing. Most important, when I found homeopathy, I felt like I had finally come home. As a result, I chose to pursue homeopathy as a career.

Levels of Involvement

A little learning is a dangerous thing;
Drink deep, or taste not the Pierian spring:
There shallow draughts intoxicate the brain,
And drinking largely sobers us again.
—Alexander Pope

There are many levels of student involvement in homeopathy. Students often begin at the first level and progress from one stage to another over time. Some progress smoothly, while others stop at certain stages for years before progressing through the journey. Some are happy to stay at one stage and never move on. The following are the five levels of involvement:

The Appreciator

Some students begin homeopathic training and then drop out, realizing it's not right for them. There can be many reasons for this, but ultimately there is a lack of resonance between homeopathy and their own nature.

Though such individuals don't wish to study homeopathy further, they often develop a deep appreciation it. Homeopathy can enliven their work and leave them changed. They might refer friends, family and patients to homeopathy, undergo homeopathic treatment themselves or work with someone who practices homeopathy.

The Experimenter

The experimenter if on who tinkers or dabbles in homeopathy, without any real commitment. This casual practice of homeopathy can be learned in a few hours of self-study or a weekend course. At this level, the usage of remedies is mostly focused on first aid. Examples include the usage of Arnica montana after trauma or Aconite napellus for shock.

Casual homeopathy can be practiced at home or in a medical office. In simple home care, the practitioner is generally treating friends and family. In an office setting, the medically licensed practitioner is primarily focused on his original field of study but wishes to experiment with homeopathy.

The Acute Practitioner

This level of practice is focused on acute prescribing. The practitioner can learn this level of prescribing in a typical 40-hour course or through more serious self- study. An example would be using the remedy Pulsatilla nigrans, Belladonna, Aconitum nappelus or Mercurius vivus in the treatment of Otitis media (ear infections).

The home practitioner uses a home-remedy kit to treat friends and family. The medically licensed practitioner uses homeopathic remedies to treat simple acute conditions. For more serious conditions, he relies on conventional medicine or refers patients to a more skilled homeopathic practitioner.

The Integrative Practitioner

This level of involvement requires a greater commitment to homeopathy. In a course lasting 100-250 hours, the practitioner learns a limited number of "constitutional remedies" that can be used in the treatment of deeper chronic conditions. These remedies generally cannot be learned by simple self-study, but require a more intensive training program (whether in a classroom or by distance learning). An example of treatment at this stage is usage of the remedy Natrum muriaticum to cure a patient whose syndrome of illness includes chronic migraine headaches, constipation, intermittent herpetic infections and a tendency toward depression.

For non-medically licensed practitioners, this stage involves integrating homeopathic practice with their other work. For medically licensed practitioners, this level involves the deeper integration of conventional and homeopathic methods. Depending on the situation, a practitioner might choose one modality of treatment over the other, or he might combine them. For some practitioners, the mixing of allopathic and homeopathic treatments can lead to confusion. More serious cases need supervision by an experienced homeopath or should be referred. The key is to know one's limits. (Some medical practitioners find it very difficult to integrate conventional and homeopathic practices and ultimately decide to move on to the next level: homeopathic practitioner.)

Homeopathic training in naturopathic schools is currently at the level of the Integrative Practitioner. Medical and osteopathic doctors can become licensed to practice homeopathy in certain states (Arizona, Connecticut and Nevada). Licensure as a homeopathic physician is not required for an MD/DO to practice homeopathy in other states. At this stage, reimbursement from insurance companies for homeopathic treatment is also possible.

The Homeopathic Practitioner

At this last level, which involves a greater degree of integration and commitment, the practitioner becomes known as a homeopath. The study of classical homeopathy is every bit as complex as that of conventional medicine. Practitioners who are serious about homeopathy can expect to devote a minimum of 500 didactic hours to the subject (although homeopathy more accurately requires a lifetime of study). At this stage, distance learning courses are insufficient without accompanying clinical training. An example of this level of practice would be the usage of the remedy Stramonium in the cure of a child with attention deficit disorder, night terrors, rage attacks and Tourette's disorder.

Homeopathic practitioners may elect to practice homeopathy exclusively or to have a more deeply integrated practice. (Some practitioners choose to separate their conventional and homeopathic practices to avoid confusion.) What differentiates practitioners who only practice homeopathy from integrative practitioners is a stronger commitment to homeopathy and a well-established identity as a homeopath. At this point, a homeopath is advanced enough to pursue certification. To become recognized as a homeopath and to avoid isolation, it is increasingly important to enter the homeopathic community.

Choosing a Program

Everywhere, we learn only from those whom we love.
—Johann Wolfgang von Goethe

There are many homeopathic schools and programs to choose from. Students must shop around for a training program in which they are comfortable with the faculty and the style of learning. They should consider several issues.

One of the first decisions is whether to choose a distance-learning program or a classroom-based program. Many students find they learn best in an interactive classroom. Others prefer self-learning at their own pace. Those who plan on studying homeopathy seriously and choose a distance-learning program must be aware that didactic training (see Chapter Four) is not enough. Quality clinical training (see Chapter Five) is critical to becoming a good homeopath.

Faculty is another important dimension in choosing a training program. According to an ancient saying, "When the student is ready, the teacher appears." The problem is that the student does not always recognize the teacher. The best teachers are not necessarily the most popular. An ideal faculty includes both good teachers and good practitioners. Early in training, it is more important to find a good teacher than a good practitioner. As training progresses, the reverse becomes true.

Some programs rely on a single teacher; others have a faculty. With single-teacher programs, it is critical that the student feels comfortable with the teacher. In programs with a faculty (featuring a few or several teachers), students are exposed to a variety of styles and perspectives. Students who choose a single-teacher program should attend seminars and pursue other educational experiences that will expose them to different ideas and learning styles. This helps to avoid teacher cloning and ensures that students develop their own style.

Mentorship is another key aspect of training programs, especially for those enrolled in distance-learning programs (see Chapter Three). Mentorship provides guidance on the homeopathic journey and helps students integrate their learning. Good mentors challenge and push students beyond their self-defined limits. They are not necessarily the students' favorite teachers.

A student cannot learn advanced homeopathy on his own. Clinical training provides the vital bridge between didactic training and actual practice. A live teacher not only shows the student how to practice, but also brings the teachings of homeopathy into the consciousness of the times.

Both quality teaching and quality administration are vital for effective homeopathic learning to occur. One is generally not sufficient without the other. (For more on effective homeopathic teaching, see Chapter Seven; for more on effective homeopathic administration, see Chapter Ten.) Certified and licensed training programs usually offer quality teaching and administration. In North America, programs are certified through the Council for Homeopathic Education (see Appendix B). Licensure of schools is obtained through each individual state. However, not all states permit licensure of homeopathic schools.

Finally, when choosing a training program, students should bear in mind two distinguishing traits of adult learners: They need to put what they learn into practice, and they need to be self-directing. It is important to find a program that meets both needs.

Developmental Stages of Growth as a Homeopathic Student

All growth is a leap in the dark, a spontaneous,
unpremeditated act without benefit of experience.
—Henry Miller

Learning is not a linear process. There is a constant motion forward and backward. Learning has a rhythm and is full of surprises and mystery. A student can feel stuck for some time and suddenly move forward with great speed and inspiration. Most important, learners go through cycles and stages of development. These developmental stages are differently described in various educational traditions. In Montessori education, for example, there are sensitive stages of a student's learning process that have greater meaning and where greater growth occurs. In homeopathic education, it is helpful for students to be aware of such stages (see below). This helps them know where they are in their training and to help normalize their experiences.

The psoric miasm is the world of the homeopathic learner (see Introduction). This is the stage of establishing identity, curiosity, initiative, hopefulness and optimism, expectation, knowledge development, confidence, nostalgia and trying. Here the student learns the work of homeopathy, learns how to learn and forms an identity as a homeopath in relationship to the world (Van der Zee 2000).

In mythology, this stage is closely paralleled by the hero myths. Carol Pearson explains this as follows:

> Heroes take journeys, confront dragons, and discover the treasure of their true selves. Although they may feel very alone during the quest, at its end their reward is a sense of community: with themselves, with other people and with the earth. Every time we confront death-in-life we confront a dragon, and every time we choose life over non-life and move deeper into the ongoing discovery of who we are, we vanquish the dragon; we bring new life to ourselves and our culture. We change the world.

Passionate Love

Initially, students often feel a great love for homeopathy. They are passionately involved in their training, and they have a sense of euphoria and freedom. Many describe the experience as having searched for something for a long time and having finally come home. This joy often lasts through the first year of training. Students go out and tell others of their discovery and are often surprised at the cold reception they receive.

Impostors

Some students feel like impostors when they begin their training. They feel that they lack the skills and self-confidence to become homeopaths. This can create considerable anxiety. As these students compare themselves to their seemingly more capable peers, some consider quitting. But when they express their feelings to others, they find many new students feel the same way.

Advancing and Retreating

Most new students oscillate between pushing forward and pulling back. They embrace the familiar while longing for the unfamiliar. When bored and too comfortable, they take risks in learning and seek new ideas and ways of being. Such leaps forward involve frenetic external learning fueled by great bursts of energy. After arriving in unfamiliar territory, however, students soon become uncomfortable. As the discomfort increases, they retreat to the familiar. To their surprise, they find that things have changed; their old ways are much less satisfying than before. Eventually, they become restless and the cycle begins again. There is a back-and-forth rhythm in this process. A few students are relentless plodders on their journey, but even they develop a rhythm in their learning process.

The pace of learning varies from student to student. Each student requires "rest periods" on the journey. At such times, knowledge can be integrated and assimilated. Then the student can again push forward. Though students often feel like they are spinning wheels and stuck during rest periods, they are actually doing a great deal of inner work and preparation for the next step.

Rest periods also provide quiet time for self-reflection, when the student can examine where he has been, where he is, where he is going and how he feels. Students often are uncomfortable with silence, yet silence is one of the most important opportunities for learning. Research has shown that adult learners learn best when they reflect on their learning (Huang and Lynch 1995). Regular reflection requires discipline. Unless students schedule time for reflection during training, it might not occur.

Depression

In the second year of training, students often fall out of their first-year euphoria and become depressed. They now realize that there is much more to homeopathy than they initially understood, and they feel overwhelmed. Some feel they have only scratched the surface and that the task before them is insurmountable. They consider abandoning their training.

Students need to recognize that the second-year blues are a natural stage of their growth, and that "this too shall pass."

Homeopathic Student Syndrome

One way that anxiety manifests in training is through the Homeopathic Student Syndrome. This is a neurotic phase of learning in which students develop all of the conditions and remedy states that they read about. It is very common for beginning students to walk up to a teacher after a remedy lecture and report that they "know that this is their remedy." A key moment in training occurs when students finally realize that all of the remedies exist as potentials within themselves. In good homeopathic teaching, these potential states become activated within a student when they resonate with the remedy. The concept of the wounded healer/student was first described by Carl Jung (Jung 1977; Geggenbuhl-Craig 1971). He examined the importance of accepting our wounds and weaknesses as healers/students. He saw this as a critical step on the journey to becoming a healer. Self awareness of these wounds helps each healer to become more compassionate in their work. To have suffered oneself makes one more compassionate for others' suffering. Clients also resonate more with healers who accept their limitations and weaknesses.

Beginner's Luck

When students begin their clinical work, they often experience the same sort of passion they felt at the beginning of their didactic work. Initial successes are commonly accompanied by euphoria, but these can be followed by a series of failures that lead to a great sense of frustration. Ultimately, students learn to become more detached from the results of their work and to respond more evenly to their successes and failures.

Letting Go

Some learners struggle with letting go of their attachments. This is an ongoing process that occurs at all phases of the training. Early in training, they must give up a previous professional identity and accept the identity of a homeopath (see "Establishing an Identity" below). Later in training, there is a need to let go of their teachers in order to move forward on their own. When letting go, it is common to feel uncomfortable, anxious and ill prepared for what lies ahead. Supervision and peer support are critical in moving through this process.

Ending Well

The ending phase of training is important and deserves greater emphasis. It is a good time for self-reflection and integration of what has been learned. It is also a time to end relationships with homeopathic clients one has treated during training, and to move into more collegial relationships with one's former teachers.

Endings are often difficult. They are filled with emotions such as grief, joy, fear and excitement. Students can develop dependency relationships with their teachers and peers that make it particularly hard for them to leave. Individuals who have problems ending relationships will have the most difficulty with this phase of their training.

Whether one attends a formal graduation or creates a private ceremony, it is important to mark the end of training and celebrate it. This provides a sense of closure that is essential before one can move on.

After training ends, there is a new beginning. It is time to give back in service what one has learned, but there will also be continual opportunities for renewal and regeneration. Students often maintain periodic contact with their teachers and administrators. Through this contact, they measure their progress and receive validation for their accomplishments.

Establishing an Identity

*We only become what we are by the radical and
deep-seated refusal of that which others have made of us.*
—Jean Paul Sartre

The first task in training to become a homeopathic practitioner is to establish an identity as a learner of homeopathy. We are not born as students. We do not become students by enrolling in a school. It is a role we grow into. Only we can make ourselves into students and make ourselves learn. It is not a passive process.

The second task is to establish one's identity as a homeopath. Some students find it challenging to let go of a past professional identity and accept a new identity as a homeopath. This task is particularly hard for medically licensed practitioners. Resistance from allopathic colleagues can make the process more difficult. It is important not to be isolated. Supervision, mentorship and peer support can be immeasurably helpful in this process.

The process of establishing one's homeopathic identity can be frustratingly slow. It is commonly thought to take, on average, ten years for professionals to fully integrate what they have learned as students. This process is faster for some and slower for others.

The last task is to establish an identity as a member of the homeopathic profession. Typically this occurs at the end of training. This means developing strong ties to the community of practicing homeopaths, accepting responsibility for one's therapies, following a code of professional ethics, and making contributions to the field of homeopathy. Professionalism is key to earning credibility and respect from patients and peers alike. This is increasingly important in our highly mobile society.

Establishing a professional identity is often difficult for non-medically licensed practitioners. Homeopaths who have not had conventional medical training have little social status in contemporary culture. They have a harder time gaining the acceptance of their community and the respect of their medically licensed peers.

Moving Beyond Your Teacher

At times it may flatter the teacher when his students are proud
of him. He who is a true teacher must rather wish that he may
be proud of his students. If the work of the novice is to praise
the master, it will be necessary that the student himself some
day become one.
—Theodor Reik

A homeopath must establish self-identity. To do so means to let one's teachers go. According to a well-known saying, "If you meet the Buddha on the road, you must kill him" (Kopp 1972). It is tempting for some students to become disciples of their teachers and to use them as crutches. These students imitate their teachers and become clones, rather than becoming uniquely who they are.

Ultimately, students must move beyond their teachers. Every tradition warns against trying to put someone else in charge of one's journey. Each student must find his own answers; over time, he must learn to internalize authority. This is part of the individuation process and a crucial step in establishing self-identity as a homeopath.

Obstacles to Learning

I have learned throughout my life as a composer chiefly
through my mistakes and pursuits of false assumptions,
not by my exposure to founts of wisdom and knowledge.
—Igor Stravinsky

All students encounter obstacles to learning that prevent them from moving forward on their journey. Learning problems occur when students respond inappropriately to the learning process. The problems can be internal or external and can take many forms. They are not caused by teachers, schools or patients, but originate within the student.

Learning obstacles must be overcome before true learning can occur. The key is to become aware of and work through them. Learning problems represent opportunities for individuals to discover things about themselves and how they relate to the world. Working through such problems also helps students become more mature and sensitive to patients and fellow practitioners. One way to help identify learning obstacles is to keep a learning journal (see Chapter Four).

Following is a list of some common learning obstacles:

Prejudice

Prejudice is perhaps the main obstacle to learning. It lives within the student who maintains, "I am right and you are wrong." Prejudice is an outgrowth of closed-mindedness and closed-heartedness. It prevents the student from listening effectively to others or making room in his heart for others. Beginning students who have just begun taking cases often claim to "know" the right remedy shortly after beginning the case. They stubbornly try to prove their choice is "correct" while shutting off all other possibilities. The remedy to prejudice is wonder, which is the capacity to be open to life's myriad possibilities.

Rigid Thinking

Directly related to prejudice is the problem of rigid thinking. Rigid thinkers often tend to see things in black and white, and believe there is only one "correct" answer. Rigid thinking prevents appreciation of ambiguity, openness to the world or appreciation for the richness of our patients' lives. The educator Sara Lawrence Lightfoot said, "Part of teaching is helping students learn how to tolerate ambiguity, consider possibilities, and ask questions that are unanswerable." The remedy to rigid thinking is an open mind and non-attachment to one's ideas.

Poor Self-Image as Learners

Many students arrive in homeopathic training with baggage from previous learning experiences. Contemporary education often closes more minds than it opens. A recent school survey showed that 82 percent of children entering a school system at age six had a positive image of their learning ability. Of students surveyed at age 16, however, only 18 percent had a positive image of their learning ability (Rose and Nicholl 1997). Somewhere along the way, many students get the message—from teachers and/or from other students—that they are "too dumb to learn." This seems to happen most often to female students, many of whom find the label difficult to overcome. (The majority of homeopathic students are women, while the majority of homeopathic teachers and administrators are male). Homeopathic students need a positive image of their learning ability and a positive attitude toward learning. The remedy to a poor self-image is self-confidence.

One key to developing self-confidence is to avoid comparing oneself to other students. All students have strengths in various areas and weaknesses in others. Some have studied for many years before entering a formal training program, whereas others are rank novices. Each student begins training at a different level and should focus on his or her own individual growth over time.

Students can also gain confidence by envisioning themselves as successful learners. Then, when someone praises their work, students need to listen to the praise, believe it, and feel pride in knowing that they have mastered the subject.

Fear

Anxiety always accompanies the move from the known into the unknown. As much as we want to learn, learning demands change and change is something we fear.

One of the most common recurring dreams in adults is of being back in school. In these dreams, the student is not able to find a class, has forgotten a class or has forgotten an exam. These dreams are accompanied by great anxiety. This underscores the universality of these fears. The traditional educational system is structured to generate anxiety in its students.

Students face many anxieties on their homeopathic journey. They fear failing, inadequacy, being overwhelmed and not understanding. They worry that their training will not be good enough, that they will be drawn into issues they would rather avoid, that their prejudices will be challenged or that they will look foolish in front of their peers. Some allopathically trained students fear committing allopathic career suicide by practicing a "fringe" form of healing. (This is less of a problem than it used to be.)

Before they can move on with their training, students must learn to master their fears without becoming paralyzed by them. The remedy to fear is courage. It requires courage to learn and step outside the boundaries of what is considered "normal." Love for the subject is also a powerful antidote for fear.

Overreaction

Some students overreact to their learning failures. They do poorly on one exam or struggle with one case and then generalize this to mean that they will never learn homeopathy and should quit. Other students have one negative experience with a teacher and feel they should leave their training program. The problem here is impatience.

Many students expect to learn homeopathy overnight or in a series of weekend courses. They soon become frustrated with the difficulty and complexity of homeopathic learning. This is particularly a problem for medically licensed practitioners who wish to add homeopathy to their current practice. They have the expectation of being able to learn the field quickly with minimal work. The remedy to impatience is patience, tolerance and compassion for both oneself and others.

Student/Teacher Mismatch

Another cause of resistance to learning is a teacher-student mismatch. Most often, this happens when there is a lack of resonance between the student's learning style and the teacher's teaching style. It can also arise from personality conflicts. Every student will be uncomfortable with some teachers and teaching styles.

The remedy here is diversity. Mismatches are much less of a problem in program with diverse faculty members. Another solution is to seek out peer teaching and peer learning. Working within a supportive community of peers can be one of the most effective learning experiences in a homeopathic training program.

The Wrong Path

After a while, some students realize that homeopathy is not for them. Homeopathic education is perhaps more demanding than they had anticipated, requires more of a commitment than they are willing to make or simply doesn't fit who they are. The remedy to this problem is to become well informed about homeopathic education before entering a training program. Prospective students should talk to homeopathic practitioners and interview faculty members about what to expect.

Techno-Stress

Many fields are participating in the information explosion, homeopathy among them. As a result, the pace of education today has become increasingly frenetic. Many students who are not comfortable or familiar with information technology experience information overload and "techno-stress." Conversely, students who love technology can face the problem of "techno-dependence." These individuals become so wrapped up in the technology that they lose the human dimension of the work.

Both issues represent obstacles to learning. Ideally, students will become comfortable with technology and find balanced ways of integrating it into their work. The remedies here are self-pacing, self-reflection and taking pauses in training to evaluate whether one is using technology appropriately. Accelerated learning techniques (see below) can also be quite helpful.

Keys to Didactic Training

Two things seemed pretty apparent to me. One was,
that in order to be a Mississippi River pilot a man had
got to learn more than any one man ought to be allowed to
know; and the other was, that he must learn it all over again
in a different way every 24 hours.
—Mark Twain

Following are some pointers that will make it easier for the beginning student to move through didactic training:

Common Is Common

There are over 3,000 homeopathic remedies to learn. As a psychiatrist, I only had to learn about 50 psychiatric medications, and in much less depth than homeopathy requires. Comparatively, the homeopath's task is immense.

It helps to know that certain remedies are better studied and more commonly prescribed than others. Certain remedies are also more commonly utilized in certain cultures and regions of the world. This can greatly simplify the work.

Seeing the Remedies in the World Around You

It is helpful for students to begin seeing the remedies in the world around them. This makes learning homeopathy much richer and brings it alive. Everything that one does and experiences in the world is an opportunity to live homeopathy first hand. This is true, whether it is opera, punk rock, poetry, sculpture, politics, botany, pharmacology, mythology or psychology. For example, when studying the remedy Tuberculinum, images of this remedy can be found in the literature (*The Magic Mountain* by Thomas Mann), music (Frederick Chopin and Bela Bartok), poetry (Edna St. Vincent Millet) the opera (La Boheme) and the cinema (*Tombstone*). All of life becomes a classroom and a teacher. As a homeopath, seeing homeopathy in the world around one makes it much easier to see it within one's patients. As students, we must see what we are learning in ourselves before we can see it clearly in our patients.

It Takes One to Know One

Homeopaths can only see remedies in their patients to the extent that they see them in themselves. Students contain the potentiality of all remedy states within themselves. An important aspect of learning materia medica (compilations of symptoms related to particular remedies) is developing a resonance between the internalized side of remedies within one's psyche and the images provided by one's teachers.

All students have both shadow remedies and ego remedies they struggle with in their work. Shadow remedies represent those parts of their own psyches with which they are uncomfortable or which they have disowned. These represent the students' blind spots. They are the remedies students never think of in their work or have the most difficulty learning. Energetically, these are fields of energy that repel.

Ego remedies represent the parts of themselves with which students are most comfortable. Students frequent think of these remedies in their work and tend to over prescribe them. Energetically, these are fields of energy that attract.

To become better prescribers, students must explore both their shadow and ego remedies and the areas of themselves that these represent. Only in this way can they be more conscious in their work.

Facts You Must Know

There are certain facts (such as keynotes) about remedies that must be memorized and learned. Some students argue that they can always look this information up and only need to learn the essences or key themes of the remedies. This is insufficient as it greatly slows down the work. Without knowing the pertinent data about remedies, it is difficult to be effective as a homeopath. The dilemma for homeopathic educational institutions is answering the question, "How much is enough?"

Data Is Not Enough

Students need more than data or information. They also must perceive the heart of the remedies, the golden thread that runs through all the facets. Some describe this as central theme or essence. This cannot be taught, but only caught.

The Law of Polarity

For beginning homeopathic students, "polarity" is often one of the most difficult concepts to grasp. The law of polarity says that something can be true about a remedy while the opposite is true at the same time. For example, the remedy Sulphur is listed in both the ideas "Ambitious" and "Indolence."

Students must learn that remedies are often paradoxical. Prominent physicist Niels Bohr once said, "The opposite of a true statement is a false statement, but the opposite of a profound truth can be another profound truth." The challenge to the student is to embrace "both and" rather than "either or." Good teachers demonstrate this skill by holding the tension of the paradox without premature resolution. Provings are conducted by administering homeopathic substances to healthy volunteers and then recording their symptoms over time.

Experiencing Remedies Firsthand

An important method of learning homeopathy and bringing it alive is to experience it directly. This can be done in a variety of ways. One is to engage in homeopathic treatment during training (see below). Another is to participate in "provings" (homeopathic research). Provings are conducted by administering homeopathic substances to healthy volunteers and then recording their symptoms over time, a powerful way of "proving" to oneself the power and validity of homeopathy. Many provers have said that they did not really understand homeopathy on a gut level until they participated in a proving. A third way of directly experiencing remedies is to see remedy images in film, literature, opera, meditations and dream work. These experiences can be helpful in immersing a student in a remedy so that it helps the remedy become alive for them. Successful students are observers of life.

Student Preparation

Those students who come to class prepared are much better able to integrate the material. Most training programs require preparatory homework prior to class. This is a way to ensure that all students are operating at a common, minimal level of understanding about the basic concepts.

Accelerated Learning

Learning is not a spectator sport.
—Anonymous

Knowledge is doubling every two to three years in almost every occupation and homeopathy is no exception. The world is changing rapidly and life is becoming increasingly complex. With the large amount of data and information that must be learned in homeopathic training, accelerated learning techniques can be quite useful. These techniques allow deeper comprehension and quicker mastery of the materia medica and repertory. If adapted to the specific learner, the techniques can reawaken the joy of learning.

Dr. Lozanov founded accelerated learning in Bulgaria in the 1960s. Since then, many excellent books have been written on the subject (Rose and Nicholl 1997, Buzan 1984, Buzan 1996, Scheele 1999, Dennison 1989, Ostrander and Schroedr 1979). Increasingly, students are turning to Lozanov's techniques for assistance.

One key to accelerated learning is individualization. Individuals learn at different rates and in different ways. Students must individualize their study habits to make them more effective and enjoyable. There are three styles of learning: visual, auditory and kinesthetic (Rose and Nicholl 1997). Visual learners learn well by video and reading, have good visual recall, focus on facial expressions in their work and do best when they are shown material. Auditory learners rely on listening, music, storytelling and speaking what they learn aloud. They have good auditory recall. Kinesthetic learners learn best through activity, dancing, body language, writing, flash cards and group interaction.

It is important for students to identify their own learning style and then find techniques that fit that style. Learning problems between students and teachers often stem from mismatched teaching and learning styles. For example, a student who is predominantly kinesthetic will have trouble learning from a teacher who is predominantly visual in his or her teaching methods.

Multiple Intelligence Theory, devised by Howard Gardner (Gardner 1983), breaks down learning styles even further. According to Gardner, there are seven types of learning intelligence: linguistic (William Shakespeare), logical (Albert Einstein), visual (Pablo Picasso), physical (Thomas Edison), musical (Ray Charles), interpersonal (Mother Teresa) and intrapersonal (Emily Dickinson). Again, it is helpful for students to identify their learning strengths and to play to these strengths in the learning process (Dardnjer 1995). For example, students who are strong musical learners might write a rap song about a particular remedy to facilitate learning, while visual learners might create mind maps, and linguistic learners might try to verbalize what they have learned to others. Students often possess more than one type of learning intelligence. They should challenge their brains with as many types as possible. This will enable them to approach their homeopathic work from a much broader viewpoint.

Whatever the specific accelerated learning technique, relaxation can be quite helpful for students in preparing the way for learning. Tension negates learning, while relaxation opens the learning channels. Movement exercises and breathing exercises have been shown to be effective in this regard (Dennison 1989). Music, especially baroque, is particularly helpful in facilitating learning.

There are also many accelerated learning techniques to help with memorization: Connecting a memory with an emotion often fixes a memory more deeply. Multi-sensory memories, in which memories are experienced through more than one of the five senses, are more effectively learned. We also tend to better hold onto memories associated with unusual events, stories, poetry or music. Other helpful memory techniques include acronyms, learning maps and categorization (Rose and Nicholl 1997).

Keys to Clinical Training

However much thou are read in theory,
if thou hast no practice thou are ignorant.
—Sa'Di

The journeyman phase is the part of education that traditionally lies between apprenticeship and mastery. Apprenticeship is not sufficient in itself. True learning requires going out into the world and facing all types of life experience. In homeopathy, the didactic student is the apprentice and the clinical student is the journeyman.

Clinical training has its own set of challenges. When participating in clinical training, students must cope with their patients, their clinical supervisor, administrative conditions and their own internalized professional ideals. This entails learning homeopathic skills, attitudes and knowledge, as well as developing a professional identity as a homeopath. All clinical students must find how they can best learn from their teachers and how to best present material to their supervisors and teachers. Emotional issues are inevitably mobilized in this process. Some key issues are identified below:

Practice, Practice, Practice

More than anything else, practice distinguishes successful students in homeopathic training programs. Those who practice what they learn incorporate and solidify their knowledge much more quickly than others. Within safe limits, it is important to begin practicing early in training. At first, practice might be limited to first aid prescribing. Later on, the limits can expand to include acute prescribing, and, finally, prescribing for more chronic conditions. Supervision, though often difficult to find, is critical to solidifying one's practice.

Acting "As If"

Students often initially feel like impostors. It is not uncommon for them to feel that patients are guinea pigs to their incompetence. Acting as if they do belong in the role of a homeopath early in training is the key to working through this stage. Gradually, as students expand their knowledge and skills, they will go from acting the role to recognizing themselves as the real thing.

Patients Are the Best Teachers

Ultimately, the best teachers are our patients. In treating patients, students must be open, honest and willing to listen. An important question for every student to ask is, "What does this patient have to teach me?" Self-reflection is a key to this knowledge.

Developing Interpersonal Skills

First-year students in homeopathic training need to develop sound interpersonal skills. The key to this is active listening. Active listening should be distinguished from passive listening where the student is the passive recipient of what they hear. Active listening is more than hearing words. It requires a concentration that most of us don't utilize in our daily lives. Hannah Merker describes it as "just a mind aware." The poet William Butler Yeats said, "Listening is the nearest of all arts to eternity." Active listening is hard work. It requires concentration that most individuals do not apply in everyday life. At first this can be exhausting. Students often become fatigued by the end of the day during clinical training, as they struggle to stay present with their patients. The exhaustion disappears over time as students get used to active listening.

Active listening can be especially difficult for allopathic practitioners and mental health professionals. They must let go of old habits and learn to listen to patients in new ways.

Clearing the Energy

During clinical work, one case must be fully cleared away before the student can begin the next. Case taking is an intense process requiring much energy, unbending intent and immersion in the energy of the case. Cases can blend together throughout the day, and it becomes critical to refocus and balance oneself between clients. A fresh perspective is particularly important when revisiting an unsuccessful case one has followed for a long time. Refocusing can help the homeopathic practitioner think about the case in a new way.

Students must find their own ways of renewing themselves and beginning fresh with each case. This comes more easily if they are taking care of and nurturing themselves during training. For example, I often juggle between clients. Juggling requires a defocusing and clearing of the mind. It also helps the mind to refocus on the whole. It is impossible to successfully juggle and to focus on any particular ball.

Dealing with Failure

One great challenge, particularly in the early stages of clinical work, is handling perceived failure. Failure can take many forms. A student might fail to find a remedy that acts, fail to be fully present while taking a case, fail as an unprejudiced observer or fail to establish a relationship with a client. How a student deals with such issues affects his or her identity as a homeopathic practitioner. Each student must find a sustaining source that will help him or her continue when things look bleak. Spouses, mentors and good friends can help provide this sustaining source.

Overcoming Fear of the Unknown

Students generally hold to what they know. In clinical training, they tend to consider and prescribe only remedies well known to them. They round up the usual suspects in choosing remedies or use the same rubrics (listings of remedies associated with a given symptom) repeatedly in their work. It takes a conscious effort to break out of this mind set and open up to the unlimited possibilities that homeopathy offers.

Making the Most of Supervision

Often students are not allowed to choose their supervisors. They seldom think about making the supervision process work for them. However, supervision can be one of the most important aspects of training, and a few small considerations can make things run more smoothly.

Students who do have a choice should interview their prospective supervisor. They should consider the person's level of receptivity, sensitivity and safety. Supervisors vary greatly in style and experience. In choosing a supervisor, it is often useful to talk to others who have had the same supervisor. Remember, however, that each supervisory relationship is unique, so one shouldn't make too many assumptions.

In sizing up potential supervisors, consider the following:

◎ What is their experience level?

◎ How do they supervise?

◎ What is their style?

◎ What are their expectations?

◎ What have they liked about their favorite students?

◎ How can a student best prepare for supervision with them?

◎ How are students evaluated (if applicable)?

◎ Who will see the evaluation forms (if applicable)?

◎ Who do they report to?

◎ What types of records do they keep?

◎ What is held confidential about students and their work?

◎ Do they prefer written notes, audio tapes or videotapes of supervisory sessions?

◎ What are the prerequisites for supervision?

◎ How should a student inform clients that he/she is are being supervised?

◎ How can they be reached in an emergency, and what constitutes an emergency?

◎ How should disagreements be handled in supervision?

◎ Do they want to see the student's clients?

◎ Are they willing to make mistakes?

◎ What are their boundaries for supervision? Will they go so far as to take a student's case?

◎ What level of medical knowledge do they have?

◎ Do they provide useful feedback?

◎ How responsive are they to the student's concerns?

Supervision is targeted more toward helping one grow as a homeopath than toward finding the right remedy. If a student poorly takes a case, there is little a supervisor can do in finding a good remedy. Good supervision involves mentorship, ethics guidance, coaching, practice analysis and support.

Supervisory learning is much more than conveying technique. True learning requires engaging both the heart and the mind. One of the hardest things about learning under supervision is that one must expose one's emotions, weaknesses and core resistance to learning. This is true for both students and supervisors. At one time or another, most students have strong emotional reactions to the process. They might feel that the work is too hard, that they are confused or that they don't know what to say during sessions. Students might have strong attractions or negative reactions to certain patients. It is hard to feel comfortable enough to reveal these kinds of thoughts and feelings to one's supervisor. The supervisor's challenge is to make the student feel safe enough to do so. Students shouldn't feel that such openness will reflect negatively on their evaluations.

When entering each supervisory session, students should be prepared with a list of topics that they would like to cover. They should feel comfortable raising questions, expressing opinions and disagreeing respectfully. After the session, there should be a review of what happened. Students should consider the following Important questions: Am I learning what I need to learn? What did I forget to say? What was I reluctant to say?

At this time, students will find it helpful to distinguish between their "internal" supervisor and their "internalized" supervisor. The internal supervisor is the student's thinking about what is going on in the work. This often consists of bits and pieces gleaned from various teachers, mixed with ideas unique to the student. The internalized supervisor is what the student believes the supervisor wants him/her to think. When the internal and internalized supervisors conflict, supervision can fall apart. This often occurs when students project their own issues onto their supervisors.

Certification

Certification is an important step in the development of the homeopathic student. In the past, most homeopaths knew each other and knew who was good in practice. As homeopathy has grown, this sort of familiarity has become impossible. Increasingly, homeopaths rely on certification as a means to demonstrating minimum quality standards, establishing credibility and promoting the growth of the profession. The certification process helps students take another step toward establishing their identity as a homeopath. A listing of certification organizations can be found in Appendix J.

Purchasing the Tools

People who are greedy have extraordinary capacities for waste—
they must, they take in too much.
—Norman Mailer

Beginning students struggle with "homeopathic gluttony." They're tempted to purchase every homeopathic book, tape and software program on the market and to try to cram it all in. They also feel an urge to sign up for every homeopathic conference, even those who are quite advanced. Mostly, this stems from impatience (see Chapter Two).

Generally, it is best to wait. There will be plenty of time later in training to purchase materials and attend conferences. Beginning students who attend advanced-level conferences often feel confused and frustrated by information they are not yet prepared to process. When embarking on the journey, it is best to stick with the basics until one has solid footing on the path. A recent study of homeopathic students revealed that 80 percent had purchased materials (extraneous to those required in their curriculum) in their first year that they later regretted purchasing. Some students especially regret purchasing computer software prematurely. Many homeopathy schools encourage students to wait about a year before purchasing homeopathic computer software.

The Importance of Homeopathic Treatment

Healer, heal thyself.
—Anonymous

Students who have been in homeopathic treatment or who engage in homeopathic treatment during their training make better homeopaths. They have more compassion for their patients. They have a better understanding and appreciation of the homeopathic process. Homeopathic treatment improves the mental health and helps to clear the perceptions of students. This thereby improves the quality of their work. Some leaders in homeopathy feel that this should be a required part of training, while others contend that requiring it would make it less valuable.

Learning Is Hard

I must admit that homeopathy has never let me down;
I have failed when I did not have sufficient facts.
Homeopathy is a life-long study,
it requires the burning of the midnight oil,
but it is worthwhile.
—Dorothy Shepherd

Learning homeopathy is difficult. It is a complex field, every bit as difficult to master as conventional medicine or acupuncture. It fully engages one's being, rather than simply the intellect.

Learning is a verb. It is active, hard work. Effective learning does not come from passive absorption, but from wrestling with everything one is exposed to. It requires the focusing of attention and active listening. New learning must be integrated with what one already knows. Only in this way is knowledge given "roots." Learning also means opening oneself to new ideas, to one's patients and to the world.

It is helpful to realize that true learning is often more about remembering than about learning something new (Bennis, 1989). As learners, we unearth and uncover that which we already know. Galileo said, "You cannot teach people anything. You can only help them discover it themselves."

Planting Seeds

Life is lived forward, but it is understood backward.
—Soren Kierkegarrd

Teachers plant the seeds of learning in their students. Learners often do not understand or appreciate this at the time. These seeds may take years to bear fruit or to flower. It is only in retrospect that students recognize the greatness of some of their teachers. Students often feel frustrated that they are unable to learn more or to integrate their knowledge completely during their training. Yet they often have learned much more than they realized.

What students need and what they want are often very different. Ultimately, teachers must focus not on what students want, but on what they need to help them to grow. Good teachers are able to help students appreciate that their needs must take priority over their wants.

Many teachers teach best at a certain level. Their skills might be most suited to beginning students, advanced students or students in clinical training. Students sometimes find that teachers they did not learn well from early in their training become some of their best teachers at later stages.

You Are Never Alone on the Journey

> *Furthermore, we have not even to risk the adventure alone, for the heroes of all time have gone before us. The labyrinth is thoroughly known. We have only to follow the thread of the hero path, and where we had thought to find an abomination we shall find a god. And where we had thought to slay another, we shall slay ourselves. Where we had thought to travel outward, we will come to the center of our own existence. And where we had thought to be alone, we will be with all the world.*
> —Joseph Campbell

Learning homeopathy can be a lonely and isolating process. Yet, students are never alone on their homeopathic journey. All the great homeopaths of all time are with them in their work, lending support and encouragement. Knowing this can help students persevere through the difficult moments in their training.

Gratitude

> *Once I was young, but now I am old. Take this third edition as the old man's testament to his many students and younger colleagues, for your success rejuvenates your old teachers.*
> —Lilienthal's introduction to the third edition of
> *Homeopathic Therapeutics*

It is important to give thanks to our teachers, both those in the present and those who came before. Gratitude is a way of renewing our spirit as students. It both validates our teachers and administrators and helps them cope in one of the most difficult of professions. Even a small degree of positive feedback can considerably brighten the life of an educator. Gratitude can be given through indirect methods, such as evaluations, or through direct feedback. It is difficult for students to find the time to fill out evaluation forms, and yet even a little commentary can provide tremendous service. Giving one's teacher an apple is another way to show one's gratitude.

The apple signifies not only the words of the teacher bearing fruit, but also the potential of the apple seeds to sprout, grow and nurture others.

In Albert Camus' autobiography *The Last Man*, he writes to his teacher, Germain, when he receives the Nobel Prize:

> When I learned the news of my award, my first thought, after my mother, was for you. Without you, without the loving hand you extended to the poor little child that I was, without your teaching and your example, nothing of this would have happened. I do not make much of this sort of honor. But it at least presents an occasion to tell you what you have been and always are to me, and to assure you that your efforts, your work, and the generous heart that you offered me are always alive within one of your little schoolboys who despite his age, has not ceased being your grateful student. I embrace you with all my strength.

Chapter Two

The Art of Learning Homeopathy

It is the supreme art of the teacher to awaken joy
in creative expression and knowledge.
—Albert Einstein

Homeopathic education concerns more than simply learning to become a homeopathic practitioner. Education involves healing, wholeness, empowerment, liberation, transcendence and finding and claiming ourselves (Palmer 1998).

As with teaching and leading on the homeopathic journey, learning homeopathy is as much an art as it is a science. This art can be described as a series of qualities, knowledge and skills that must be both called forth from within and discovered from without. Qualities are ways of being in the world. They reflect our underlying attitudes about our work, ourselves and our world. Knowledge is the perception of truth. It requires awareness and mental clarity. Skills are the means by which we apply what we have learned. Skills require applied excellence.

Qualities of Good Homeopathic Students

*We have learnt that nothing is simple and rational except
what we ourselves have invented; that God thinks neither in
terms of Euclid nor of Riemann; that science has "explained"
nothing; that the more we know the more fantastic the world
becomes and the profounder the surrounding darkness.*
—Aldous Huxley

Homeopathic students must learn skills and knowledge on their homeopathic journey. More important, they must learn the attitudes essential to being a good homeopathic learner (Kreisberg 1998). Awareness of these qualities (the art of homeopathy) can take the student a long way toward becoming an effective learner.

The qualities of good homeopathic students are identical to those of good homeopathic practitioners. They are similar to the qualities of good homeopathic teachers and leaders. Yet they are unique as well.

Listed below are qualities commonly seen in successful students. They cannot be sought but they can be cultivated (see also Banner and Cannon 1999).

Patience

*Only with winter-patience can we bring
the deep-desired, long-awaited spring.*
—Anne Morrow Lindbergh

An irony of learning homeopathy is the feeling that one must know everything about homeopathy before one can even start. Beginning students often want it all, and they want it now. Yet their impatience can be an impediment to their learning.

Many students suffer from homeopathic gluttony (see Chapter One). They cannot get enough of homeopathy. They become obsessed with their learning, buying every book available. Their restless pursuit of knowledge leaves them unbalanced, and they eventually burn out or become ill. The door to learning opens inward. The harder one pushes on the door, the more it closes.

It is critical that learning remains in harmony with other aspects in the student's life. Homeopathic students need to practice patience. They must develop thoroughness in their work that belies hurrying. The homeopathic journey demands a lifetime of study. Good students patiently remain for the long haul.

Compassion

> *One looks back with appreciation to the brilliant teachers,*
> *but with gratitude to those who touched our human feel-*
> *ings. The curriculum is so much necessary raw material,*
> *but warmth is the vital element for growing and for the*
> *soul of the student.*
> —Carl Gustav Jung

Compassion defines good healers and is central to the experience of being a homeopath. Unfortunately, this quality is systematically trained out of most students in contemporary medical education. Medical schools frequently focus on scientific objectivity and provide no room for authentic sharing of one's humanity. This is especially true of the emotional side of students' lives.

Compassion cannot be taught; it must be discovered (Rachel Naomi Remen, MD, in Glazer 1994). It rises from the experience of empathy, the realization that all suffering is like our suffering. For people to feel compassion, they must be connected with others. One part of compassion is the ability to resonate or be in tune with others while maintaining one's own distinctness. This is different from sympathy, where students lose themselves in the difficulties of others.

Compassion comes from a place of authenticity. To learn and practice homeopathy effectively, it is necessary to be authentic in the work. When students begin their homeopathic training, they are often wearing many masks that have been carefully built up from the past. These masks can only be removed with courage and some pain. Many have been wearing the masks for so long, they have forgotten that they are wearing them. Through mirroring (see Chapter Five), homeopathic clients can help students see behind their masks.

A Search for Wholeness

> *That is what learning is.*
> *You suddenly understand something*
> *you've understood all your life, but in a new way.*
> —Doris Lessing

True learning requires that one engage all of oneself in the process. It means bringing one's humanity into the work. This requires intimacy with one's perception, one's experience, one's feelings, one's heart and one's spirit.

The Latin word "educare" is the root of "education" and means "to lead forth the hidden wholeness." For many students, this can be a fearful process as it touches on new and sometimes uncomfortable ways of being with their patients and themselves. One of the great challenges in homeopathic education is to help students see the whole rather than the part.

Much of contemporary medical education teaches students to narrow down and to use only parts of themselves. This makes them skilled technicians but not real healers. Allopathic education fosters the worldview of seeing life through a material lens—the world is a place where matter is to be owned, manipulated and used. In such a world, value is lost. When education is separated from wholeness, the result has been described as "flatland" (Ken Wilbur in Glazer 1994). Ultimately, to heal and to educate mean much the same thing. In homeopathy, one must own the split-off parts of oneself and use all of oneself in the work.

Good education fosters a lifelong journey into wholeness. It is impossible to engage fully in the work of being a homeopath without transforming and changing oneself in important ways.

Fascination with the Little Things in Life

God is in the details.
—Espinoza

Learners of homeopathy must have the capacity to see the very small. They must be fascinated with the minutiae or the details. What is unusual, strange, rare and peculiar in homeopathy often represents what is most important in understanding and experiencing our patients. From this perspective, the little facts about remedies become as important as understanding their broad pictures. The dance in learning becomes the movement back and forth between the little things and perception of the whole.

Self-Discipline

Learning is not attained by chance,
it must be sought for with ardor
and attended to with diligence.
—Abigail Adams

Self-discipline is order that one imposes on oneself, a way of building an internal structure to one's life. Learning homeopathy requires much concentration and focused thought. Those who work hard and are diligent develop a deep sense of inner commitment to the process and the journey.

The initial enthusiasm and euphoria will only carry students so far. It is very difficult for adult learners to engage in a program of two to four years without a deep sense of commitment. It is hard to predict what will occur in one's life, years from the present. Self-discipline can sustain students through the vicissitudes of the journey.

Some students deny the importance of self-discipline, focusing on their intuition to carry them through their work. My experience has been that students who rely too much on intuition in their work become frustrated and eventually drop out of training. They undervalue what they have learned.

Much of self-discipline has to do with a willingness to identify one's weaknesses as a learner of homeopathy and work on them (see Chapter One). It is important for students to play to their strengths, but also to work continually on their weaknesses.

Initiative

There is no learning without your wanting it
and your starting it.
—Nathaniel Cantor

Beyond self-discipline lies initiative. Students must take initiative and responsibility for their own education. Initiative is the antidote for laziness and inertia. It keeps students going despite the roadblocks life throws their way. Initiative is born from the passionate love of the subject.

Initiative also creates adventure in learning. Homeopathy is a relatively young field of study and homeopaths have only scratched its surface. Discovering more about homeopathy requires initiative, courage and a willingness to run risks. Learning is chaotic and involves moving into the unknown. It necessitates tolerating uncertainty and ambiguity. Good students quickly become comfortable with the chaos that learning entails.

Initiative is not motivated by competition. When students compare themselves with other students (either through striving to be better than or feeling less than), they lose the openness of heart, mind and spirit that true learning entails. This ultimately leads to increasing preoccupation with performance and a movement away from the "Great Subject" that is homeopathy. Competition is always about power, unless it is competition with oneself.

Students with initiative see evaluations as learning opportunities. They do not rely on exams just to test their knowledge, but also to test themselves.

Excitement

> *Study, learn, but guard the original naivete.*
> *It has to be within you, as desire for drink is within*
> *the drunkard or love is within the lover.*
> —Henri Matisse

Learning requires excitement—action and passion about the subject and the learning process. It has been said to be like love: there must be some ongoing source of fascination, mystery and magnetism. The most powerful learning can then become like play.

Most students begin training with an initial feeling of passion and exhilaration. The challenge is to maintain this feeling over time. Excitement helps sustain students on the homeopathic journey.

What helps students maintain excitement is playing to their interests. Some students become excited about repertory, others about materia medica, while still others find their passion in case taking and case analysis. It's hard to stay excited while one is struggling with the learning process. Students should study and learn what excites them. This excitement can sustain them through dull parts of training. Studies have consistently shown that students remember best that which they are intrigued by. Good curriculums often alternate homeopathic subjects throughout the day, with the hope that all students will find something especially interesting to them.

Success in learning, demonstrated perhaps by a good evaluation or test result, generates excitement. When setbacks occur, it helps to remember one's successes and maintain a positive attitude.

Finally, excitement occurs most when the student and the subject feel most alive. Students can accomplish this by seeing the remedies in the world around them and connecting what they learn with their life (see Chapter One).

Enjoyment

> *It is paradoxical that many educators*
> *still differentiate between a time for learning*
> *and a time for play without seeing the*
> *vital connection between them.*
> —Leo Buscaglia

Learning must be fun, and it is best accompanied by laughter. One of the keys for this is to bring play into learning. Good teachers know how to be playful, and learning in their class is a pleasure.

A childlike attitude is key to making the learning process fun. Children have a natural love for learning. Play is a principal way in which children learn about life in all its complexity and wonder. As they grow, this frequently gets trained out of them. Students have to combat the negative popular beliefs that it is silly, unscientific or foolish to be at play during learning.

Wonder

> *It is the state of wonder that creates*
> *the human desire to learn.*
> —Socrates

Wonder is an attitude that students hold within themselves. It keeps them open as learners. It is more than curiosity or pondering. Curiosity and pondering come from an openness of the mind. Wonder comes from an openness of the mind, heart, imagination and spirit. When people hold wonder in their heart, it means that they are open to all of life and lie in wait to ambush and pounce on the "great things" of life. It is a childlike place, full of surprise, where they are filled with the possibilities of life. Wonder is the place where students sit when they realize that each client has a gift to offer them. Zen teachings describe this as "beginner's mind."

Wonder keeps students asking the questions they should be asking. It is important not to take what one learns on faith, but to ask why and seek explanations for everything. Wonder is the most important attitude that homeopaths carry in case analysis. The life of Samuel Hahnemann (the founder of homeopathy) provides a powerful example of wonder. He constantly had the courage to be open, experiment and try new things. Wondering is a defining quality of homeopathy. It separates homeopaths from allopaths. Allopaths ponder, whereas homeopaths wonder.

The opposite of wonder is prejudice. Prejudiced learners believe that they know more than others; that they are right and others are wrong. Prejudiced students do not feel wonder and are not paying attention to themselves and the world around them. They've closed down; and a closed mind cannot learn. Each student must try out new knowledge and play with it. Students can only wonder as far as they allow themselves to grow.

Developing the capacity to wonder is a central task for a homeopath. The homeopathic journey can become a thrilling adventure filled with wonder.

Aspiration

The type of mind which homeopathy needs and which is susceptible to homeopathy is not the type which waits to be told by science or some authority what to do. The right minds for homeopathy will be attracted by the vision of it, by the spirit of adventure in the realm of principles and potentials.
—R.E.S. Hayes

Part of what helps students survive a rigorous and difficult training program is to have a vision that sustains them. This vision provides a road map and compass for what lies ahead. It involves setting learning goals and having the determination to pursue those goals throughout homeopathic training. In this way, students can define and grow into their professional identity.

This personal vision should be established at the beginning of training. In part, it is an image of having completed one's training and having become a homeopath. It also consists of a series of professional goals. Aspiration cannot be given; it must come from within. It can be helpful to study the aspirations of others in creating your own.

This vision serves as a compass. It nurtures students during training and is a source of strength. It also orients them when they fall off course. It should be periodically revisited throughout training. For optimum learning to occur, the student's vision should be in harmony with the school's collective vision.

The vision must be larger than the individual. Students should imagine themselves going beyond what they are required to study and learn. Their vision should encourage them to surpass who they are and their circumstances.

Aspiration is separate from ambition. Ambition is self-centered and power seeking. Aspiration is coupled with ideals. It comes from a place of responsibility to those who teach you and to those who have come before. It also relates to the responsibility of leaving a legacy for those who follow.

Imagination

To accomplish great things,
we must dream as well as act.
—Anatole France

Imagination opens the door to knowledge. During the process of integrating knowledge, students need to reflect on and play with what they have learned. Imagination brings creativity to learning. It makes the concrete abstract and the abstract concrete. It enlivens learning and can make the ordinary magical.

Through imagination, students can see where they are on their homeopathic journey. Imagination also helps them envision what it is to be a homeopath.

Imagination can be cultivated. The key is to become free from the internal censor. The internal censor is that part of the human psyche that strives to limit the imagination, keeping things safe and encouraging the mind to stay with the tried and true. When students can free themselves from it, training becomes a laboratory in which they experiment with truth.

Although the imagination is a powerful tool for the student, it must always be grounded in the here and now. In analyzing a case, for example, it is important to use the faculty of the imagination, while staying focused on what the patient says and how they act.

Civility

I disapprove of everything you say,
but I will defend to the death your right to say it.
—Voltaire

Good students are civil. To be civil, means to be a citizen of a larger learning community. Civility is thinking not just of oneself, but also of others and their needs. Civil students acknowledge the right of others to speak, to be heard and to think in their own way. Their actions do not hurt others around them. They maintain self-control. Civil students treat others with respect and kindness. Homeopathy is a small profession. It is important to be nice to other students, as fellow students of today will be colleagues of tomorrow. Civil students are punctual, polite and well mannered. They remember that teachers and administrators were also once students.

Honesty

He who conceals his disease cannot be cured.
—Ethiopian saying

Honesty is the foundation of trust between the student, the teacher and the administrator. Honesty has both external and internal components. Externally, honesty relates to telling the truth to others. This requires openness and sincerity. It means taking responsibility for one's work and representing that work fairly. To grow effectively, students also need honest evaluations from their teachers and peers.

Internally, honesty is concerned with telling the truth to oneself. Internal honesty requires that students know themselves and be able to evaluate themselves accurately. It means knowing their weaknesses and strengths. Honest self-evaluation becomes critical to a student's continuing journey as a homeopath, especially after training is completed. Students can only be honest with themselves if they are also honest in their work. Most students have difficulty with self-evaluation. Good teachers assist them in becoming more effective at self-evaluation.

Humility

The more we study, the more we discover our ignorance.
—Percy Bysshe Shelley

Homeopathy is a "Great Thing." It is vast and unbounded. To be fully in its presence brings a feeling of humility. This sense of humility is coupled with respect. As long as students stay focused on the subject, and not on themselves, humility is possible. Nothing shuts down true learning faster than arrogance and pride.

Knowledge Is Central to Good Homeopathy

No man can reveal to you aught but that which already lies half-asleep in the dawning of your knowledge. The teacher who walks in the shadow of the temple, among his follow-ers, gives not of his wisdom but rather of his faith and his lovingness. If he is indeed wise he does not bid you enter the house of his wisdom, but rather leads you to the threshold of your own mind.
                                                —Kahlil Gibran

Good students develop a thorough knowledge of their subject. Because the field of homeopathy is so broad, this can be a challenge. Homeopathy is potentially daunting, as it touches on the study of all life. The key isn't to learn it all, but to learn enough to continue ones' education on ones' own after graduating from a formal training program.

Students also must develop knowledge of themselves. Self-awareness is a critical factor in the practice of homeopathy. For example, self awareness helps to prevent the freedom from prejudice that's central to good case taking and case analysis.

Lastly, those who study homeopathy must develop knowledge of the homeopathic community and profession. Only then can they integrate themselves into the homeopathic community on completion of their train-ing. This community provides nourishment and a sustaining source through the vicissitudes of practice.

Most students can learn anything they choose if they have sufficient self-discipline and aspiration. Good learners are not born; they are made. This is also true of good homeopaths.

Learning How to Learn

They know enough who know how to learn.
                    —Henry Adams

Most of the heart of becoming a homeopath is learned only after the student finishes homeopathic training. The most important task in train-ing is not learning homeopathy, but learning how to learn homeopathy. Students must know how to study and observe on their own, for doing so will be a continual process in their career.

It is hard to convince students of the importance of self-learning. Self-learning requires commitment and self-discipline (Landis 1990). The process of homeopathic training is concerned with uncovering the homeopath that is already within the student. In this way the learning of homeopathy is caught rather than taught. Through self-learning, students move from teacher dependence to active learning.

Practicing Self-Observation and Self-Reflection

> *Truth is within ourselves; it takes no rise*
> *From outward things, what'er you may believe.*
> *There is an inmost centre in us all,*
> *Where truth abides in fullness; and around,*
> *Wall upon wall, the gross flesh hems it in,*
> *This perfect, clear perception—which is truth.*
> *A baffling and perverting carnal mesh*
> *Binds it, and makes all error; and to know*
> *Rather consists in opening out a way*
> *Whence the imprisoned splendour may escape,*
> *Than in effecting entry for a light*
> *Supposed to be without.*
> —Robert Browning

Homeopathic training is both an outer and inner journey of discovery. It is not possible to go through homeopathic training and come out the other side unchanged. Changing one's perception and finding alternative ways of looking at the world forces the student to grow. Self-observation and self-reflection are critical parts in facilitating this inner journey. Sharing ones inner experience with one's peers, dream work, mentorship groups and retreats all represent opportunities to further this inner work.

True understanding comes only from reflecting on one's experience. Students learn to trust their intuition or gut instincts. This is an important tool in homeopathic work. Like any tool, it can be over-utilized and overly relied upon. It is important to balance this with sound study and external knowledge.

Skills of the Homeopathic Learner

The man who can make hard things easy is the educator.
—Ralph Waldo Emerson

Students must not only possess certain knowledge and qualities to be effective learners of homeopathy, but also certain skills. Skills make the journey easier. They help you avoid the obstacles and pitfalls along the way. Although these skills can be effectively taught and learned, all students must create their own "skill tool kit" that uniquely fits them. Necessary skills include but are not limited to the following:

Individualizing One's Learning

There is no royal road to learning.
—Euclid

Each student learns differently. There is no right way to learn. It is important to find the style and approach that uniquely fits the student. The skill is to honor one's uniqueness and individuality in learning. This requires a willingness to continually experiment.

Students also find that their learning needs change over time. Learning methods that were effective at one stage of training might not be useful later on. At each stage of the journey, students should reassess their learning style and seek out new and more effective methods that match their current needs.

Working within a Community

Never doubt that a small group of thoughtful and committed citizens can change the world. Indeed it is the only thing that ever has.
—Margaret Mead

A great survival tactic for students is to become part of a supportive learning community. Such a community provides shelter amid the storms of learning. Education is often a lonely process. (This is particularly true for students in distance-learning programs.) A student often feels that he or she is the only one struggling with certain material and is astonished to find that others are sharing the same struggles.

It takes two to learn. This is true whether a student learns from a patient, a current teacher or those who have gone before. Much of learning is collaborative and reciprocal. Students often learn better when working together, finding that the learning increases exponentially. Student learners expand beyond their individual capacities when they are in community. They are lifted higher. Community also adds human interest to learning, thereby making learning easier.

A student can be part of a learning community through a class or by pairing off with other students in stable dyads, triads or tetrads. They can also join study groups, although it is critical that students in the group are at similar learning levels for the group to survive. The Internet also offers many possibilities for the development of an extended homeopathic learning community.

Learning communities offer opportunities for the learner not just to receive, but also to give something back. Teaching others can be a critical step in integrating and assimilating knowledge. This can be the beginning step that helps learners to become teachers themselves. Learning communities enable students to teach and to experience other students' strategies and "tricks" in learning. They teach the skill of interdependence, which is critical to professional development once the student is out in practice.

Attending graduations are an important part of working within a community. Not only can these be inspirational, but they also help students see where they are on their respective homeopathic journeys.

Tolerating Ambiguity

> *In their everyday work, therapists, if they are to relate to their patients in an authentic fashion, experience considerable uncertainty…the capacity to tolerate uncertainty is a prerequisite for the profession. Though the public may believe that therapists guide patients systematically and sure handedly through predictable stages of therapy to a foreknown goal, such is rarely the case: instead therapists frequently wobble, improvise, and grope for direction. The powerful temptation to achieve certainty through embracing an ideological school and a tight therapeutic system is treacherous; such belief may block the uncertain and spontaneous encounter necessary for effective therapy.*
> —Irving Yalom

Most students want certainty and abhor change. They wish their teachers to provide them with the "right" answers. This is particularly an issue at the beginning of training, when students require a solid foundation on which to build. New students are often certain about homeopathic prescriptions, defending them vehemently, although they have been studying for only a short time. They are disconcerted when different faculty members offer different points of view about something. Ultimately, the faculty must be similar enough to share a common foundation, but diverse enough to help students develop their own uniqueness.

Homeopathy is not only a science, but also an art. There is much uncertainty and ambiguity on the homeopathic journey. It is critical for the homeopathic student to become comfortable with this ambiguity and to celebrate it as a reason to go deeper in their work and understanding.

Taking Advantage of the Unexpected

> *When I was six years old, growing up in Pittsburgh, I used to take a precious penny of my own and hide it for someone else to find. It was a curious compulsion; sadly, I've never been seized by it since. For some reason I always "hid" the penny along the same stretch of sidewalk up the street. I would cradle it at the roots of a sycamore, say or in a hole left by a chipped off piece of sidewalk. Then I would take a piece of chalk, and, starting at either end of the block, draw huge arrows leading up to the penny from both directions. After I learned to write I labeled the arrows SURPRISE AHEAD or MONEY THIS WAY. I was greatly excited, during all this arrow-drawing, at the thought of the first lucky passer-by who would receive in this way, regardless of merit, a free gift from the universe. But I never lurked about. I would go straight home and not give the matter another thought, until, some months later, I would be gripped again by the impulse to hide another penny.*
> —Annie Dillard

Unexpected events occur throughout the learning process. These surprises often represent the most significant episodes in learning (Speak and Mocker 1984; Spear 1988). They cause the student to take an unanticipated turn in their learning journey. Most often, these events have a strong emotional component and are synchronous in origin. The key is for students to learn to take full advantage of these events when they occur, seeing them as opportunities rather than events to get around.

Stalking

In summer I stalk. I have to seek things out. I can stalk them in either of two ways. The first is not what you think of as true stalking, but it is the Via Negativa, and as fruitful as actual pursuit. When I stalk this way I take my stand on a bridge and wait emptied. I put myself in the way of the creature's passage.
—Annie Dillard

Homeopathic training often requires single-minded intensity. It necessitates total immersion and absorption in the field and in one's clients. It is a place where there are no distractions, where one puts all of one's being. This intensity is well encompassed in the idea of stalking. What one stalks as a student is the "Great Subject" of homeopathy. Students must constantly be on the lookout for learning opportunities. This necessitates a willingness to embrace change and diversity.

In *Winnie the Pooh* by A. A. Milne, Pooh bear stalks a woozle. Piglet later joins him in the search. They have never seen a woozle before, but they know that it might be dangerous. As they proceed on their search, they come across tracks in the snow that they follow. Eventually, a second set of tracks appears with the first set, and they realize that there are now two woozles. They proceed with even more caution and suddenly discover four sets of tracks. Piglet becomes frightened and decides to return home, while Winnie the Pooh bravely continues. After awhile Pooh sees Christopher Robin, who has been watching him for some time and asks Winnie the Pooh what he is doing. Pooh replies that he is stalking woozles. Christopher Robin laughs and says that he has been watching Pooh go round in circles following his own tracks.

In stalking, it is important to always remember what one is stalking. This changes as the homeopathic journey progresses. What begins with a search for external knowledge leads eventually to greater self-awareness. What begins with a search for the "right" remedy in our casework leads to seeking wholeness and health. When students encounter the fiercest monsters on their journey, they encounter themselves.

Seeing/Perceiving

> *The secret of seeing is, then, the pearl of great price. If I*
> *thought he could teach me to find it and keep it forever I*
> *would stagger barefoot across a hundred deserts after any*
> *lunatic at all. But although the pearl may be found, it may*
> *not be sought. The literature of illumination reveals this*
> *above all: although it comes to those who wait for it, it is*
> *always, even to the most practiced and adept, a gift and a*
> *total surprise.*
> —Annie Dillard

There are many ways of seeing, feeling and listening in a case. A key to effective clinical work is to develop one's own perception. The best homeopaths have developed skills that allow them to perceive in diverse yet complementary ways. Some of this is reflected in the capacity to perceive what is unique and individualizing in life. A lover can spot their beloved in a crowd in an instant, just as an experienced homeopath can spot the remedy or perceive what is central to the case.

Perception involves both analysis and synthesis. In synthesis, one takes much disparate information and brings it together in a meaningful whole. In analysis, one breaks down a large amount of data into its component parts and underlying ideas. A student must be comfortable with both skills and able to move back and forth between them.

Taking Responsibility for Learning

> *A teacher is a guide and director; he steers the boat,*
> *but the energy that propels it must come from*
> *those who are learning.*
> —John Dewey

Many students believe that it is the teacher's responsibility to make them learn. It truth, it is the student's responsibility. Students are their own best teachers. It has been said that you do not get an education, you make one. Students summon from within themselves the qualities that make education productive (Bannor and Cannon, 1999). They must feel free to follow their own learning in whatever direction it leads.

Accepting and Providing Good Feedback

The greater one's love for a person, the less room for flattery.
The proof of true love is to be unsparing in criticism.
—Moliere

Communication is an essential building block for good learning. It is critical to practicing effectively as a homeopath. Listening to feedback is a major part of good communication. Good students actively seek feedback. They see their mistakes as learning opportunities. They ask for specific, descriptive feedback and then reflect on what they have understood from that feedback.

It is often difficult for students to receive feedback without feeling defensive and criticized. Feedback can be perceived as personal attack, rather than as professional critique. It can elicit strong emotional reactions, including shock, denial and resistance. Students need to truly listen to feedback, rather than attempting to defend their position. In listening to feedback, it is helpful for students to seek alternatives and not answers. Students must also make sure they have properly understood the feedback and are not projecting their own issues onto the evaluation. Summarizing one's understanding of feedback can be quite helpful.

Students must not only receive, but also give feedback. Teachers and administrators rely on student feedback to learn and grow. Students must put discipline and energy into providing good feedback, but this is critical to the development of the school culture. Learning to give feedback is also important for homeopathic practitioners, teachers and leaders.

Critical Incident Review

Where there is no vision, the people perish
—Proverbs 29:18

A technique called "critical incident review" can help students identify the skills, qualities and knowledge essential to the art of homeopathy. During this process, students review critical moments in their homeopathic learning experience (Brookfield 1990). This occurs individually or within a community of peers. Important questions to consider include the following:

◉ At what moment did the student decide to pursue learning? What inspired the student at that time? What was the student's vision? Does the student hold the same vision now?

◉ Who are the student's models of good learners? What makes these models good learners? What are the qualities that inspired the student? Which of these qualities does the student share, and which ones does the student need to develop?

◉ At what moments has the student felt her or she was learning best? What made the learning particularly effective? What teaching qualities were employed at those times that made learning effective?

◉ At what moments has the student felt he or she was learning worst? What made the learning particularly ineffective in these moments? What are the student's learning weaknesses? How are these weaknesses coupled with their strengths?

When Does the Student Become a Teacher?

In seeking knowledge, the first step is silence,
the second listening, the third remembering,
the fourth practicing and the fifth—teaching others.
—Solon Ibn Gabirol

For many students, teaching is an important learning method. The standard educational quip in medical school is, "See one, do one, teach one, administrate one." Teaching can begin early in training as students assist one another and join as "study buddies" who informally teach one another. The key is to teach at a level at which you are both knowledgeable and comfortable (see Chapter Three). There are many opportunities for giving introductory talks and entering beginning-level study groups in most communities.

Some students choose to be perpetual students, always staying in the role of learner and never becoming practitioner or teacher. There comes a stage in one's self-growth where it is necessary to give something back. Learners are like cups: Knowledge can be continually poured in, but at a certain point the cup overflows. Unless the cup is continually emptied—whether through teaching, practicing or leading—the student cannot absorb any more knowledge. Volunteering in homeopathy can be another important way of emptying the cup, giving something back and making room for further growth.

Chapter Three

The Art of Teaching Homeopathy

The Call to Teach

> *When you do know something about the reality*
> *of the world that those who stand in ignorance*
> *do not know, then you can't not educate.*
> —Betty Powell

Teachers do not choose to teach, they are called. The call comes from the deepest parts of themselves and the deepest aspects of what they teach. For many teachers, to deny this is to deny their inner nature, the teacher within.

When teaching in class, teachers experience moments of epiphany that make them much more than they are. The deepest parts of the teachers' heart are called forward in the teaching process. Teaching opens the heart and makes one vulnerable. It takes great courage to keep the heart open in this way. Teaching is an act of courage and a lifelong art. This is illustrated in such movies as *Mr. Holland's Opus*, *Stand and Deliver* and *The Pride of Miss Jean Brodie*.

There is a natural progression from learning to teaching. Teaching is the next step in self-growth and in forming a professional identity. To teach is to learn twice. There is no better way to learn.

Teaching is very different from practice. Practice in homeopathy can be an isolating and lonely experience. Teaching is more public than practice and occurs at the intersection of personal and public life. Some choose teaching as a means to break out of their isolation.

Teachers are found in the student's life at every stage of growth and individuation. Yet, at a certain stage in that growth, the student can no longer find a teacher. For some students, this is a time when they seek desperately for the next teacher on their journey and can feel disappointed. For others, it is a time to start being a teacher themselves.

It has been said, "Those who can, do; those who can't, teach." Although this is occasionally true, to be an effective homeopathic teacher, one has to have experienced homeopathy deeply. Most often this experience has been in practice. The interplay between teaching and practicing can help one grow tremendously as both a practitioner and a teacher. The best teachers are not necessarily the best practitioners. What is critical is that they are homeopathic learners.

It is important not to confuse academic success with teaching ability. Teachers who struggled in their own learning process may make better teachers because they understand their students' struggles. Good teachers are always growing. There is always another step in the teaching journey.

The most important thing to teach is a deep love for homeopathy. This is expressed in the language, actions and heart of the teacher. The teacher's main challenge is to help students have the courage and heart to become homeopaths. Yet not all students become practitioners, nor should teachers insist that they do so. There are many ways to serve homeopathy outside homeopathic practice.

Good teachers strive to see transformation in their students. An effective homeopathic teacher wants to see students grow not only as homeopaths, but also as individuals.

Teaching Models

> *Believe me, we homeopaths are not what you have been taught to think; we have no secrets; we aim all of us, each according to his ability and in his own way to advance the true interests of our beneficent art, and our most earnest desire before God and man is to teach all we know to all knowledge seeking lovers of truth…*
>
> —James Compton-Burnett

Teaching is a form of service. Whom do teachers serve? Do they serve themselves, their students or their subject? Teachers must struggle with these questions and find answers for themselves.

The following are several models that teachers adopt.

The Teacher-Centered Model

Much of the current teaching in healing is allopathically oriented. The allopathic world is a one of objectivism, where things are broken down into their component parts. It is a world of theoretical knowledge, deductive reasoning and inert ideas.

The allopathic teaching model is teacher-centered. In this model, truth is traditionally handed down from the authorities (teachers) to the amateurs (students). The class often becomes like a dictatorship. Students are treated as children by their all-wise and all-knowing parent/teachers. Consequently, students often feel belittled, controlled and ignored. Teachers in this model often feel isolated from their students and resent their students' dependency and rebelliousness. Students and teachers are much more likely to project thoughts and feelings from their own childhood onto one another. The other problem with this model is that there is little self-development or self-learning.

The Student-Centered Model

Another model of teaching is the student-centered ("isopathic") model. Here the focus is more on active learning. The classroom emphasizes honoring the students, and they become the center of the class. A disadvantage of this approach is that it can lead to chaos in the classroom, with many side-tracks and a meandering flow. Students often lack clear direction, purpose or vision in this model. Inspiration or deep motivation to learn can also be lacking. Teachers in this model often feel peripheral and powerless. The class has a life of its own and is out of the teacher's control. Isopathy, though sometimes an effective method of healing and teaching, does not go deep enough.

The Subject-Centered Model

Homeopathy, by its own nature, requires a subject-centered teaching model. This style of teaching originates from a love for homeopathy. Here, a community of learners surrounds the "great subject" that is homeopathy (Palmer 1999). This great subject is much more than what they are. The poet Rilke once said, "Community is held together by the power of the grace of great things." (Rilke 1986).

Great subjects require teachers and students to practice humility and honesty when working with them. The best teachers point to homeopathy and then get out of the way. They act as a bridge between the student and the subject. They are detached enough to enable the student not to confuse the teacher with the message.

Levels of Teaching

Not only is there an art in knowing a thing,
but also a certain art in teaching it.
—Marcus Tullius Cicero

There are three levels to teaching. The first and most superficial is teaching to know. This level focuses on relating knowledge, facts and data to the student. Students absorb this material and memorize it.

The second level lies deeper and concerns teaching to learn. This requires a deeper understanding of the material. Here students learn how to learn about new remedies and explore homeopathy on their own. Teachers must awaken a thirst for knowledge.

The third and deepest level of teaching is teaching to "be." This is where students learn how to be homeopaths. It is about establishing an identity. Teachers must awaken a longing to become a homeopath.

All these levels are important, and the art of teaching is to address all of them simultaneously. Good teachers are comfortable moving back and forth between these levels. Although the subject is homeopathy, good teaching concerns all of life. Students must know something about pathology, anatomy, physics, biology, anthropology, chemistry, zoology, botany, mineralogy, psychology, pharmacology, sociology and many other fields.

Getting Started

Much have I learned from my teachers,
more from my colleagues, but most from my students.
—From the *Talmud*

There is a certain amount of arrogance in believing that if you are a good practitioner, you are also an effective teacher. Good teaching must be learned and practiced. Teaching homeopathically means finding a method of teaching that is similar to that which is being taught (see Introduction). Subject-centered teaching is an important step on that journey.

Some teachers feel that they cannot teach unless they have studied teaching for years. It is not necessary, however, for every good teacher to have a master's or doctorate in education. The best teachers learn how to teach from their students.

Many potential teachers are hampered by the fear that they lack sufficient knowledge and skills to be effective. They may feel that they don't have what it takes. However, if teachers wait to begin teaching until they "know all the answers," they will never begin. Most good teachers, like most good students, are made and not born. Homeopathic teachers must work to develop the skills, attitudes and knowledge that will make them good. During this process, it's helpful to remember that students can learn as much from a teacher's failure as they can from his/her success. Good teachers show students how to find answers for themselves.

Some practitioners begin teaching immediately, on an introductory level. They see teaching as an opportunity to consolidate their knowledge and skills. They start with introductory talks or by teaching beginning-level study groups. (See Appendix C for opportunities in your area.) Other practitioners feel comfortable teaching only after many years of practice, when they have had a chance to carefully refine their thoughts, feelings and experiences.

One way to ease into teaching is as a student teacher. A student teacher practices in a classroom with an experienced teacher who can offer guidance and immediate feedback. Student teaching is a way to get comfortable in the teaching role.

Another way is acting "as if." A group of prominent spiritual teachers was once asked to name the skill that was most helpful to their success. They said it was to act "as if." When teachers begin, the group explained, they must act as if they are great teachers. Gradually, they go from acting the role to living it. Effective teachers must be authentic to themselves.

Learning to teach homeopathically is a life-long process. There is always a next step on the journey.

Stages of Development as a Teacher

In some ways, growth resembles a game of leapfrog.
As soon as we've got past one puzzling question,
we discover we're faced with another.
—Jean Grasso Fitzpatrick

As with learning and leadership, teaching development can be viewed miasmatically (see Introduction). Miasms are part of the growth process and can be used to describe the stages of growth and development on the homeopathic journey (Van Der Zee 2000). Carl Jung called this individuation, the process of self growth and becoming more of who we truly are (1977). Teaching and practice represent the sycotic (middle stage) aspects of the homeopathic journey. This is the stage of exploring endurance, empathy, tolerance, freedom from prejudice, the shadow and the unconscious, forgiveness, honesty, self-appreciation and self-condemnation (Van Der Zee 2000). In this phase of the journey, the teacher and practitioner encounter hidden and unaccepted parts of themselves (shadow) that are brought to the surface to be examined. Underworld mythology best describes this process.

There are a variety of predictable phases in teacher development:

Initial Euphoria   There is often a series of initial successes in teaching. At first, most teachers feel euphoric and fall in love with what they do. The first blush of enthusiasm can carry teachers for some time. However, it is not sufficient to sustain a teacher through the difficult aspects of the work.

Self-doubt   It is not uncommon for euphoria to be gradually replaced by feelings of incompetence, doubt and depression. Teachers begin to feel overwhelmed and realize that teaching is hard. This letdown often follows the first negative evaluations from students. Some teachers get trapped in this stage and never escape. Teaching is an experience in which one commonly feels lonely, anxious, alienated and abused (Jersild 1955). All teachers eventually fail and ask if it is worth it.

Impatience   Teachers often feel impatient with the rate of their students' growth and development. They can become pessimistic, feeling that the task is impossible and that they will never make a difference in their students. At such times, it's helpful to remember the "butterfly effect." Chaos theory teaches that a butterfly spreading its wings in Asia can have profound effects on the weather in North America. Small changes can make a big difference. A small accomplishment in the teacher's eyes might appear to the student as a breakthrough transformation. Teachers plant seeds. The seeds may not bear fruit for some time.

Burnout

Burnout is another common stage in teaching. It is especially prevalent among teachers who need control and seek perfection in their work. These teachers feel they must anticipate every problem or they are failing. They feel that they must not seem uncertain or hesitant and cannot ever be confused. Teachers who seek perfection are afraid of taking risks in their teaching, and their teaching often becomes about performance. They lose the capacity to teach from all of themselves-utilizing their mind, heart and spirit. Perfection in teaching is elusive. Teaching is a messy and turbulent process.

One of the keys to avoiding burnout is teaching from an undivided self. Effective teaching necessitates authenticity and utilizing the whole self in the work. Students don't trust teachers that hold something back or who do not fully engage them. When teachers attempt to hold something back, this takes considerable energy, depletes the energy reserves and contributes to the burnout process. The other crucial aspect to preventing burnout is teacher renewal (see below). Teachers must honor themselves as well as their students.

Teaching at Your Limits

It is for us to make the effort.
The result is always in God's hands.
—Mohandas Gandhi

Teachers are limited by their level of knowledge and level of skill. New teachers are often teaching at or beyond their limits. The workload is very heavy in terms of preparation, while the learning curve is steep. New teachers often feel anxiety over whether they will perform well. This eases over time as they mature and grow in experience.

Sometimes, experienced teachers also teach at their limits. This happens when they are asked to teach something outside of their expertise or comfort zone. This can take courage, but it's not unusual for teachers to feel they've done their best work when teaching a subject for the first time. Teachers often are most creative and grow the most when challenged by their subject and their students. Conversely, teachers who have taught the same subject for many years can become jaded and stale. Their classes seem rigid; the class material, canned. It is important that the teacher always strive to keep the material fresh and enlivened.

Teachers who teach infrequently often have difficulty getting to know their students. In such circumstances, "teaching" is often replaced by "speaking." To connect with students prior to class time, teachers can review the students' school application materials, speak to other faculty members or simply talk to the students themselves.

Obstacles to Teaching

Obstacles are things that show what men are.
—Epicetus

"Obstacles to cure are factors that hinder the progression of treatment toward a curative response" (Hahnemann). Teachers experience "obstacles to teach" in much the same way. Below is a partial listing of the common obstacles to teaching.

Adult Learners

We should be careful to get out of an experience only the wisdom that is in it and stop there; lest we be like the cat that sits down on a hot stove-lid. She will never sit down on a hot stove-lid again—and that is well; but also she will never sit down on a cold one anymore.
—Mark Twain

Methods that are effective in teaching children frequently do not work well with adults (Jolles 1993), yet these are the methods most teachers are familiar with and use in teaching adults.

Adults are less open and more suspicious than children. Many have had negative experiences in learning that make them mistrust education. They have underlying preconceptions and judgments about the learning process. This mistrust can cause a strong resistance to learning.

In teaching adult learners, surroundings are important. Children are comfortable in most settings, regardless of temperature, lighting, etc. Adults require more rigid control of their learning environment. For example, negotiating temperature settings can become a critical issue in some adult-learning classrooms.

Students have traditionally been brought up in classrooms filled with fear. This includes a fear of teachers, fear of administrators and a fear of appearing stupid. For some this leads to a hatred of learning, which makes it difficult to approach a school again as an adult. It can take them a long time to re-establish trust. It is essential that the teacher build a safe space for their students. This safe place must be free from fear where students feel free to explore and grow. This becomes a sacred space and time with predictable boundaries, teachers, curriculum and rules.

Adult learners need clear-cut goals and objectives for learning. They need to know "What's in it for me?" This requires logic in the learning process that is much less necessary in teaching children.

Adults, unlike children, generally hate surprises. They want teachers to tell them what is expected in clearly defined terms from the outset of the training program, even to the small details. Adult learners need road maps of what to expect. Without this, they experience much anxiety.

Both adults and children require repetition to learn, although studies have shown that adults require this more so (Boud 1987). Only through repetition can material become fully integrated. It is a challenge for teachers of adult learners to constantly find new ways to repeat the material while still keeping it fresh and alive.

Lastly, adults have much more life experience than children. Good teachers utilize their students' life experience as a learning tool in their classrooms. They do this in part by grounding new material in the students' experience.

Overcoming the Fear of Teaching

Knowledge is the antidote to fear.
—Ralph Waldo Emerson

Fear is one of the greatest obstacles to teaching. John Scotus Erigena was a philosopher in the court of the Holy Roman Empire. His students turned on him and stabbed him to death because he tried to get them to think. This is an extreme example, but it represents every teacher's unconscious fear of rejection. Teachers worry that if they push students too hard or appear too vulnerable the students will destroy them.

Fear shuts down the learning and teaching process. It cuts teachers off from themselves, their students and their subject. Fear prevents teachers from being connected to the organic process that is teaching and learning. Teachers sometimes attempt to hide their fear through arrogance and a need for rigid control of their class.

Teachers have obvious fears, such as being disliked by students, being bad at teaching and losing their job. Much of this revolves around performance. Because teachers have invested their ego in their work, they often feel they must perform well for their students. Much of their energy is devoted to protecting themselves from student criticism. Some teachers avoid teacher evaluations as a way of not hearing what they don't want to hear. Ironically, teachers cannot see the fear in their students until they first see it in themselves (Palmer 1998).

Teachers also experience more subtle fears, including fear of conflict, fear of diversity and fear of change. Conflict is inevitable in teaching. It arises when divergent viewpoints meet and clash. Some teachers avoid discussion in their classrooms because they are uncomfortable with conflict. Fear of diversity is evident in teachers who believe only their own ideas are valid. They appear disrespectful of others ideas and beliefs, but actually are threatened by them.

Fear of change is deeply rooted in many people. It is tied to the fear of losing one's identity. For teachers who strongly identify with their own ideas, changing those ideas means losing their identity. Training programs in homeopathy cause change and transformation in both their students' and teachers' lives in ways they never expected. Fear and anxiety often accompany this process.

The fear of change also manifests in a fear of experimentation. When teachers have taught for a while, they often stay stuck with the same teaching methodology and are reluctant to change it. Yet good teachers must constantly grow. One technique that ensures growth is to make a certain percentage of one's teaching each year experimental and research focused. This gets the teacher to try new ideas, methods and ways of being with students. It's a good way to keep one's teaching alive and growing.

Although fear is an inevitable part of the teaching process, teachers do not need to identify with it or become the fear. One option is to channel ones' fears and anxieties into one's work. Another is to share one's anxiety. When teachers share their fears and anxieties with their students, it helps the students become more comfortable with their own fears and anxieties. Often when a teacher is afraid of something in class, it is a red flag that the issue needs to be attended to and given voice.

"Problem" Students

Some people are molded by their admirations,
others by their hostilities.
—Elizabeth Bowen

Every teacher has certain students who are difficult and challenging to teach. A student one teacher finds difficult might not seem so to another teacher, but some students represent a challenge to nearly all teachers. Typically, "problem" students take up more of the teacher's time than their peers. The dilemma is how to give challenging students extra time without shortchanging the rest of the class.

It is important for teachers to analyze what types of students most challenge them. Typically, teachers blame the student as the "problem." They feel that the difficult student will never learn and is wasting their time. Teachers who believe that a student will come to no good can make a self-fulfilling prophecy of it.

It is difficult for a teacher to face what they bring to the equation. "Problem students" often represent shadow aspects of teachers that they have disowned and projected onto others. One of the only ways they can see their shadow is by having it mirrored back to them in someone else's behavior. Difficult students can provide a "gift" in this way. These students are often projecting their own problems with authority onto their teachers.

Typically the most difficult students are those who do not engage in the learning process. They never seem to "get it" and don't put out much effort. They seem to be only seeking gratification of their immediate needs. These students can be a great source of frustration for their teachers. They are often bored in class and can be quite disruptive. Teachers can become obsessed with these students to the exclusion of the rest of the class. They also may give up on these students before giving them a chance, assuming that they are hopeless.

Silent students can also represent a challenge. This is particularly true in classes that are discussion focused or where class participation is a required part of the grade. Silence might just reflect shyness, but can also indicate a passive-aggressive anger that is unexpressed.

It is important to honor each student's silence. Silent students can be fully engaged in the learning process, yet choose not to speak. Often, silent students are carrying on a full inner dialog with their teacher that is not outwardly expressed. There are also cycles within the learning process that require more silence and introspection. Learning journals provide these students a way of expressing themselves without being forced to speak in class (see Chapter Four).

More difficult are students who tend to dominate the class and class discussions. Such students often draw the resentment of their peers. They are perceived as attention hogs that intrude on their classmates' space.

Rules for speaking in class, especially in class discussions, can help prevent any one student from dominating. Teachers can also take dominant students aside privately to explain that they must learn to hold themselves back so that others will have an opportunity to speak. Rather than confronting the student, a respectful discussion of the problem and possible solutions works best. It helps to give the student specific behavioral feedback about speaking in class. For example, the teacher might suggest that the student only speak after three other students have spoken, or wait 10 seconds to process an idea before speaking (Brookfield 1990). As the student makes progress, it is important to acknowledge his/her efforts.

To curb dominating students in class discussion, the teacher can assign roles to individuals in the discussion groups—such as observer, heart keeper (one who monitors the emotional content of the discussion), moderator, etc. Although artificial, roles can help to contain more dominant students and to encourage more quiet students to speak. Another technique is let the class decide how to deal with dominant students. This approach is generally more confrontational. Here the teacher may point out that one student's dominance is only with the tacit permission of other silent students. As a last resort, the teacher may have to ask the dominant student to leave.

Some dominant students have a user mentality and feel entitled to more attention than their peers. They attempt to exploit the teacher's knowledge and time with little awareness of the impact of their behavior on the teacher. They often will call the teacher at home or keep the teacher for long periods after class. Often this arises psychologically out of a need for dependency on the teacher. With these students, the teacher must set careful boundaries and avoid becoming their codependent.

Manipulative students seek special favors from their teachers. They look for opportunities to control the relationship, eventually making the teacher feel used and resentful. Careful boundaries must also be set with these students, and the teacher must not be willing to give away his/her power.

Tensions Between Professional Homeopaths and Medically Licensed Homeopaths

There is often tension in the homeopathic community between professional homeopaths and medically licensed Homeopaths. Some teachers and administrators fear that this tension will play itself out in the classroom and represent an obstacle to teaching. Consequently, they may choose to only teach to one group or the other. This tension is less of a problem than commonly thought.

It is my experience that these groups have much to teach each other. Rather than creating tension and obstructing learning in the classroom, combining these groups can be beneficial. Medically licensed practitioners bring a great deal of medical knowledge, discipline of training and clinical experience to the classroom. At the same time, they have a great deal of unlearning to do—including unlearning of prejudices, attitudes, rigidity of thinking and other undesirable habits they have inculcated over time. Non-medically licensed practitioners bring freshness, optimism, critical thinking and openness to the classroom. Yet they lack medical knowledge and clinical experience.

Teachers Are the Target for Projection

He who can does and he who cannot teaches.
—George Bernard Shaw

Teachers are often the targets for their students' unconscious projections. Students' issues with authority can be projected onto the teacher. This can create an obstacle to teaching because these students lack awareness of this process and react to their teacher as if they were some distant figure from the past. This may occur despite the actions and behaviors the teacher displays.

One student in my class was consistently challenging and often disruptive. Intermittently, he would mistakenly call me Frank. One day, we discussed this and he stated that he had no idea why he did this. When I asked him who in his life was named Frank, he replied after some thought that his father had carried that name. He then told me how angry he had been at his father while growing up because his father was authoritarian and physically abusive. He admitted that he sometimes saw me in that way. Following the conversation, he became much less challenging.

Homeopathic treatment can be very important in this regard. Although not required in most training programs, homeopathic treatment can significantly reduce resistance to learning and help students work through their unconscious projections.

Resistance to Learning

> *The best teacher will be he who has at his tongue's end the explanation of what it is that is bothering the pupil. These explanations give the teacher the knowledge of the greatest possible number of methods, the ability of inventing new methods, and above all, not a blind adherence to one method, but the conviction that all methods are one-sided and that the best method would be the one which would answer best to all the possible difficulties incurred by a pupil, that is, not a method, but an art and talent.*
> —Leo Tolstoy

Reasons for resistance to learning by students are manifold. Teachers must attempt to sort out the causes of the resistance. In didactic teaching, the teacher must speak to each resister individually and understand where he/she is coming from. Student applications should be shared with all faculty members at a school, so that they better understand the students they are teaching. Teachers should admit to students that some resistance to learning is normal and within their rights.

Student resistance to learning often arises early in training and even in the application process. The reasons for resistance include, but are not limited to, the following (Brookfield 1990):

◎ Not all students are ready for homeopathy. Some students do not realize what they are getting into when they embark on a homeopathic education. It is often more than they bargained for. This is especially true of medical professionals who expect to learn homeopathy in a few weekend courses. They are often dismayed when they realize that learning homeopathy is every bit as difficult (if not more so) as learning allopathic medicine. Some allopathic medical professionals also succumb to their fears that they will be committing career suicide by practicing a "fringe form of healing. This is less of a problem than it used to be. The antidote to this problem is for teachers to better prepare students at the outset of training programs for what lies ahead.

◎ Many students struggle with a fear of change and the unknown. This can be paralyzing and can prevent them from being present in the classroom. The antidote is for teachers to achieve a balance between challenging students and supporting them. Good teachers also model a willingness to embrace change.

◎ One cause of resistance to learning is a teacher-student mismatch. Most often, this happens when a student's learning style and a teacher's teaching style clash. The antidote is diversity. Teachers who use only one teaching style are more prone to this problem than those who vary their teaching styles.

Mismatches can also arise from personality conflicts. A supportive community of peers makes a crucial difference through the facilitation of Peer learning and Peer teaching (Topping 1988; Goodlad and Hirst 1989).

◎ Many students are insecure about their ability to learn. They may have heard and internalized negative messages about themselves as learners from previous teachers. When I was in fourth grade, for example, my music teacher told me that I had one of the worst voices that she had ever heard. Following that, I never sang. As an adult, I took singing lessons as a way of overcoming my negative self-image as a singer and discovered that my voice was actually average. The antidote here is to create situations in which students succeed at learning. Breaking down homework and exercises into smaller pieces can be helpful. It is also important for the teacher to consistently acknowledge and affirm their students' progress.

◎ Students go through periods of relative stagnation and frustration in their learning process. This can cause them to feel that they are not progressing, when they are actually integrating and processing material already learned. The antidote is to let students know that these slow periods are necessary to their learning.

◎ Students can become resistant to learning when they feel that the current subject is irrelevant to their education. Every student is attracted to certain subjects and repelled by others. Many teachers have found that the least popular subjects in the homeopathic curriculum are history, Organon (Hahnemann's philosophy), repertory and small group process. The antidote lies in diversifying and integrating the curriculum, rather than presenting each subject by itself. Teachers also must explain why each subject is relevant to homeopathic education and practice. Lastly, teachers must teach from a place of excitement and adventure. Even the most "boring" subject can be great fun in a class with a good teacher. The challenge to teachers when they teach the same subject repeatedly is to make it new each time.

◎ Sometimes the level at which the class is taught can be either too simplistic or too advanced. Students become frustrated and tune out at either end of the spectrum. Generally, good teachers try to target a class a little above the average level of the students. A homeopathic curriculum often covers a great quantity of material quickly, and students may feel that the teacher is pushing too far, too fast. Informational overload is a common problem. It is important that the teacher be realistic about what students can accomplish. Similarly, more advanced students can feel bored and frustrated with a class that is too introductory. Mixing up the curriculum by putting more advanced material even in the beginning of the curriculum can help. Over time, classes normalize so serious students are at the same level by the end of a training program.

◎ A less common cause of learning resistance is confusing or bad teachers. The antidote is good administration. It is the administration's responsibility to ensure that the quality of teachers is sufficiently high for learning to occur. All teachers teach certain subjects and certain students more effectively than others. Teachers must be able to listen to criticisms of their teaching with openness and grow accordingly.

Unlearning

You have learnt something.
That always feels at first as if you had lost something.
—George Bernard Shaw

Teachers often require "unlearning." This is especially true of those who have had formal training in teaching. In the process of their previous education, these teachers have developed their own private truths with learning and teaching. Good teachers must be willing to suspend those beliefs and attitudes about homeopathic education and approach this in a fresh way. Ultimately this takes courage.

Jealousy

Wherever there are beginners and experts,
old and young, there is some kind of learning going on,
and some sort of teaching. We are all pupils and all teachers.
—Gilbert Highet

As students grow and expand beyond their teachers, jealousy can arise. Some teachers manifest their jealousy either consciously or unconsciously by trying to inhibit their students' growth. Such students might live in a teacher's shadow until the teacher retires or dies. For these students, resentment builds up over time. The other strategy some teachers adopt is to work that much harder in an attempt to stay ahead. This can lead to burn out. Rather than succumbing to jealousy, teachers need to accept their students' growth, promote collegiality and surrender the need for exclusive mastery.

Handling Negative Evaluations

Teachers commonly experience significant doubt after their first bad student evaluations and to want to flee. For many teachers, it is easier to handle poor evaluations from peers and administrators than from students (Brookfield 1990). They often magnify the negative student evaluations and ignore the positive ones. The challenge is to not become defensive.

In dealing with negative evaluations, teachers should consider the following: All teachers have good and bad days. All have certain subjects, classes or levels of students with which they struggle. It is often true that the most significant learning occurs with pain. When teachers are experimenting and growing, there will be both successes and failures. It is better to have occasional failures than to never risk growth. Negative evaluations can also represent the student's obstacles or learning resistance.

Types of Students

Few students are of one plain, decided color;
most are mixed, shaded, and blended;
and vary as much from different situations,
as changeable silks do from different lights.
—Lord Chesterfield

Teachers should be aware of where their students are on their learning journey. Without such awareness, teachers can become frustrated and disillusioned when students drop out of training or suspend their studies.

81

Not all students are meant to become "homeopaths. There are many levels of practicing homeopathy, including occasional first-aid prescribing, acute prescribing, integrative medicine and full-time constitutional prescribing (see Chapter One). Good teachers will help students find the level that best fits their needs, while pointing the direction to further studies when they are ready.

The seasons of the year provide a useful metaphor to describe the various degrees of commitment and attachment to the learning process. Four basic types of students pursue homeopathic training. These types reflect students' level of attachment to previous training and teachings.

Spring Students

These students will leave after a brief exposure to homeopathy. Many are exploring homeopathy superficially and will eventually decide that it is not right for them. Others are "shoppers" who will move from one training program to another without ever committing. There are also spring students who have strong attachments to previous training and learning that they are unable to release. Still others are unable to overcome their doubts and prejudices and may experience such a fear of change that they are unable to move forward. For them, arrogance and ego can be part of the problem.

Summer Students

The second category of homeopathic students includes those who will stay but never fully integrate homeopathy. They are along for the ride but never invest in homeopathy. Many of these individuals are unable to let go of previous careers. Those trained in conventional medicine may be unable to integrate allopathy with homeopathy. Although they catch the vision of homeopathy, they are unable to live it fully. This can be very frustrating, and these students complain of feeling caught in a no man's land between different forms of healing. Other students in this category have strong resistance to learning that they are unable to overcome (see Resistance to Learning section).

Fall Students

These students grow painfully but steadily over time. Learning is difficult, yet a vision and love for the subject keeps these students going through the process. In a very real way, fall students must earn what they learn. Gradually, they establish an identity as a homeopath.

Winter Students

The last category includes students who take to homeopathy like a duck to water. They feel born to it. Although there may be struggles on the homeopathic journey, there is never any doubt that this is what they want to do. They identify with homeopathy early in the process. One student said, "I can't not learn homeopathy. It is who I am." Although some of these students may interrupt their studies or do other things, they are pulled back to homeopathy because it is where they feel at home. Homeopathy as a "Great Subject" transforms these students.

Teaching Styles

The best method for a given teacher is the one
which is most familiar to the teacher.
—Leo Tolstoy

There are as many effective styles of teaching as there are teachers. Teaching should spring from the teacher's own nature. Contemporary education is always developing teaching methods du jour. Adopting these methods forces a teacher to teach the way others teach, with no allowance for individualization.

Teachers must teach from all of themselves, especially from their hearts. They can only engage their students if they capture their hearts. One must teach from an undivided self (Palmer 1999). Only then can students bring everything they are into the learning process.

One way of classifying teaching styles is by kingdom. Kingdoms are an important contemporary concept in homeopathic case analysis. Within this schema, there are three types of teachers: mineral, plant and animal.

Mineral Teachers

Mineral teachers are structured, organized and orderly. They plan their classes far in advance. They often give their students detailed notes. These teachers can be very skilled at plumbing the depths of a subject. Their pace is slow and steady, and they rely less on brilliance in their work, than on persistence. They are reliable and can be very conscientious. They exhibit a very fine discrimination and can display great depth in their thinking. Their students often have a solid understanding of the material. Mineral teachers are able to show the whole picture to their students and gently bring them to the heart of the matter.

Students sometimes find mineral teachers boring. They can experience their classes as dull, methodical and lacking imagination. The emphasis on organization can lead some students into an overly rigid and schematized view of homeopathy. These teachers can also seem non-nurturing.

Plant Teachers

Plant teachers often connect more with their students' feelings. Classes wander and weave in and out of their subjects, ultimately creating a single bright tapestry. Students often experience such classes as musical. The various harmonies and melodies lead students into a richer appreciation of the subject. Plant teachers are focused on the growth and development of their students, and seeing that they are well-nurtured. They often work through the heart center (emotions) and teach through modeling.

Students may find plant teachers confusing and get lost in the pattern. They may complain of lack of structure and guidance. The nurturing qualities of these teachers can be perceived as stifling. Students might also complain of a lack of dynamic purposeful energy.

Animal Teachers

Animal teachers can be very dynamic. They are direct, emphatic, persuasive and forceful. They can exude animal magnetism that captivates their listeners. They can be quite charismatic. Students in their classes often catch their passion and enthusiasm for the subject.

Students can find animal teachers threatening. A classroom can become an unsafe and dangerous environment. Students often find these classrooms chaotic. Animal remedies have strongly conflicted energy that often crystallizes into polarities. Students of animal teachers often feel torn between these polarities. Animal teachers can be distracting to students of the opposite sex. In addition, there is often more competition between students in their classes. Some students experience these teachers as manipulative.

Ultimately, teaching styles reflect the characteristics of the teachers. All three types have strengths and weaknesses. Through awareness, the best teachers learn to play to their strengths and to minimize their weaknesses.

Building Trust

Students have been conned for so long that a teacher
who is real with them is usually seen for a time
as simply exhibiting a new brand of phoniness.
—Carl Rogers

Trust is essential between teacher and student. Learning cannot occur until trust has been established. To earn students' trust, teachers must prove their credibility and authenticity (Brookfield 1990). Students tend to trust teachers who are willing to be learners themselves.

Credibility is the critical competence that students expect from their teachers (Freire 1970). This encompasses knowledge, skill and the essential qualities of good teaching. It is important not to sabotage credibility with false modesty. Yet teachers must also be willing to own up to their mistakes.

Authenticity occurs when a teacher's words and actions are congruent (Moustakas 1997). This happens when the individual's inner and outer teachers become one. Authentic teachers allow themselves to be human and teach from all of themselves. They listen carefully to their students' problems and issues. They take each of their students seriously and encourage their criticisms. Some teachers use an autobiographical metaphor to reveal aspects of themselves unrelated to teaching (Tarule 1988). This helps them become more authentic to their students.

A sure way to generate mistrust in a class is to play favorites. Inevitably, teachers find some students more likable than others, but to favor those students over others is nothing less than prejudice. Teachers can do this unconsciously when they make scapegoats of less-favored students.

Importance of Modeling

What the teacher is, is more important than what he teaches.
—Karl Menninger

Living the principles and truth of homeopathy is what brings people to it. One has to walk the talk. This is especially true for teachers. What one teaches in words is a mere fraction of what one teaches by living example. This is a great responsibility. There is a story of a famous Indian holy man who saw a mother and daughter for help with the daughter's addiction to sweets. He sent them home for two months and then had them come back. When they came back, he sternly admonished the daughter to stop eating sweets, and she left much chastened. After the visit, one of his students asked him why he waited two months. He replied that he first had to give up sweets himself.

Students use their teachers as role models as they shape their own identity. Students take those parts of their teachers that they resonate with and incorporate them into themselves. Most commonly internalized by students are their teachers' attitudes. Yet even the smallest actions of a teacher can carry great significance for the student. As homeopathic education progresses, modeling becomes increasingly important (Jackson 1986).

Hahnemann (the founder of homeopathy) was both a good and bad model as a teacher in homeopathy. At his best, he displayed the spirit of inquiry, critical thinking and willingness to take on a challenge that are so vital to homeopathy. As teachers, we need to model these qualities to our students. At his worst, he was well known for haranguing and attacking others, and for pontificating from a position of power rather than humility. His pupil Franz Hartmann described him as "pouring forth a flood of abuse against the older medicine and its followers…" while others described him as "a raging hurricane." Each teacher must internalize from their teaching models those aspects which are the best and leave out those which are not conducive to good teaching.

Diversity in Teaching

There never were, in the world, two opinions alike,
no more than two hairs, or two grains;
the most universal quality is diversity.
—Montaigne

Most teachers teach in the way they were taught. Frequently, this is the only method they know and feel comfortable with. It is difficult for teachers to change this (Kennedy 1991). All teaching methods are valid, but some work better in certain situations than others.

Diversity in teaching methods is important because each learner has a particular method to which they best respond. Teachers who use diverse methods can meet the needs of many students. They individualize their teaching. Teachers cannot change their style (teaching from their own nature), but they can vary their teaching methods.

Teaching methods can be visual, oral, somatosensory (kinesthetic) and written. Good teachers use all of these approaches in their teaching. They are aware of the differing types of learning intelligence—including linguistic, logical, visual, physical, musical, interpersonal, and intra-personal (see Chapter One). Traditionally, homeopathy has been taught utilizing linguistic and logical intelligence alone.

Diversity in teaching allows for independent study, collaboration, lecturing, group discussions and role-playing. It also encourages periods of reflective analysis for students. A diverse teacher utilizes materials from a variety of areas— including art, movies, music, poetry, books, nature, drama, opera, basic sciences and philosophy. A diverse teacher uses all of life and creates a rich tapestry for students.

Sometimes teachers rely too much on their strengths and avoid their weaknesses. They should model to their students a willingness to experiment, explore, take risks and fail.

Power Issues

The true teacher defends his pupil against his own personal influence.
He inspires self-trust. He guides their eyes from himself to the spirit
that quickens him. He will have no disciple.
—Amos Bronson Alcott

Power often plays itself out in the classroom. It is important to be aware of this so as to prevent unconsciously acting them out in the classroom.

Students often attribute more power to their teachers than the teachers actually have. Projection is an inevitable fact of human relationships. Teachers can take on the role of parent, magician, judge or prophet (Guggenbuhl-Craig 1971). The counter-projection is that teachers see their students as childlike, helpless and longing for guidance.

Some teachers identify with their students' image of them as all-powerful authority. They hide behind their professional persona, needing to show who is boss and making students feel childlike and dependent. They seek followers and disciples, dominating students with their great wisdom. These teachers can make hurtful observations about students as a way of displaying their power and control. These teachers also flatter students as a way of binding them to the teacher. They attempt to convince students that they, and only they, speak the truth. Ultimately, however, students must find their own truth.

Much of contemporary education promotes "power dependence." The authority-dependent student cannot imagine being as good as the teacher. They need the teacher's permission for everything. Such students often have an unconscious need to be taken care of and look to the teacher to take all responsibility from them. They place their teachers on a pedestal and expect them to be more than mortal. They desperately try to live up to their parental fantasies, which they can never achieve. These students may react strongly when the teacher makes a mistake, which every teacher inevitably must. The teacher then becomes devalued and worthless.

The student can also try to take on a position of power themselves, which can be very threatening to the teacher. The teacher in turn must exercise increasingly rigid control.

The antidote to this struggle is the archetype of the wounded teacher/healer, historically represented by Chiron the centaur. Chiron taught Asclepias the art of healing, despite having incurable wounds himself. A teacher's wounds make him more effective as a teacher. The teacher must be vulnerable and humble in his work, open and honest about who he is. Good teachers are willing to be vulnerable and refuse to harden their hearts. They recognize that teaching is a daily exercise in humility.

The struggle is to maintain authority without moving into power. When teaching arises from a place of power, the central issue becomes performance. This is what creates anxiety in teaching. Teachers worry that they will not know an answer or will appear incompetent. If they can stay focused on the great subject that is homeopathy, they can move from a position of power to one of authority. They can let go of the need to be right and move from needing to meet their own needs to meeting the needs of the whole.

Handling Uncertainty

Teach the tongue to say, I don't know.
—Maimonides

Teachers frequently do not have the answers. Especially in homeopathy, which is as much art as science, they must learn to be comfortable with uncertainty and ambiguity. It is tempting for teachers to present themselves as more knowledgeable than they are, but they need to be able to admit their own doubts. Acknowledging that one experiences uncertainty in teaching and in practice lets students know that it's normal for them to feel unsure at times too. Teachers should also talk about failed cases, as well as the successful ones, because students should understand that the answers in homeopathy are sometimes elusive.

Beginning students typically don't like ambiguity and uncertainty. They want to know the right answer. They need to become oriented on a solid foundation. Beginning students often feel that they are totally certain about a remedy in a given case, despite their lack of experience and knowledge. Later in training, they may become more comfortable with confusion and uncertainty.

For teachers, it is helpful to remember that students are ultimately responsible for their own learning. Teachers merely point the way. Teaching self- responsibility helps prepare students for practice. In covering areas of uncertainty, the teacher can assign homework or present exercises in class to explore these areas.

Polarities are a prime example. The law of polarities states that both one thing and the opposite can be true at the same time. Many students have difficulty grasping this uncertainty-provoking concept. It should be discussed early in training to prepare students for the many other challenging concepts they will encounter in homeopathy.

Teacher/Administration Interactions

Education is that which remains after
one has forgotten everything he learned in school.
—Albert Einstein

Teachers often find themselves caught between the needs of students and the needs of administration (see Appendix One). They may question whether they owe more loyalty to their employer or to their students. Some teachers seem to always be at battle with administration. They see administration as an enemy who interferes with their work with students. For them, administration becomes an obstacle to teaching. Sometimes, administration problems are real. At other times, the teachers are working out their own authority issues through their interaction with administration.

Several strategies can be helpful here. First, it is imperative that one knows the administrators. Many teachers isolate themselves from the administration and overreact when political realities impact on their teaching. Another important strategy, if a teacher wants to survive politically, is to develop a nose for danger (Snow 1964). Teachers should choose their battles carefully. Some battles are more winnable than others. Finally, conflict with administration is often avoided by staying focused on the "Great Subject" of homeopathy.

Balancing Teaching with Practice and Research

> *The most important obligation now confronting the nation's colleges and universities is to break out of the tired old teaching versus research debate and define, in more creative ways, what it means to be a scholar.*
>
> —Boyer

Teachers often struggle to find a balance between teaching, practice and research. It is difficult to develop the skills and knowledge base necessary to do good work in all of these areas. However, there is much overlap as well. Some homeopaths find the right balance by devoting a separate time to each of these areas to prevent role confusion. For example, certain days they practice, other days they teach and another day they do research. Others homeopaths choose to pursue only one of these areas at a time in their careers.

Teacher Renewal

> *To be a teacher in the right sense is to be a learner.*
> *Instruction begins when you, the teacher,*
> *learn from the learner, put yourself in his place*
> *so that you may understand what he understands*
> *and in the way he understands it.*
> —Soren Kierkegaard

Critical to the survival of teachers is the idea of teacher renewal and development. Unfortunately, there are few resources available to support the teacher. It is not just students who need a supportive community of peers; teachers also need community. Without community, teaching becomes an isolating and lonely experience. The growth of any profession depends on dialog within a supportive community.

What makes teacher renewal more difficult is teachers' resistance to getting together or talking to their colleagues. Many teachers do not feel comfortable having their work examined. They often feel threatened when evaluated.

Yet teachers benefit from interacting with their peers. They learn from each other. Teachers are ever changing and unfolding. Continual learning keeps them fresh so that their students are enlivened in their learning. It is highly useful for teachers to visit classrooms of other good teachers. The key is to go with the intent not of learning content but of observing the teaching process.

A teacher is ever changing and unfolding and must stay constantly in the role of learner. Continual learning keeps them fresh so that their students are enlivened in their learning. It is very useful for teachers to visit the classrooms of other good teachers. The key is to go with the intent, not of learning content but to observe the process of the teaching.

It is important for teachers not to evaluate themselves based solely on student satisfaction. This is especially true for teachers who expect and need to be loved by their students. Teachers can over-invest in their teaching, attracting students to fulfill their psychological needs rather than having a healthy outside life. It is very hard for such teachers to handle the inevitable anger and hostility that arises in the classroom.

One important aspect of renewal is for teachers to periodically examine why they chose teaching. Teachers must revisit the source of their decision to become a teacher. This helps them reconnect with their passion for teaching.

It is also helpful for teachers to see themselves as students see them. They can do this by videotaping their teaching. Alternatively, listening to the comments of a trusted fellow teacher who sits in on one's class can bring new perspective to one's work.

Faculty meetings can be another vital source of teacher renewal and support. When well conducted they provide an opportunity to connect with one's peers and see the larger picture of the educational process. They also provide forums for open dialog between faculty and administration. Seminars supporting teachers and teacher training can also be very useful. The North American Network of Homeopathic Educators (NANHE) has been an important attempt to serve in this regard (see Appendix D). Teacher training should help to renew teachers and reconnect them with their desire to teach. They also should work to expand their teaching skills.

Another important aspect of teacher training is to become more aware of how students experience learning (Kolb 1984). In part this means continuing one's own learning process and experiencing learning from a student perspective (Boud, Kieogh and Walker 1985, Boud and Griffin 1987).

Lastly, homeopathic treatment is crucial not only for students but also the faculty. Not only does this keep the teacher healthy and more balanced, but it renews his/her awareness of what it is to be a patient.

Chapter Four
Didactic Teaching

Homeopathic teaching can be divided into didactic and clinical. The skills, knowledge and attitudes necessary to be an effective teacher are quite distinct in these two areas. Clinical teaching is concerned with the skills and knowledge-in-action necessary to the effective practice of homeopathy. It is mostly case based. Didactic teaching focuses on the knowledge necessary to becoming a good homeopath. It is mostly classroom based. This chapter reviews the teaching styles and techniques necessary to effective didactic teaching.

Lecturing

We should not be speaking to, but with.
That is second nature to any good teacher.
—Noam Chomsky

Of all the methods of teaching, the lecture is the most often used and abused (Brown 1980, 1987). This often stems from a teacher-centered model where the teacher is authoritarian and hides behind the podium. For many teachers, lecturing feels more comfortable and safe. These teachers "speak to" rather than "teach to" their classes.

However, lecturing does play an important part in homeopathic education. Following are some valid reasons to lecture (McKeachie 1986):

◎ To establish broad outlines of a body of material or to introduce new material
◎ To set guidelines for independent study
◎ To model intellectual attitudes you want to promote
◎ To encourage learners' interest in a topic

The Effective Lecturer

The effective lecturer needs to keep several things in mind. The average student attention span for lectures is about 15-20 minutes (Bligh 1972; Brown 1980; Rogers 1989). After that, students get bored, and their attention wanders. To keep lectures short and interesting, teachers can ask students what they know about the subject beforehand and then focus their presentation on new material. Afterward, they can continue to explore the subject through discussion groups and critical incident exercises (incidents in their lives related to the lecture's theme).

Teachers need to make their lectures as stimulating as possible. They should not deliver a lecture as if their audience was irrelevant. For example, reading lectures eliminates the elements of surprise and wonder so necessary in the art of teaching. Teachers also maintain eye contact and ask questions of their audience to keep them engaged. Teachers must personalize their presentations. Students connect strongly with personalized descriptions. Drawing on examples from cases, one's own life, film, sports, TV, poetry and mythology can all help to bring a lecture alive. Giving examples is one of the teacher's most powerful techniques.

Storytelling

> *And sermons are less read than tales.*
> —Matthew Prior

A good teacher tells stories. A story captures the imagination. It connects the heart of the learner with the heart of the subject. Stories teach through metaphor and analogy. Many concepts cannot be precisely defined (Wittgenstein 1953) and are best expressed through stories and legends. This is especially true in the healing arts. Learners also remember stories long after they have forgotten the facts of the lecture.

In *Lincoln Talks*, Abraham Lincoln explains why he tells so many stories: "They say I tell a great many stories. I reckon I do; but I have learned from long experience that plain people, take them as they run, are more easily influenced through the medium of a broad and humorous illustration than in any other way; and what the hyper-critical few may think, I don't care."

There are "little" stories and "big" ones. The little ones illustrate our lives and our personal experiences. It is important for the teacher to honor these stories as they arise in teaching. For example, the student who excitedly raises their hand and describes their grandmother who is a strong image of the remedy being presented. Part of the healing process for many students in letting go of their old educational baggage is to tell their stories. This is a critical step at the outset of a training program and is often accompanied by much emotion. Many students are in recovery from previous trainings and teachings and have a desperate need to give this voice.

"Big" stories are drawn from the culture of homeopathy. These larger stories help connect students to the homeopathic community and to feel part of its rich tradition. An example is the story of Constance Hering and his proving of the remedy Lachesis. Hering became interested in the use of snake poisons while he was working in Surinam. Clarke describes the story after the natives brought him a surukuku snake from the Upper Amazon in his *Materia Medica*:

> At last one was brought in a bamboo box, and those who brought it immediately fled, and all the native servants with them. Hering stunned the snake with a blow on the head as the box opened, then, holding its head in a forked stick, he pressed its venom out of the poison bag upon sugar of milk.
>
> The effect of handling the virus and preparing the lower attenuations was to throw Hering into a fever with tossing delirium and mania-much to his wife's dismay. Towards morning he slept, and on waking his mind was clear. He drank a little water to moisten his throat, and the first question this indomitable prover asked was "What did I do and say?" His wife remembered vividly enough. The symptoms were written down, and this was the first installment of the proving of Lachesis. The natives crept back one by one next day, and were astonished to find Hering and his wife alive.

Class Discussions

> *Gramma said when you come on something good,*
> *first thing to do is share it with whoever you can find;*
> *that way, the good spread out where no telling it will go.*
> *Which is right.*
> —Forrest Carter

Class discussion actively involves students in the educational process. Discussion is both democratic and participatory. It places teachers and students on more of an equal level. Class discussion is where some students learn best. For good teachers, class discussion is like music, and they are like conductors.

Beginning teachers are frequently surprised by the difficulty of leading a class discussion. Like good lectures, good discussions require significant preplanning. Typically, teachers use lectures to introduce new topics or ideas, and discussions to allow the class to expand upon the new material. Beginning teachers beware: Students will complain if there is too much group discussion and may interpret this as a sign of a teacher's laziness or lack of expertise.

Why Have a Discussion?

Following are some good reasons to utilize a discussion format (Brookfield 1990):

◎ To engage students in exploring a diversity of ideas on a given topic

◎ To assist students in discovering new ideas

◎ To emphasize the complexity and ambiguity of issues

◎ To help students recognize the assumptions underlying many of their fixed ideas

◎ To utilize and model active listening

◎ To increase students' emotional connection to an issue

◎ To demonstrate to students that their voices are heard

◎ To help build community

The best discussion topics are more controversial than factual. Students often prefer group conformity, and it can be difficult for them to let this go. Many students are unwilling to voice dissenting opinions, but teachers must encourage and model this behavior. With controversial topics, dissenting opinions are inevitable. Another technique that can be helpful is to give them small bits of information that are disturbing or create cognitive dissonance (Daloz 1986). Cognitive dissonance occurs when two opposing ideas conflict in the mind of a student. For example, a patient may be saying one thing but their body language says another (see Chapter One).

Getting Discussions Started

Getting discussions started can be difficult. Teachers often feel they have to push their students to respond. One approach is to ask good questions. The questions must be neither too general nor too specific. Another approach is to focus on critical incident reviews. This gives students the opportunity to explore significant experiences they've had concerning the topic. Alternatively, teachers can begin a discussion with a controversial statement by a leader in homeopathy.

The following types of questions encourage learning discussions:

◉ Questions that both support and challenge (I hear you when you say X, but why is it that aren't saying Y?)

◉ Questions that stimulate reflection (Tell me more about X?)

◉ Questions that summarize (You have told me A, B, C and D. Is this an accurate portrayal of what you thinking and feeling?)

◉ Questions that reframe and reformulate (When you say X, perhaps it can be understood in the context of Y?)

◉ Ethical questions (What is the value of X? How can it be understood in terms of ethics or morals?)

◉ Questions that move the discussion deeper (Can we take X to a deeper level? How can we understand X more deeply?)

◉ Questions that clarify (What do you mean when you say X?)

Accepting the Silent Student

Some students are not comfortable talking. The teacher should acknowledge this at the beginning of the discussion and honor their silence. Not all discussions need to be aloud to be educationally valid (Rogers 1989). For this reason, teachers shouldn't grade on class participation. If students feel forced to participate, they are more likely to focus on performance and competition, rather than on learning.

Learning journals can be helpful to silent students (Modra 1989; Lukinsky 1990). Here students speak from their heart in a private journal that they submit directly to the teacher. They write about significant learning experiences in class and feelings that they have during their education. In their journals, they write as if they are speaking directly to the teacher. This can be a powerful way for students to participate fully, yet at a distance.

Managing Emotions, Chaos and Group Dynamics

Discussions are often full of emotion (Lewis 1986). It is important for the teacher to recognize this and be comfortable with the emotion expressed, without trying to shut it down. Students often let down their defenses in discussions and can be vulnerable. The teacher must act as guardian, keeping the discussion focused on the topic and avoiding personalization of comments.

Because discussions can be chaotic and are never alike, the teacher feels much less in control than when lecturing. The teacher can provide order in the chaos by asking some participants to summarize the discussion every 20 minutes.

Familiarity with group dynamics can also help teachers facilitate class discussion (Robbins and Finley 1995; Corey and Corey 1987). Managing disagreement—perceived by some students as aggression—can be especially problematic. Teachers should model a willingness to explore disagreement in a supportive context. During this process, individual students must not be allowed to dominate the class (see Chapter One). Everyone must be given a voice.

Whether a discussion group is large or small, the teacher needs to facilitate the discussion without getting in the way of it. Individuals in the group should not feel that they have to perform for the teacher. The class must be kept open. Good teachers have the capacity to turn questions back to the group without answering themselves. They trust that the group can find the answers. They remain focused on the larger group and interweave individual issues back into the whole. These teachers also have the capacity to place small issues into a larger context.

Size Is Significant

Group size is important. Larger groups provide anonymity but less opportunity for sharing. Three-person groups are generally the most difficult, as two members of the group often pair with each other against the third. Even-numbered groups are generally most stable, whereas odd-numbered groups tend to be more creative.

Smallish "mentorship" group discussions are particularly effective. Here a faculty member meets with a small subgroup of the class in an informal and intimate setting. This is an opportunity for students to ask questions they might not otherwise ask. It also can be a place where students let down their defenses and share their feelings. Students often reveal their aspirations in this setting, and this helps them see where they are in their learning process.

Role-Playing

An actor can remember his briefest part well into senescence
and long after he has forgotten his phone number and where he lives.
—Jean Kerr

Role-playing exercises are experiments with truth. They provide students an opportunity to gain a strong visceral sense of their learning (Milroy 1982). Role-playing helps students simulate and prepare for the difficult, complex situations they might face in practice. It also prepares them for situations and issues that they fear or are avoiding.

Role-playing is an excellent technique for teaching case-taking and case management. For this purpose, focusing on critical incidents is very important (Brookfield 1990). Critical incidents represent key moments in the students' practice and experience of homeopathy. These are times when the student has experienced much emotion or been in crisis. Working through critical incidents can be a great facilitator of learning.

The key to successful role-playing is authenticity and trust (Milroy 1982). Students are often fearful of being on stage and of how others will react to their "performance." There are risks involved in role-playing, and the teacher must explain to the students why it is important to take these risks. There are also risks for the teacher. Teachers should not involve their classes in role-plays unless they are confident and familiar with the material.

In setting up a role-play, there should be just the right amount of material. Too much detail constricts the acting of the students and does not allow them the spontaneity to make the role-play uniquely theirs. Too little material creates confusion for the student, which often results in them projecting too much of their own "stuff" into the role-play.

During role-plays, some students take on the role of observer. These individuals give both positive and negative feedback once the role-playing is completed. Their comments should come after the actors have had a chance to talk about their feelings about the experience. Providing time for self-reflection and analysis is critical. Videotaping lets students see themselves in action and allows more careful analysis.

Building Community

> When the representatives were debating signing the Declaration of Independence, John Hancock said, "We should be unanimous; there must be no pulling in different ways; we must all hang together." Then Benjamin Franklin added the punch line, "Yes, we must indeed all hang together, or most assuredly we shall hang separately."
> —Anonymous

A strong homeopathic community is critical to the survival of homeopathic schooling (Rowe 2000). Teachers must foster the growth of a learning community (see Chapter Eight). One way they can do this by providing opportunities for students to get together and connect. Shared homework, class discussion, role-playing, retreats and class exercises all facilitate community building. What destroys community is competition, which rears its ugly head when students compare grades and evaluations.

Peer teaching also facilitates community building (Whitman 1988). This typically occurs in small subgroups of two, three or four students. Such "learning partnerships" can be essential for some students in completing their training program (Robinson, Saberton and Griffin 1985). Learning partnerships provide opportunities for students to share common interests and more deeply explore homeopathic issues. Individuals in these subgroups can serve to balance each other.

Emotional Communication

> A teacher who can arouse a feeling for one single good action...
> accomplishes more than he who fills our memory with
> rows on rows of natural objects, classified with name and form.
> —Goethe

Learning is a very emotional process. Students learn most from feeling. Studies show that what students retain in their memory is that which has the greatest emotional charge. When they speak about learning, they often become emotional. Students draw emotional support from the learning community in which they grow. A teacher's role is to transmit the experience of being a homeopath, complete with feelings, skills and knowledge.

Emotions are just as important to a teacher's work as critical thinking (see below), yet some teachers are uncomfortable with emotion. Consciously or unconsciously, they attempt to suppress emotions in the classroom, or are comfortable only with certain emotions. Stifling emotions blocks the educational process. Teachers must strive to honor both negative and positive emotions.

Students experience a broad range of emotions:

◎ Anxiety, lack of confidence and embarrassment are most common among beginning students. These emotions can be crippling and provide an obstacle to learning. It's the teacher's responsibility to instill confidence, hope and courage in their students.

◎ Sadness and grief can arise as students open up to new ideas and let go of previous certainties. This is lessened if students couple this with the joy of new learning.

◎ Anger can emerge when students resist change or perceive their teachers and administration as callous. This is less of an issue when classes are organized and taught homeopathically, rather than allopathically (see Chapter Eight).

◎ Jealousy surfaces in response to competition and perceived teacher favoritism. Good teachers help to normalize a student's experience and turn competitive feelings into being with the students themselves.

◎ Gratitude can be an important step for some students in opening their hearts and expressing appreciation to homeopathy and their teachers.

◎ Finally, joy and freedom often are the product of learning deeply and completing one's studies.

Good teachers are supportive—and not surprised—when feelings crop up in the classroom. They are aware of the developmental stages of learning and the emotions that accompany them. These teachers model ways of handling emotions in class so students will feel comfortable and know how to react when their patients express emotions.

Practicing Critical Thinking

If you would be a real seeker after truth,
it is necessary that at least once in your life you doubt,
as far as possible, all things.
—Rene Descartes

Critical thinking is concerned with openness and alertness of the mind (Mezirow and Associates 1990). Critical thinkers question what they are taught and trust their own experience, insights and intuition. This is true even if they go against dominant ideas and values. Critical thinking is freedom from prejudice. The founder of homeopathy, Samuel Hahnemann, was one of the best examples of a critical thinker. Critical thinking results in deep understanding and knowledge. It involves constructing new knowledge and reconstructing information, rather than simply memorizing it. Critical thinking is important in all aspects of the homeopathic curriculum (Meyers 1986). Critical thinking helps students develop good mental habits, including clarity, logic, relevance, application, comparison, contrast, explanation, hypothesizing and consistency (Paul 1986).

Teachers are seldom aware of how to teach critical thinking. The best way is by example. Good teachers think critically themselves. They help their students to come to their own answers rather than passing along some predetermined doctrine.

Good teachers also have attitudes that support critical thinking. They are open to others' ideas, confident in their ability to problem-solve, curious, constantly searching for deeper meanings, and willing to think "outside the box" (Baron 1988; Ennis 1986). Teachers who encourage critical thinking ask thought-provoking questions that open their students' minds. They are not tied to a particular methodological stance in teaching.

Many teachers have found that "peer teaching" fosters critical thinking among students. Students engage in peer teaching as teacher's assistants (TAs) or as members of small groups in which they question each other about the class material. Either way, teaching other students improves their capacity to learn. Brookfield (1990, p. 85) states: "When all students engage in critical thinking, the classroom takes on the appearance of a community of learners working together to enhance each other's thinking and learning."

Learning from Failures

Flops are a part of life's menu and
I've never been a girl to miss out on any of the courses.
—Rosalind Russell

In teaching *materia medica* (descriptions of what is characteristic about individual homeopathic remedies) one must focus on successful cases. Only in this way can students see how remedies work. Too often, however, teachers get so caught up in illustrating successful remedies that they don't talk about the dark side of homeopathy—the failures. Students who only see beautifully cured cases in training leave with the expectation that their cases will all be cured when they begin practice. They are not prepared for the partial cures and failures that are inevitable for any practitioner, and become frustrated and disillusioned. Exposure to failures and how to learn from them during training can prevent unrealistic expectations and frustration later on. Teachers must be willing to present the negative outcomes along with positive ones.

Repetition

After people have repeated a phrase a great number of times,
they begin to realize it has meaning and may even be true.
—H. G. Wells

Teachers often forget that it takes many repetitions to fix a concept in students' minds. The challenge is to keep the material fresh each time it is presented. This can be achieved by presenting the material in different formats and combinations.

Teaching homeopathy is like preparing the remedy "homeopathy." The ideas must be succussed (given energy) and potentized (strengthened) repeatedly. With each repetition, each idea is brought to a new level of potency and the students increase their inner awareness of it. In the end, students and faculty take that remedy and internalize it. They prove homeopathy. They prove it for themselves in its majesty, its wonder, its power and its love.

Balanced Presentation of the Old and the New

If a man keeps cherishing his old knowledge,
so as continually to be acquiring new,
he may be a teacher of others.
—Confucius

Students need ample exposure to the words of the homeopathic masters. After all, the masters provide the foundation of our work. However, Hahnemann, the ultimate master, was constantly seeking new knowledge and kept expanding and reworking his theories. As teachers, we must do the same.

Our challenge is to strike a balance between teaching the old thought and exploring the new ideas in homeopathy. Rather than teaching only one traditional approach to our craft, we should share new approaches with students and teach them to think critically about what they learn. Otherwise, students' thinking becomes fixed and they become disciples of a particular dogma. Sharing new ideas also connects students to current thinking and brings the material more alive. If teachings do not fit the consciousness of the times, the material will not be assimilated.

Predominance of Women in Homeopathic Training Programs

As we left the building the students [males] had formed them-
selves into a double line, through which we passed, mid jeers
and groans, coarse jokes and shouts, pelted with bits of wood
and gravel.
—Elizabeth Cady Stanton

Women currently far out number men in homeopathic training programs. Women have always been attracted to homeopathy (Winston 1999). In addition, many educators feel that women ultimately make better homeopaths than men.

From the teacher's standpoint, it's important to understand and appreciate how women experience adult and post-graduate learning This includes such issues as emotional vs. cognitive aspects of learning, sexism in the classroom, sex role stereotyping, the importance of relationships, the need to build community, balancing family and studies during training and safety issues. Good teachers are aware of these issues and work to make their teaching more effective for women students. It is interesting to note that despite this, many teachers in homeopathy are male. One of the administrative challenges in creating a faculty is to find a male/female balance.

Evaluations

You can get all A's and still flunk life.
—Walker Percy

For many students, the most anxiety provoking part of learning is evaluations. Some find it difficult to separate issues of self-esteem from evaluation of their work. Some are devastated by any critical comments. Students often take evaluations too seriously and overreact to them. With this in mind, teachers must write evaluations with care. Well-done evaluations support students, acknowledging their positive strides, and at the same time challenge them.

Some teachers are no happier to give evaluations than their students are to receive them. They feel that evaluations interfere with the learning process, and they point to studies that consistently have shown that course evaluations do not predict success in professional practice (Jencks and Riesman 1977). Most professions place too much emphasis on short-term memory at the expense of long-term understanding (Wurman 1989). Nonetheless, evaluations are part of the political reality of education. Students must be prepared to face licensure and certification evaluations on completion of their training. Evaluations are also a learning tool for the serious student.

Developing effective evaluations is an art. The goal is to emphasize assessments that mimic what it is like in the practice of a homeopathic practitioner. The most useful evaluations look at not only knowledge, but also clinical skills and competency. Unfortunately, there has been little written on adequate evaluation of case taking and case analysis.

A good evaluation process has the following ingredients (Brookfield 1990):

◎ **Clarity**: Evaluations need to be understandable to the student.

◎ **Consistency**: Teachers must be consistent in their evaluations. This prevents student favoritism or student scapegoating and helps to prevent the projection of the teachers own issues on to their students.

◎ **Promptness**: Feedback should be given as quickly as possible, while the evaluation is still fresh.

◎ **Regularity**: Students should be reevaluated at periodic intervals. Different challenges arise at various points in the training process and must be evaluated separately.

◎ **Opportunity for discussion**: Teachers must be available to discuss evaluations with students and justify their comments.

◎ **Individualization**: Each evaluation should be unique, based on the performance of the individual student.

◎ **Support**: Students only feel safe in the evaluative process if they are simultaneously supported by both faculty and administration. Support is an important difference between authoritative (subject centered model) and authoritarian (teacher centered model) teaching.

◎ **Educational objective**: Evaluations should answer the questions, "How can I do this better? What can I do as the next step?" Teachers should focus on what students can learn from their comments rather than on judging their students.

◎ **Humor**: Students take evaluations very seriously. Adding a little respectful levity can help dispel tension and stress.

In forming evaluations, teachers are torn between preparing students for certification and licensure evaluations and addressing their educational needs. Ultimately a balance must be struck between these two poles. It is hoped that as certification and licensure exams improve, these two poles will increasingly come together.

Self-evaluation is another critical component of the evaluation process. When students arrive in practice, they must have the capacity to evaluate their own work and practices. Teachers can show students how to critique and evaluate their own work in a mature fashion.

Peer evaluations can also be useful. Students need to be prepared to handle criticism from others. Some students are comfortable with peer review, whereas others find it quite threatening. Teachers can help set an objective, non-threatening tone during peer review.

Finally, teachers need to re-experience what it is like to be evaluated themselves. Teacher evaluations are critical to good teaching. It is often hard for teachers not to react defensively to student evaluations. However, they should model mature self-reflection to their students. Only in this way does the evaluation process become more collaborative.

Homework

I like work: It fascinates me. I can sit and look at it for hours.
I love to keep it by me: the idea of getting rid of it nearly breaks my heart.
—Jerome K. Jerome

Homework can be very productive for students. It is an opportunity for teachers to encourage self-learning and critical thinking. Varying homework over time encourages students to be creative. Homework is also an opportunity for faculty to assess, apart from examinations, how students are doing.

There are two kinds of homework: regular and periodic. Regular homework is the work students do to prepare for class. Examples include reading about remedies, practice cases and repertory exercises. Periodic homework is the more extensive work students do to complete special projects assigned intermittently. Special projects allow students to explore subjects in depth and to bring together disparate elements of learning. Examples include writing up cases, essays on comparative materia medica (comparing remedies), evaluations of comparative rubric analysis (comparing the occurrence of remedies for a given symptom) and exercises such as asking students to live as if they were in a remedy state for 24 hours.

How much homework one should give depends on the program and the students. There is a delicate balance between class time and homework. Too much homework promotes student burnout. Too little homework prevents student growth and integration of knowledge. No matter how much homework they assign, teachers should give students individualized feedback on their work.

Handouts

If you emphasize everything, you emphasize nothing.
—Anonymous

Students love handouts. Some prefer extensive handouts that allow them to just sit back and listen. Others prefer skeletal notes in which they can fill in the details. As a rule, teacher handouts should be succinct and stick to the main points. Handouts that are too extensive can be a problem for students who learn and process information by writing it down. Too much information can also make it difficult for students to know what is most important.

Teaching Materia Medica

> *Dr. Kent teaches* materia medica *by making it live, not by crowding the memory with keynotes, red tape, and worthless catch phrases, but by making each remedy an individual so real that when we meet the patient we recognize him by his photograph…*
>
> —Maybelle M. Park (Kent's student)

Good *materia medica* (descriptions of individual homeopathic remedies) lectures often are the highlight of training for homeopathic students. There are many ways to teach *materia medica*, from lectures to problem-based learning (see Chapter Nine). Appendix I details a historical discussion of *materia medica* teaching methods from the American Institute of Homeopathy convention on education in 1894. Whatever the method, it is essential to balance learning the data with understanding the heart of the remedy. The teacher's challenge is to present the facts of the remedy in an interesting way, and then to bring the remedy alive for the student. The student can then feel the remedy and grasp it as more than just a collection of data.

Some teachers teach *materia medica* from the part to the whole. They begin with the important data about a remedy, often based on the provings, and then carefully weave together the disparate elements into one rich tapestry. Other teachers teach from the whole to the part. They begin with cured cases and work backward to explore the remedy and understand all of its disparate elements. Each method has strengths and weaknesses.

Helping students see the remedy in the world around them is an important part of effective *materia medica* teaching. Seeing remedy states in movies, opera, books, historical analysis, poetry, art and mythology can bring the remedy alive and put it into a context that is meaningful to students. It also helps the student see and perceive the world in a new way.

Effective teaching of *materia medica* demands a partial knowledge of geology, botany, zoology, taxonomy, toxicology and other related fields. It requires knowledge of the substance from which the remedy is derived in its natural world. It also necessitates an understanding of remedy relationships and remedy families. Teachers often neglect to impart to students a thorough understanding of how a remedy state develops over time, including the appearance of remedies in childhood, adolescence, adulthood and old age.

Some training programs focus the teaching of *materia medica* on polychrest (common) remedies, and quickly run through smaller remedies at the end of the training. The advantage of this approach is that it makes the learning of *materia medica* more manageable for students and gives them a solid foundation. It is easier for students initially. The disadvantage is that it can be very hard for students to let go of a "polychrest mentality." Increasingly in their practice, they tend to fall back on remedies that they know and are comfortable with. This can lead to rigidity in thinking and practice.

Other schools value each remedy more equally in teaching. They spend more time on remedies that are considered less common, feeling that all remedies are potential polychrests. This is harder for students initially because the amount of material is overwhelming, but ultimately it leads to more flexible and skilled practitioners.

A practice database is helpful in teaching *materia medica*. Via their database, teachers can cross-reference all of their cured cases and make information readily available for teaching purposes. One advantage of a large faculty is having a greater pool of cured cases from which to draw. Databases also prove enormously helpful in practice-based research.

One of the challenges of *materia medica* is the large amount of data that must be learned. Accelerated learning techniques can be helpful (see Chapter One). So can class exercises in which the material is integrated into fairy tales (see Appendix F), creative arts and poetry. Music also creates magic and consecrates feelings in the class.

Another problem in teaching *materia medica* is the creation of provings. Experienced teachers often do a mini-proving of the remedy being taught. However, this can be disconcerting and destabilizing for beginning teachers, until they learn how to separate living the remedy from being a vehicle for the expression of the energy of the remedy. This is similar to the distinction between sympathy and empathy in homeopathic practice. In the former case, the teacher merges with the subject, whereas in the latter case, the teacher participates in the subject yet remains separate and distinct.

There are many methods of effectively teaching *materia medica*. The central keys are flexibility in the approach and a capacity to bring the material alive for the students.

Teaching Research

Do not be too timid and squeamish about your actions.
All life is an experiment.
—Emerson

Early in training, many students identify themselves as either research-ers or clinicians, and there is often tension between these two types of stu-dents. Clinicians carry the tradition of established and proven knowledge and enforce standards of theoretical and technical knowledge. Clinicians are not so interested in making new contributions. In contrast, researchers tend to develop new ideas and question older ones. They are destroyers of tradition. Their curiosity drives them beyond what they know.

Without research, a homeopathic training program becomes a trade school that trains competent technicians in homeopathy. The ideal school can teach both types of students and help them demonstrate respect for each other.

Types of Research

Research has traditionally been defined as the pursuit of knowledge for its own sake. In 1990, however, the Carnegie Foundation for the Advance-ment of Teaching issued a report examining the modern definitions of research (Boyer 1990). The report's categories of scholarship define various types of research: scholarship of discovery; scholarship of integration; scholarship of teaching and learning; and scholarship of practice.

◎ **Scholarship of Discovery**: This refers to pure research, in which knowledge is pursued for its own sake. Traditionally, pure research has been considered the most important form of research. In home-opathy, it includes basic science research, research demonstrating the validity of homeopathy using conventional paradigms and prov-ing research.

◎ **Scholarship of Integration**: This form of research integrates knowl-edge. Here, researchers have the capacity to bridge disciplines and look for new relationships between the parts and the whole. They find patterns of meaning that cannot be seen through a focus on individual subjects.

◉ **Scholarship of Teaching and Learning**: Educational research examines how professionals learn and effectively teach in their disciplines. It has been much neglected.

◉ **Scholarship of Practice**: This form of research pertains to clinical practice. It explores the qualities, skills and knowledge necessary for effective practice.

Ways to Teach Research

One way students can learn about quality research is by working on research projects or theses. Teachers need to supervise such projects closely. Though research content (basic science research, clinical research and proving research) is important, teachers should also emphasize attitudes conducive to good research. When the projects are completed, students can share their finding with peers through research presentations.

Another way to teach research and experience it firsthand is by participating in provings. Many teachers and students have felt that they understood homeopathy on a much deeper level after they were involved in provings. They also have benefited by taking part in ongoing clinical or basic science research in the training program.

When mentoring students in research, teachers should consider the conclusions of a 1987 study by Bland, Hitchcock, Anderson and Stritter. The authors identified the following 11 factors as important in the development of researchers in training programs:

◉ In-depth knowledge of the subject or research
◉ Training in research methodology
◉ Socialization to the research profession
◉ Experience with research mentors
◉ Inculcation of scholarly habits
◉ Supportive research network
◉ Productive colleagues and peers
◉ Involvement in multiple simultaneous research projects
◉ Adequate time devoted to research in training
◉ Research related activities both inside and outside of training programs
◉ Training environment supportive of research

Teaching Repertory

If you love homeopathy it will love you; such is its natural clarity.
We owe no obedience to man, not even to our parents
after we are old enough to think for ourselves.
We owe obedience only to Truth.
—James Tyler Kent

Teaching repertory (a compendium of remedies associated with particular symptoms) is one of the hardest challenges for homeopathic teachers and the greatest source of frustration for beginning students. Students also find repertory work tedious. Repertory teaching often is flat and unimaginative. Students need to be taught the diversity of repertories and repertorization methods. However, it is critical that students use the same repertory in class exercises and clinical training. Otherwise, there will be much confusion.

The most challenging aspect of teaching repertory is helping students to convert symptoms into repertory language. This conversion can be practiced in class exercises but is more effectively taught through carefully integrated casework. Another central challenge is to help students understand and feel the layout and design of the repertory.

Integration of repertory teaching into other aspects of the curriculum can be helpful. Case-based repertory analysis is an important tool. The key for students is practice and repetition. Some students have an aversion to or fear of the repertory. For them, repertorization is an onerous task and something to be avoided. Teachers must find a way to make repertorization come alive for these students. They should help these students to see repertorization as a learning exercise and a way of furthering their learning process. Creative repertory exercises where rubrics are analyzed in comparative *materia medica* can be helpful.

Other students gravitate strongly to the repertory. They may over-utilize it and develop a dependency. Teachers must help these students understand the repertory as one tool among many and illustrate the dangers of over-reliance on the repertory. Because of these dangers, some training programs do not teach repertory until later in training.

An important aspect of this problem is the usage of computers to repertorize. Computer repetorization tends to move students towards a more mechanistic model, analyzing in pieces rather than seeing the whole and focusing on data and information. Some tasks are much better done by computers and others by humans. It is important for teachers to balance the strengths and weaknesses of computers for their students in all aspects of their training.

Teaching Case Taking, Case Analysis and Case Management

A school should not be a preparation for life.
A school should be life.
—Elbert Hubbard

Case taking, case analysis and case management do not lend themselves well to lecture format. Students need to learn these skills through extensive clinical training (see Chapter Five). Becoming adept at these skills requires unprejudiced observation, clear perception, the capacity to find what is unique in a case, patience and wonder.

Modeling is the most important method of teaching case taking, case analysis and case management (see Chapter One). Students carefully observe their clinical teachers and copy their behaviors and attitudes, both consciously and unconsciously. Lecturing plays a role in introducing these subjects, but theories often are not meaningful to students until they see them in practice. Other techniques that can be useful are role-plays, group exercises and class discussions. (Competencies associated with case taking, case analysis and case management are well summarized in Appendix E.)

Teachers take note: Training programs often fail to instruct students in the following aspects of case taking, case analysis and case management:

◎ Knowing when to take on a case and when to refer

◎ Communicating to clients about the nature of homeopathic treatment

◎ Evaluating the resources available to clients in making important changes in their lives

◎ Knowing when to obtain collateral information in case taking

◎ Balancing homeopathic treatment with other allopathic and alternative modalities

◎ The importance of obtaining medical reports

◎ Discussion of prognosis and the development of case-taking forms

◎ Understanding "obstacles to cure"

Many clinical training programs focus on initial case taking and case analysis and do not provide students an opportunity for long-term case management. Consequently, when students get into practice they often are unprepared to manage cases over time. To prevent this problem, teachers need to focus students on expectations and prognosis in treatment. This includes teaching them about the pace and rhythm of healing, as well as how healing occurs. Students also must learn how to evaluate their results in terms of homeopathic philosophy.

Teaching Ethics

Physical science will not console me for the ignorance of moral-
ity in the time of affliction. But the science of ethics will
always console me for the ignorance of the physical sciences.
—Pascal

Homeopathic schools often only give lip service to the important topic of ethics. This happens because teachers are not entirely comfortable with the subject and don't know how to properly teach it. Given their own lack of ethical training, they might also feel ill-equipped to model good ethics for students.

Why Ethics Is Important in Homeopathic Training

Because the public has grown increasingly cynical about the ethics of professionals, other professional training programs have placed much greater emphasis on ethics. Homeopathic training programs must do the same. It is especially important for homeopaths to assure the public that they have been well-trained in ethics because the homeopathic profession is not as well-established or well-accepted as some other professions. At this point, unfortunately, most homeopathic professionals are unable to articulate their ethical standards.

Some educators relegate ethics to a policing role, but the goal in ethical education is much more than eliminating the small fraction of homeopaths who practice unethically. It is also to help practitioners who are conscientiously trying to ethically deal with the increasingly complex problems they face.

Why Teaching Ethics Is Challenging

One of the challenges in teaching ethics relates to the question, "Who is the expert?" The teacher is no more the expert here than any student. When it comes to ethics, medically licensed students have no real advantage over non-medically licensed students. Everyone comes with a rich variety of ethical experiences to share with each other.

Teachers may resist teaching ethics for several reasons. Some feel that adult learners are fully formed and that it is not possible to change their ethical conduct. This is simply not true (Ozar 1993). The development of professional ethics is an ongoing process. One's ethical values are constantly changing and growing as one develops as a practitioner. Another objection is that while necessary, ethics cannot be taught but only modeled. It is certainly true that role modeling is an important method of teaching ethics. However, to be truly effective it must be done consciously. This can only be done if students are made aware of ethical issues.

Ethics does not lend itself well to lecture, but is best taught through discussion. It is not effective to simply tell someone how to act. Written essays, case evaluations and role-plays can also be quite helpful.

Keys to a Good Education in Ethics

What are the goals of an ethical education for homeopathic professionals? David Ozar describes six objectives (Ozar 1993):

Enhanced modeling of ethical learning: Teachers should see the presentation of cases as an opportunity to teach ethics to their students. This is mostly a matter of increasing faculty awareness and emphasizing the importance of teaching ethics in a problem-based learning format.

Increased awareness of ethical issues in professional practice: Students often are unaware that ethical issues are at stake in their casework. A guided discussion in the classroom can help increase their ethical awareness. Types of ethical issues that need to be addressed include:

◎ Whom does the homeopathic practitioner serve?

◎ What are the central values of the homeopathic profession? What are its boundaries?

◎ What is the ethical relationship between homeopaths and their clients? What is the ethical relationship between a homeopath and other homeopaths? What is the ethical relationship between homeopaths and the homeopathic community?

◎ Are homeopaths ethically responsible for educating the public about health?

◎ What is the relative priority of a client's well-being?

◎ What is the homeopath's commitment to service?

◎ How competent must homeopaths be in their practice?

Strong moral reasoning skills: This skill is perhaps the most difficult to teach. Students struggle with an inadequate ability to reason ethically

(Rest 1982, 1983). The most useful method of developing this skill is through written essays in which students demonstrate their ethical reasoning in evaluating a case. In their essays, students should not only consider "What is the ethical standard here?" but also "How should I implement the ethical standard?" and "What should the ethical standard be?"

Basic understanding of the nature of a profession and of professional obligations: Being a member of a profession means having certain obligations defined by a dialog between the professional group and the community (Ozar 1993). A guided discussion format is a good way to teach students about professional obligations. The discussion can explore what to do when professional obligations conflict with an individual's morals, ethics and values, as well as the dilemma of conflicting professional obligations often faced by homeopathic practitioners who are medically licensed.

Skill in utilizing and applying ethical decisions in practice: Many students have a fundamental understanding of ethical concepts but struggle when trying to apply them in practice. This can become an increasing problem as the complexity of one's life and one's practice increases. Another problem is conflict between legal issues and ethical issues. Generally, legal issues should be taught separately from ethical ones. It is important to help students keep these two types of issues separate in their thinking. These issues are best addressed through clinical training as they arise in case work as well as in clinical supervision.

Improved communication skills in articulating ethical issues in professional practice: It is crucial that students not only have sound ethical reasoning and be able to apply it in practice, but also that they be able to articulate their reasoning to others. They must be able to define their ethics. Increasingly, it is becoming important to share one's ethical reasoning with other professionals and the community. An example includes the issue of when to refer a client to another practitioner. This issue has both legal and ethical implications.

Ultimately ethics must be integrated into every aspect of the homeopathic curriculum. A training program's entire faculty should become ethics educators and role models for students. Faculty and administrators need to be always conscious of the impact of their ethical behavior on their students. They also should discuss these issues with each other on an ongoing basis, seeking commonalty and new ways of presenting ethics material.

Teaching History

Human history becomes more and more a race
between education and catastrophe.
—H. G. Wells

For some students, especially in our present-focused American culture, history is a dead and dry subject that must be survived. Fortunately, there are also students who see historical images as essential to understanding where they are and what they have become. These students have developed a historical consciousness. They know that history can provide the larger context that is so necessary in the development of freedom from prejudice.

Historical consciousness must be taught and modeled to homeopathic students. Teachers need to stress the great debt we owe to the homeopaths that have lived and served before us.

It is important in teaching history to bring it alive. History is not concerned with facts, but people. Good history teachers use colorful, descriptive language to bring historical figures to life in the student's imagination. They also draw parallels between contemporary life and historical truths (and often ask students to explore these parallels in essays). In addition, they are aware of the cyclical nature of history, its ebbs and flows. They use this awareness as a bridge to look to the future.

A few remarks on content: Homeopathic history should begin with the development of healing in Western Civilization. Only in this way can Hahnemann be fully understood in his historical context. The ongoing dialectic between rational and empirical medicine, between allopathy and homeopathy also must be fully explored. Finally, it is important for teachers of homeopathic history to describe the development of homeopathy not only in their own country, but also around the world. This helps students become less myopic. (Content for historical teaching is outlined more completely in Appendix E.)

Teaching Communication Skills

Communication is a continual balancing act,
juggling the conflicting needs for intimacy and independence.
—Deborah Tannen

Communication skills are seldom introduced into professional training programs. However, it is increasingly important that a professional be able to communicate well in their practice, and to communicate their skills to others. They must be able to communicate well with patients, other homeopathic practitioners, allopathic practitioners, the media and the public.

In part, teaching communication is teaching how to teach. Students should be taught that learning and teaching are different sides of the same coin. Teaching and communicating then become an integral part of their practice, even if they never formally teach.

An important aspect of communicating well is being aware of boundaries. Student must learn to recognize and respect the boundaries between themselves and clients, other homeopathic practitioners, teachers and other students. Good teachers model appropriate boundaries for their students, but boundaries should also be discussed in class.

Within a training program, communication skills can be developed in a variety of ways, from peer teaching to faculty modeling to role-plays focusing on communication problems. Most importantly, however, students build good communication skills from exposure to good clinical teaching (see Chapter Five).

Teaching Philosophy

Let no young man delay the study of philosophy,
and let no old man become weary of it;
for it is never too early nor too late
to care for the well-being of the soul.
—Epicurus

Given that the principles of homeopathy have remained unchanged for 200 years, philosophy is the single most important subject that homeopathic educators teach. It, more than anything else, defines who homeopaths are.

There are many effective methods of teaching homeopathic philosophy. Lectures and discussion groups can be quite effective, but it's more useful for students to see the application of philosophy in practice. For example experiencing the Law of Similars first hand by participating in a proving, brings homeopathic philosophy alive and to a whole new level. Often philosophy is taught at the beginning of a training program and not touched on again. It is better for students when philosophy is integrated into every aspect of the curriculum. They should see the homeopathic principles in action throughout their training.

Clearly, philosophy must begin and end with the *Organon* (the fundamental text of homeopathy written by Samuel Hahnemann). Appendix I contains a historical discussion of the teaching of the *Organon*, from an AIH convention on education in 1894. The most recent translation of the *Organon* has brought it more dynamically alive for students (Hahnemann). Besides becoming familiar with the *Organon,* students must be able to contrast homeopathic philosophy with allopathic philosophy and other philosophies of healing.

Teaching Medical Competency

> *Medicine contains a compendium of the successive and contradictory mistakes of medical practitioners, when we summon the wisest of them to our aid, the chances are that we may be relying on a scientific truth the error of which will be recognized in a few years time.*
> —Marcel Proust

Medical competence in the practice of homeopathy is the minimum set of knowledge, skills and attitudes necessary to prescribe homeopathy in a fashion that is effective and safe for the client. A full examination of the teaching of medical competency is beyond the scope of this book, but I would like to touch on it briefly. (For more information on minimum medical competencies and standards, see Appendix E.)

Medical competency is generally an issue only for training programs that teach non-medically licensed practitioners. Most homeopathic training programs expect students to get their medical training elsewhere, through basic college courses on anatomy, physiology, pathology, pharmacy and first aid. The problem with this strategy is that students have difficulty integrating their medical and homeopathic knowledge bases into any type of unified whole. To solve this problem, there is a new but growing trend to integrate medical material into the homeopathic curriculum.

Students must have enough medical training to be able to pick out the common symptoms of illness and to distinguish what is unique and individualizing about a case. They also must be aware of conditions that are urgent and emergent and should be referred. This requires knowing their limits.

Students should develop an appreciation not only of allopathic medicine, but also of alternative medicine. This includes an understanding of allopathic drugs, herbs and dietary supplements. This requisite knowledge should be sufficient to help them become comfortable working with other practitioners, whether they be homeopaths, allopaths or practitioners of some other form of alternative medicine.

Though it is seldom emphasized, a homeopath's medical training should also include some study of the psyche. Important topics in this area include maps of the mind, familiarity with psychological development, psychological responses to stress, psychological terminology and an appreciation of family and group dynamics (Heaton 1998).

Mentorship

Everything that happens to you is your teacher.
The secret is to learn to sit at the feet
of your own life and be taught by it.
—Polly Berends

Mentoring is a crucial component of homeopathic training and can be useful in all phases of training. Mentorship should be distinguished from supervision. Supervision is mostly case focused, whereas mentorship is mostly process focused.

In Homer's *Odyssey*, Mentor was entrusted with the education of Odysseus's son, Telemacheus. Mentor served as both a guardian who protected Telemacheus and a wise teacher who educated him in the ways of the world. In homeopathic training, mentors help to hold up a mirror so students can see where they are on the homeopathic journey and become inspired to take the next step. Mentors help to bring out the full potential of their students.

Good mentors offer information, challenge assumptions, provide vision, lend an ear and a helping hand, guide the learner to set realistic expectations and goals, encourage the learner to network with the community and help the learner to see the larger picture. They also help students integrate career and family life. Mentoring is a powerful growth experience for both the mentor and the homeopathic learner.

True mentorship is not as concerned with transferring knowledge to the learner as with facilitating a learning relationship. Mentors of old were authority figures that homeopathic learners modeled themselves after; mentors of today are facilitators of learning. They see themselves as resources for their students and share the responsibility for learning. According to Brookfield, effective mentoring is characterized by voluntary engagement of both partners, mutual respect, collaboration, critical reflection and empowerment of the learner (Brookfield 1986).

Diversity in mentorship is very important in training. Cross-cultural mentoring, cross-gender mentoring, cross-generational mentoring and cross-medical discipline mentoring can all promote the growth of a homeopathic community. Finding the perfect match between mentor and homeopathic learner is less important. A mentor often has much to offer, even if the homeopathic learner is not fully comfortable. Exposure to a diversity of mentors also reduces the risk of mentor cloning. As the number of homeopathic women practitioners grows, the demand for female mentors will steadily increase.

Mentoring can occur face-to-face or via chat rooms, phone conferencing and e-mail. It is not unusual for mentoring to begin face-to-face and transition into a long-distance relationship. In long-distance relationships, however, it is much harder to tell what the other person is feeling and thinking.

Mentorship can also occur in a group format. Mentorship groups are often formed toward the end of professional training programs. Sometimes called "professional seminars," they are designed to help students make the difficult transition from school into practice.

All mentoring relationships have predictable phases (Schlossber, Lynch and Chickerin 1989). It is important for the mentor to be aware of these phases and their signposts during mentorship. The phases include tilling the soil, planting the seeds, nourishing the growth and reaping the harvest (Zachary 2000).

Tilling the Soil

Mentors must prepare carefully for mentorship. Homeopathic knowledge and experience are insufficient. During this phase, mentors should reflect on their motivations for becoming a mentor, get comfortable with mentoring skills, identify their own learning needs and develop an awareness of their limits as a mentor. Such self-understanding will allow them to become more committed to mentoring.

Individuals typically want to become mentors for the following reasons:

⦾ To foster their own personal and professional growth

⦾ Because they enjoy collaborative learning

⦾ To help others learn

⦾ To learn new things about themselves, their students and the organization

⦾ To challenge themselves

In evaluating whether to become a mentor, practitioners and teachers must consider whether they can make the time commitment necessary for quality mentoring. Most mentors underestimate the time commitment, and lack of sufficient time is the main reason mentoring relationships fail.

Mentorship requires different skills from classroom teaching or even supervision, and mentors need to acquire these skills before mentoring begins. Some schools offer training programs in mentorship and have mentoring programs for teachers and students. Mentoring skills include (Zachary 2000):

- **Brokering relationships:** Making the right contacts and laying the groundwork for learners to connect with other people who can be useful resources.

- **Relationship building:** Being attentive, patient and persistent in developing a relationship with the learner

- **Coaching:** Assisting individuals by filling in knowledge gaps and helping them learn to do things more effectively.

- **Good communication:** Building trust, authenticity, clarity, and effective listening.

- **Confidence building:** Encouraging, cheer leading, motivating and inspiring.

- **Facilitating:** Promoting self-directed learning.

- **Goal-setting:** Helping learners crystallize, clarify and set realistic goals; helping them envision themselves as successful homeopaths.

- **Guiding:** Clearing the path by helping students remove the obstacles to learning.

- **Conflict management:** Being able to provide mediation and anger management assistance.

- **Problem-solving:** Helping learners with strategic planning and reframing.

- **Feedback:** Giving learners written and oral commentary on their work.

To prepare students for what lies ahead, mentors must have a clear understanding of their own journey. To this end, they should reflect on their own past experiences with mentors. They also should have clarity about administrative expectations and roles.

Planting the Seeds

This phase of mentorship is more the business end, yet it is critical in building and forming the relationship. The key to successful mentoring involves taking the time to establish the human connection. Only when the relationship has been successfully built will the learning follow.

During this phase of mentorship, mentors first meet the homeopathic learners and establish rapport. Their initial contacts involve bargaining, sharing information, establishing an understanding about assumptions, setting boundaries, creating shared goals and a plan to achieve those goals, exploring confidentiality issues and ethics, outlining expected stumbling blocks on the journey and defining successful completion criteria.

This is a good time to talk about underlying expectations formed from previous mentoring and teaching experiences. The conversation must be collaborative: Learners must be involved in planning how and what they will learn. Ultimately, mentors and learners must reach a consensual agreement as to how they will meet the work goals.

Simple ground rules must be established. These might include beginning and ending on time, communicating openly and candidly, respecting differences, honoring each other's expertise and experience, safeguarding confidentiality and putting interruptions aside. Consequences should be established for when ground rules are broken.

As each learner is unique, a mentor must prepare anew for every mentoring relationship. It is important to assess the homeopathic learner's idiosyncratic learning style and adapt one's teaching style accordingly. In order to know where to begin, the mentor also needs to determine where the learner is on his/her homeopathic journey. The best embarkation point is where the learner finds himself/herself at the present moment (Lindeman 1989).

Nurturing the Growth

This is the longest phase of mentorship. Learning must be nurtured or it becomes mechanistic and rigid. The three keys to nurturing a homeopathic learner's growth and development are support, challenge and vision (Daloz 1999).

Mentors provide support by establishing and maintaining a safe learning climate. This requires that the mentor demonstrate respect and authenticity. Other nurturing behaviors include respectful active listening, consistency, providing a learning structure, positive expectations, acting as an advocate (publicly and privately), admitting ignorance when one does not know and being open to feedback. Good mentors give themselves and learners permission to make mistakes and then create ways to learn from the mistakes together.

Mentors must also challenge the homeopathic learner to grow. This requires setting tasks, assigning homework and setting standards. Good mentors provide ongoing feedback to the homeopathic learner and the administration. The learning process must be monitored to ensure that the homeopathic learners' goals are being met.

Finally, mentors should provide and sustain a vision for the homeopathic learner. They do this most effectively through modeling what it is to be a homeopathic practitioner. Figuratively speaking, they hold up a mirror that helps students see themselves more accurately. Open, accurate and honest feedback is a vital part of this process. This mirror function is a great advantage of mentoring over classroom teaching. It helps students see where they are and chart their course on the homeopathic journey.

During this phase, mentors often benefit by keeping a written record of the mentorship experience. This allows them to work through feelings and meaningful learning. A written record can also serve administrative purposes and help with accountability. This record can take the form of "process notes," in which details are less important than process.

Though mentors should seek to develop a strong, nurturing relationship with learners, they should set careful boundaries to keep the relationship focused on the homeopathic work. Some students seek to make their mentor their counselor or therapist. They may start confiding serious personal problems or ask their mentor to take on the role of homeopathic practitioner. Such issues are beyond the scope of mentorship. These students should be referred for counseling or to their homeopathic practitioner.

Reaping the Harvest

It is often difficult to tell when a mentorship should end. Students can develop a dependency on their mentors that makes ending the relationship difficult. As a rule, it's time to end when the goals established at the beginning of the mentorship process have been met. It's easier for everyone if the conditions for termination have been established at the beginning of the mentorship.

This end phase of mentorship is an opportunity for much growth and self- reflection for both the mentor and the homeopathic learner. It is a time to harvest what has been learned and to move into a more collegial relationship. For the student, it is an opportunity to give back in service what he/she has learned.

It is important for mentor and learner to mark the ending and celebrate it together. This models how to end well with clients and in other aspects of homeopathic work. Inevitably, endings are emotional processes filled with grief, joy, fear and excitement. Individuals who have difficulty ending relationships will have the most difficulty with this phase of the work.

Even after the harvest, however, the journey is not complete. There is always another step. The opportunities for renewal and regeneration are continual. Mentors can be an important resource for their former students long after the mentorship has ended. Students often maintain periodic contact to receive validation for their accomplishments and to measure their progress.

Quality didactic training is crucial in the development of a good homeopathic practitioner. However, this is even more true for quality clinical teaching. Many teachers excel at didactic teaching but struggle when it comes to clinical teaching. The next chapter strives to identify those qualities that underlie successful clinical teaching.

Chapter Five

The Importance of Clinical Teaching

I hear and I forget.
I see and I remember.
I do and I understand.
—Chinese Proverb

Due to its long neglect in homeopathic education, clinical training remains stuck in infancy. Training programs vary greatly with some treating clinical training as an afterthought, while others integrate it fully into the curriculum. Many schools graduate homeopaths who never actually enter practice. This is usually caused by a lack of clinical training. Many professions are criticized for poorly preparing professionals for practice (Brown 1988; Carter 1983; Dinham and Stritter 1986; Edwards 1988; Grabowski 1983; Halpern 1982; Tomain and Solimine 1990). Those who finally integrate their knowledge and move forward in homeopathy are those who practice their skills from the beginning of their training.

Increasingly, certifying bodies are requiring clinical training, reflecting a growing recognition of its general importance in homeopathy. Students learn best by doing and feeling. Current research on adult learning indicates an inherent need for immediacy of application. It's not enough to learn skills; the student must be comfortable in applying them.

It is a privilege to do homeopathy, but with this privilege comes great responsibility. It is the clinical teacher's duty to ensure that a sense of this responsibility and ethics is inculcated into students. This is difficult to teach in a purely didactic format.

Ultimately, a clinical training program should be well integrated into homeopathic training. After graduation, the final leap into practice shouldn't be difficult, since the student has been performing throughout their training. Clinical training should be an extension of the didactic training. It's critical that students are fully prepared for practice. The large number of students who graduate from training programs, but never practice, is a great problem in contemporary homeopathic education. Unprepared students often find the move into practice too overwhelming.

Much of this work needs to be done in a clinical environment through a student's practice, although discussion groups can be helpful. Students must also know and understand the homeopathic community within which they will practice. Building bridges to the community and helping students connect to it before they finish their training is of major importance.

There is a common belief that medically licensed practitioners have a distinct advantage. My experience contradicts this belief. Clinical training in most medical schools is very poor and allopathically focused. Medically licensed practitioners must spend considerable time unlearning old habits and learning to open their hearts, minds and spirit.

Why Are There So Few Clinical Training Programs?

What we have to learn to do, we learn by doing.
—Aristotle

Finding clinical teachers is as challenging as conducting the training itself. Many teachers feel comfortable in a didactic format but quail at the thought of clinical training. Their own lack of training leaves them with little to work from and lacking confidence. To teach clinically means putting your work and ultimately yourself on the line. It requires a willingness to be vulnerable and examine oneself, both with and through others.

Logistically, it's hard to design clinical training programs where teachers are adequately reimbursed for their services. Often clinical training is done by volunteers, making it difficult to organize and establish formal requirements.

A deeper problem relates to the focus of homeopathy today. Most current homeopathic literature reflects a disproportionate amount of energy expended expanding our knowledge base with new materia medica, repertory and provings. Too little attention is placed on the process of homeopathy, including the development of skills in listening, perception, self reflection and awareness, ethics, freedom from prejudice and case taking. We have many tools in homeopathy but we still utilize them in an allopathic (mechanistic) way (Chappell 2000). Effective clinical training can remedy this problem.

Structure and Purpose of Clinical Training

First the patient, second the patient,
third the patient, fourth the patient, fifth the patient,
and then maybe comes science.
—Bela Schick

Clinical training is inherently complex. There are four participants: the patient, the student, the teacher and the administrator (see Appendix A). Attention and care must be placed in each of these areas for a clinical training program to be successful. Ideally, each of the four participants should be equidistant from the others, in order to maximize the effectiveness of the work. All of them must be centered on the great subject of homeopathy.

The clinical training should, as much as possible, mirror what students will experience in their daily practice. This requires diversity. The training should also help prepare students for emergencies as well as strange and peculiar situations so that they will have the confidence to handle them. Clinical training should also help students develop an awareness of the dangers and risks associated with homeopathic practice. This is part of developing an awareness of the practitioner's limits.

What is the purpose of clinical training? Is it to provide the best possible care for our patients or to provide a rich growing and learning environment for the students? This dilemma is a central challenge of clinical training. Ultimately, a training program must do both.

The Therapeutic Model

Prescribing the proper remedy is only a part of a physician's
function, a part of the treatment. He has to consider all
aspects of the case. He must know how to prognosticate, how
to readjust the patient physically, mentally and spiritually,
and how to promote and hasten a cure by all methods avail-
able, physical, psychological, mechanical, nutritional,
hygienic and so on. And he must know not only how to guide
the patient to recover his health but to maintain it.
—Dr. P. Sankaran

Most clinical homeopathic training is focused around prescribing, but a good homeopath is much more than a good prescriber (Paul Sankaran 1996). There are many good prescribers who are poor homeopaths and good homeopaths who are poor prescribers. This underscores the importance of non-specific factors in the healing process. These are common factors that cut across theories and techniques and account for change. These factors include respect, common sense, compassion, establishing rapport, instilling hope and providing the opportunity to learn new ways of thinking, feeling and perceiving. It is vital to incorporate the building of these qualities into clinical training.

Good homeopathic clinical training is quite distant from allopathic training. The closest model of practice is that of psychotherapy. Though there are differences, there is much that clinical teachers of homeopathy can learn from the psychotherapy model. Much of what follows in this chapter borrows from psychotherapeutic models. Ultimately however, homeopaths need to develop their own model and language for clinical training.

Competing Schools of Thought

What is laid down,
ordered, factual is never enough to embrace the whole truth:
life always spills over the rim of every cup.
—Boris Pasternak

A central concern in designing clinical training programs is its central philosophy or school of thought. How does a supervisor handle a supervisee who bases their practice on a different school of thought?

Differing psychotherapeutic philosophies have long competed bitterly against each other. Research shows that most of these schools have comparative efficacy (Smith and Glass 1977; Stiles and Shapiro 1986). Similar research is needed in homeopathy, although I suspect that the results would be similar. Most homeopaths (including Hahnemann) are far more eclectic in clinical practice than they are in theory.

Developing Core Clinical Homeopathic Skills and Qualities

Train up a child in the way he should go:
and when he is old he will not depart from it.
—Proverbs 22:6

A variety of skills must be developed through the clinical training process. Jolles describes four stages in the development of skills in the student (Jolles 1993). The first is the Unconscious Incompetent. At this stage, the student lacks skills and is unaware of what they don't know. These students can be a challenge due to their ignorance.

The second stage is the Conscious Incompetent. The student becomes aware of their lack of skills. When students fully arrive at this stage, they can experience frustration and despair about the daunting task ahead.

The third stage is the Conscious Competent. Though this student practices his skills effectively, he must be always mindful of what he does. Students often experience this stage as work and struggle.

The last stage is that of the Unconscious Competent. Here the skill has been fully integrated into the student's practice. Much of what homeopaths do in effective clinical practice is unconscious and they have difficulty explaining this to others (see Tacit Knowledge on page 140). The challenge for clinical teachers is to make these skills conscious so that they can be shared and taught. Ultimately, these stages come full circle as the student continues to grow.

The early stages of clinical training are especially important as students create habits that are often unconscious and may last for the remainder of their careers. It is important that students not mimic their clinical teachers, but examine each aspect of clinical practice for themselves.

Clinical teachers must not be bound by rigid adherence to technique. In stressing that clinical expertise is something external, teachers prevent students from developing their full potential. Ultimately, each student must find their own style of practice that is independent of their teacher's.

"If one only has a hammer, everything looks like a nail." With developing skills, the key is diversification. The core skills required are many, but should, at the very least, include the following:

Unprejudiced Observation

The most important of all skills is observation, both of the patient and the student him/herself. Videotaping the student as well as the patient during case-taking can dramatically increase a student's self awareness and observation skills. Role playing and case review can be very helpful in this regard. Good clinical teachers can successfully observe their students as well.

In clinical training, students must learn methods of observation that they would take for granted in other settings. There are four basic aspects to observation: nonverbal communication, verbal communication, the relationship between verbal and nonverbal communication and emotions.

Non verbal cues arise from observation of the general appearance. There are several factors here, such as clothing, grooming, eye contact, posture, mannerisms, facial expressions and eye contact. Kinesics is body language and consists of posture, facial expression, movement, gestures, breathing changes and eye focus. Personal and cultural biases often prohibit us from deciphering body language accurately (Arredon et al, 1996). Proxemics represent personal space, including distance from the homeopath, positioning in the room and touch.

Verbal expression includes such factors as volume, inflection, rate, fluency (ease of articulation and flow of words), dialect, phrasing and tone. It is important that students develop a basic understanding of socio-linguistics. Individuals from different cultures express themselves linguistically very differently. For example, Americans generally speak more loudly than individuals from other cultures.

Speech content includes idiosyncratic word usage, vocabulary, psycho babble, pauses and silence. Idiosyncratic word usage refers to clients that utilize words that have profound meaning to them, but can only be fully understood by exploration and free association. Psycho babble is a term used to describe word usage and phrasing inculcated into the patient through the process of psychotherapy, but not representative of the patient themselves. Silence is one of the most important areas here. Students often have considerable difficulty with silence and jump in too quickly before the silence has been understood. Exercises in which students practice silence in the context of an interview can be helpful.

The relationship between spoken and non-verbal language is important in that it helps the student understand a client more deeply. When there is a non-congruence between these domains, it represents an opportunity to delve deeper into the clients' world and their feelings. It reveals what is defended against. Movement harmonics and turn taking are other aspects of communication (Heaton 1998). Movement harmonics represent the synchronous rhythmic motion present in most communication. There is an expectation of reciprocal interaction and complementary movement. Dissonance represents a quality of the client's interactions with others or a lack of effective mirroring by the homeopathic student. Students watching videotapes of their own case taking can see this more clearly.

Lastly, emotional expressions are both externally observed and internally felt by the student. Feelings are catching. Body language can reflect a clue to the underlying emotional state but may also represent an underlying physical condition. For example, I recently had a patient who was wringing their hands. I interpreted this as a nervous habit, until I asked about it and discovered that this was caused by a profound coldness in their hands. Students should be aware of the interaction between emotions and speech. Speech errors are much more likely when a client is emotional. Clients jump from topic to topic when they are exploring painful memories. There is much to be learned from the language of tears and laughter.

Clear Perception

The process of perception is central to good observation. Students must examine how they perceive homeopathy, their patients, themselves, and the world. This includes clarity of perception about what needs to be cured and how to perceive the central disturbance. Students must also examine how their personal beliefs and preferences influence their perception. Teachers should encourage students to seek homeopathic treatment. Only in this way can students remove the internal obstacles to practice.

Menear describes a beautiful class exercise that researches the process of perception for students (Menear 1990). Students examine a flower from three perceptive standpoints. In the first exercise, they look at the flower while holding the thought "I am looking at the flower." In the second part of the exercise they look at the flower while removing all thoughts from their mind. Finally, they look at the flower while holding the awareness that "the flower is revealing itself to me."

Wonder

Central to case analysis is developing the capacity to wonder (Rowe 1998). The capacity to wonder gives students the courage to delve deeper in their work. It keeps students open to the possibilities of life and brings joy to their practice, while encouraging humility. Wonder can only be conveyed by a teacher modeling it for his students.

Finding What Is Unique

Equally challenging is the capacity to see what is unique and individu-alizing. Students must learn to appreciate characteristic symptoms. This is particularly a challenge for non-licensed homeopathic practitioners, who, due to their lack of formal medical training, may have more difficulty per-ceiving common symptoms. Case taking exercises can be useful in high-lighting what is strange and peculiar. Students should also recognize their own uniqueness and individuality, both as a learner and as a homeopath. Their individuality allows them to perceive the individuality of others.

Patience

Patience is a central skill for clinical students to learn. Students have a natural tendency to attempt to hurry the process of healing. This is particu-larly a problem for those with more masculine energy, who feel a need to always be doing something. Though the best teacher is often the student's own experience of failed cases resulting from impatience, this also can be effectively incorporated into clinical training.

Presentation of problematic, failed and difficult cases can be a very important part of clinical training. One problem with clinical training that leads to impatience in treatment, is the presentation of cured cases only. Students whose clinical training consists of observation of cured simili-mum type cases develop the expectation of a rapid and smooth course of healing and become frustrated when their own cases fail to follow suit.

Locus of Power or Control

Another important skill focuses on the locus of power or control within the clinical environment. At the beginning of clinical training, stu-dents often either find themselves taking complete control of the session (independent practitioner and dependent client) or relinquishing all con-trol (dependent practitioner and independent client). Medically-licensed practitioners often are more comfortable with seizing control or power (the allopathic model). Non-medically licensed students are often more com-fortable with relinquishing all control in the therapeutic environment. A good clinical teacher helps each of their students move the locus of control to the center of the healing interaction. This is where true healing occurs (interdependence).

This issue also arises in the interactions between the teacher, student, patient and administrator. Who has the ultimate authority? Who has the control? When conflict arises between student and supervisor, how do decisions ultimately get made? Working through these issues in other venues can help students prepare for clinical training.

Synthesis and Analysis

It is important that students develop both inductive and deductive reasoning skills and the capacity to move smoothly back and forth between them. A good teacher models these skills and the ability to shift from one to the other. Since many students rely on a single method of reasoning, it is important for teachers to help them develop the one they miss. Medically licensed practitioners are often more comfortable with analytical thought (allopathic training) whereas non medically-licensed practitioners are often more comfortable with synthesis. Good evaluations of clinical students by faculty should also be both synthetic and analytic.

Listening

Listening skills are paramount. Students often find it challenging to avoid imposing their own judgments, beliefs and attitudes on their clients. Listening must come from an open heart. Effective teachers model this by listening carefully to students.

A student should be taught to listen in new ways, to listen with the "third ear." This means listening not only to content, but also to the central disturbance—hearing both the language and the music of one's patients. Case taking exercises can be of great help with this.

Establishing Rapport

Rapport is the glue that holds a therapeutic relationship together and makes results possible. It's basic to a good healing relationship (Rogers 1980). Homeopaths often rely on a client's initial enthusiasm to carry them through treatment. However, without an established rapport, treatment falters, even when the remedy has been successful. When rapport is established, clients feel understood, accepted and safe. A lack of rapport engenders feelings of disharmony, lack of safety and resistance to change. Lack of rapport is the main reason clients either fail to effectively engage in treatment or leave it prematurely. Ultimately, if a training program is well designed, this clinical rapport will mirror what was established in the classroom.

The challenge is to find ways to enhance and build rapport in clinical training. This begins with the establishment of a close rapport between clinical teacher and student. It involves helping students integrate who they are with what they know. It means nurturing their basic relationship skills.

The optimum place to explore the issue of rapport is in a training-clinic environment (see Models on page 145). Case observation and supervision are less effective environments to work on this issue.

In some ways, it is easier to recognize lack of rapport than to teach it. Clues that rapport has been established include the following:

◎ When the client tells us

◎ When the client reacts spontaneously

◎ When the client reads our intentions clearly

◎ When the client can disagree with the homeopath and express a difference of opinion

◎ When the client is open and not defensive

◎ When the client feels cared for in a total, rather than conditional way

Respect is one of the most important aspects of rapport. Respect means a willingness to accept one's clients as they are while conveying a willingness to help them grow. Students must learn to convey basic respect by honoring their clients' autonomy, while expecting them to assume personal responsibility for the choices they make. Students convey basic respect through punctuality and attentiveness to their clients' concerns. They also must learn self respect by not allowing their clients to be disrespectful, such as taking too much of their time or not paying their bills.

Another part of rapport is congruence, which occurs when homeopaths openly express feelings that are flowing through them. When students are congruent, they can honestly express their most authentic reactions. Clients need to hear that the homeopath is understanding what they are saying. This is more than summarization. They do this by responding to the client's pace and responding to non verbal cues. Students must be active and expressive to establish congruence.

Rapport requires an appreciation and empathy for the patient's suffering. This necessitates a degree of graciousness and the ability to suspend one's personal reactions. Remaining open to cultural differences and a client's individuality is helpful. Lastly, rapport is established through mutual celebration of progress in treatment and reinforcing each client's strengths and understandings.

Inevitably there will be ruptures in the rapport. Students need to learn how to handle their mistakes without becoming defensive. Clarifying what happened and acknowledging the rupture are critical to repairing it. Students need to learn these skills through apologizing and providing support.

Charles Kleinke has developed a self-assessment called the Opener Scale (Kleinke 1994). Ten items are scored on a five-point scale, with a positive answer worth 1/2 point. It helps students perceive their strengths and weaknesses in establishing rapport.

1. People frequently tell me about themselves
2. I've been told that I'm a good listener
3. I'm very accepting of others
4. People trust me with their secrets
5. I easily get people to "open up"
6. People feel relaxed around me
7. I enjoy listening to people
8. I'm sympathetic to peoples' problems
9. I encourage people to tell me how they are feeling
10. I can keep people talking about themselves

Clinical Knowledge

The doctor's role is to entertain the patient while they get better.
—Marcel Proust

Several areas of knowledge are important for the student to explore in clinical training. Homeopathy involves much more than learning a set of skills. Homeopathy, unlike allopathic medicine, has a central clinical philosophy and clinical core.

It is also important for students to remember and strengthen their "humanity." Effective homeopathic clinicians use self knowledge as a tool in their work.

Clinical knowledge can be learned through clinical didactic lectures, problem-based learning methods or integration into clinical training. Specific competencies and standards are summarized in Appendix E.

Homeopathic Knowledge

The focus here is on case taking, case analysis, case management, posology and potency. Most important, this includes knowledge about analyzing what needs to be cured in each case. Students must learn how to evaluate cases for suitability to their practice. This requires knowledge of one's limits. The assessment of obstacles to cure is frequently neglected (see below). Students should also develop the ability to evaluate the strength of the vital force and the center of gravity. Finally, this involves assessing prognosis and the efficacy of treatment.

Clinical knowledge competencies are summarized in Appendix E. Important specific knowledge competencies concerning the handling of sessions include:

- Establishing boundaries
- Handling greetings
- Setting the tone of the session
- Setting and clarifying expectations
- Agreeing on a course of treatment
- Establishment of a treatment plan
- Clearing the field
- Setting and maintaining time limits
- Making a diagnosis when appropriate
- Obtaining informed consent
- Instilling hope
- Finding appropriate methods to end sessions

Most training programs effectively focus on knowledge pertaining to initial visits but neglect long-term management. Students entering practice often complain that this is the single weakest area of their training, as it quickly becomes the area where they spend the bulk of their time and energies. This includes knowledge of pacing treatment (expectations of the pace of healing) and maintaining focus in treatment. Students should develop a knowledge of how to retake a case and deal with intercurrent prescribing. More peripheral issues include the handling of homework assignments, clarifying the role of advice and support, confrontation and challenging assumptions, the appropriate use of humor and the role of silence in treatment.

Allopathic Medical Knowledge

This includes a knowledge of medical terminology, physical examination, anatomy, clinical pathophysiology, toxicology, allopathic pharmacology, nutrition and diagnostic testing. There must be a thorough knowledge of psychology and counseling theory. In particular, concepts such as projection and transference are vital. Finally, there must be a knowledge of medical reporting.

Practitioners should be able to recognize signs and symptoms of both common and dangerous medical conditions. It is important that students understand the common symptoms of diagnosed diseases so that they can distinguish them from a client's individualized symptoms. They also must be able to distinguish between emergent, urgent and routine conditions.

Alternative Medical Knowledge

This includes a working knowledge of the basic forms of alternative medicine. Factors that interfere with homeopathic care or confuse the homeopathic picture should be recognized. Basic herbal pharmacology and nutrition should be understood.

Knowledge of the Natural World

Knowledge of the natural world includes an introductory knowledge of botany, biochemistry, biology, physics, zoology and mineralogy. This can be accomplished through a survey course(s).

Knowledge of the Human Condition

It's important for students to have knowledge of human development, mythology, anthropology and sociology. They need insight into subcultures, ethnic groups as well as their own culture. They should be aware of culture shock, produced by our modern world's constant change (Vargas and Willis 1994).

Practice-Based Knowledge

Students need to learn how to conduct a business. Proper preparation for practicalities reduces anxiety and stress. If this area is neglected, students make arbitrary decisions and formulate destructive habits. Mentorship can effectively address these issues.

The following are essential to practice-based knowledge:

- Billing practices (including billing for phone time and no shows)
- Setting fees
- Establishing sliding fee scales
- Collecting payment
- Raising fees
- Handling phone calls between sessions
- Managing paperwork
- Dealing with no shows and interruptions
- Constructing patient information
- Marketing a practice
- Designing a suitable physical environment
- Writing reports and letters
- Recording cases
- Keeping appropriate records (differs from allopathic practices; should be regularly reviewed by clinical faculty)

Appropriate Use of Referrals, Consultation and Supervision

Billing is often the most problematic practice-based issue for beginning students. Students are often uncomfortable dealing with finances. Most charge too little and struggle with feelings of unworthiness regarding payment. Students often have difficulty referring to other practitioners, feeling they must take everything on themselves. Knowledge of their own limits is required for students to recognize when they're moving out of their realm of expertise and experience. Clinical teachers can help with this.

Students need to learn how to communicate effectively with clients, with peers, and with the community at large. An understanding of one's role as a professional is critical, including awareness of professional obligations within the community. This requires critical evaluation of care and the use of feedback from others.

Little attention has been placed on how to begin and end treatment, but this knowledge is critical to students, many of whom are uncomfortable and lack the knowledge required to end well. This ignorance can jeopardize the efficacy of treatment. Issues such as expectations, transitions, dependency, premature endings, abandonment, self monitoring and written records of termination should be explored. Similarly, students lacking the knowledge to properly initiate treatment will struggle with establishing the rapport necessary to successful care.

Ethics are an important aspect of practice, including issues of confidentiality, boundary issues (social, financial and sexual contacts with clients), appropriate touching and the handling of gifts in the context of treatment.

Tacit or Practical Knowledge

Tacit knowledge (also called practical knowledge) is knowledge gained by dealing with the complexities of practice. Some of the most important problems in practice are characterized by complexity, uniqueness, uncertainty and conflicting values (Schon 1983, 1987, 1991). One of the main goals of practice is wise action, learning judgment in specific situations with conflicting values and how to solve them. This requires seeing many cases and developing a repertoire of responses and techniques.

The teaching of tacit knowledge is difficult. It is best learned through practice and reflection on practice in the indeterminate zones of the work (Harris 1989; Cervero 1989). The key is to integrate problem-solving experiences with knowledge acquisition in order to use and apply knowledge in practice (Elstein, Shulman and Sprafka 1978). This can't be done with a simple course late in the curriculum.

Through reflection, knowledge is delineated, criticized, restructured and utilized in further action and experimentation. Practical knowledge involves both reflection in action and reflection about action. Reflection in action occurs in the midst of the case, whereas reflection about action generally occurs on completion of a case. Reflection about action can be taught through class discussions, supervision and training clinic environments.

Much of reflection in action is tacit knowledge, that is, knowing more than we can say or verbalize as teachers. This is composed of actions, recognition and judgments typically carried out unconsciously. Observation is the best way for students to acquire such knowledge. Construction of virtual worlds through the use of computer technology and role playing can also simulate practice while slowing it down to allow safe reflection in action.

Self Knowledge

Self knowledge is a central aspect of clinical training. A homeopath's effectiveness is reflected not only in his general knowledge about patients and the nature of the homeopathic process, but also in a new and fuller use that they make of themselves. Students must know who they are. Through careful observation of oneself, it is possible to reduce errors of judgment and prejudice. Self knowledge adds another important tool to homeopathic work. Self scrutiny takes courage (Yalom 1981), as many students would rather avoid or deny these areas.

It is important that students develop an awareness of their limits. Whether licensed or non licensed, all homeopaths have limits to their practice skills that they shouldn't exceed. Without this knowledge they place themselves, their patients and their teachers at risk.

Another aspect of self knowledge is awareness of one's psyche. This includes both shadow and hero archetypes. The hero is that part of the psyche that one is overly comfortable with and that the student sees everywhere around them. Students over prescribe heroic remedies as they often represent their favorite remedies. Clients that have traits consistent with the student's hero, will be very attractive to the student and they may have difficulty maintaining objectivity and boundaries. Students often draw on their hero/heroine archetypes first while in clinical training.

The shadow is that part of the psyche that we cannot accept and therefore deny. It is always somewhat destructive. Shadow remedies are those remedies that lie within the shadow of the student. These remedies are difficult for the student to prescribe because they cannot see them within themselves. Clients that have traits consistent with the shadow of the student can also be very difficult for them to treat.

Developing a knowledge of personal reactions (how clients effect you) is an important part of clinical training. Personal reactions are responses to clients that all homeopaths experience. Personal reactions can be emotional, cognitive or behavioral. This area can be hard for students to own up to, as the sentiments are often politically incorrect. Students may fear a negative reaction from their teachers. Good modeling by the clinical teacher here is vital. There are three types of personal reactions: idiosyncratic, shared and counter transference.

When harnessed productively, a student's idiosyncratic reactions can provide important information in both case taking and case analysis. For example, the student may react to all clients that need the remedy Medorrhinum with a wish to nurture and care for them. These feelings are not typical responses to the remedy, but are idiosyncratic to the student. In case work, these feelings can help guide the student to the remedy.

Shared reactions are commonly experienced by homeopathic students. Awareness of these reactions can help students to develop a sense of how their clients are experienced by others. For example, students commonly react to a client that needs the remedy Pulsatilla with a need to nurture and take care of them. When this issue is explored, they may realize that many people in the client's life react in the same way, and that the client's behavior is targeted at eliciting this response.

Counter transference is a personal reaction to a client that stems from unconscious forces within the homeopath. Counter transference is an important aspect of self knowledge that represents the area where students are most vulnerable. Counter transference causes a student to lose objectivity in their work and to become prejudiced. For example, a homeopathic student may have had an upbringing in which they did not feel nurtured and cared for. When confronted with a client who needs the remedy Pulsatilla and has issues around nurturing and being cared for, they feel empathy and their own issues become activated. They may react with unconscious anger (why should they get nurturing and care when I never did as a child?). This can destroy the relationship and the students' objectivity. The following factors can indicate to student and teacher that counter transference is occurring:

- ◉ Strong, inappropriate emotional responses to clients
- ◉ Feeling bored or fatigued in the work
- ◉ Irritability or tension
- ◉ Feeling compelled to talk about oneself and one's own issues
- ◉ Inappropriate feelings of failure

◉ Responding to clients in a overprotective or over solicitous manner
◉ Seeing oneself in one's clients
◉ Seeking constant approval from one's clients
◉ Strong attraction or repulsion to one's clients
◉ Recurring themes in one's reactions to clients

Through self awareness and self reflection, students develop an awareness of how their behavior affects clients. Students also need to develop an awareness and knowledge of how to work with clients who always give them what they want (needing to please the homeopath) and clients who never give them what they want (needing to sabotage treatment).

Obstacles to Cure and Resistance

Students must learn of the myriad obstacles to a cure, but this knowledge is only a starting point. They also must develop the capacity to assist clients in removing those obstacles. This entails an awareness of resistance to change and strategies that promote change. Students often embark on attempting to remove obstacles to cure before the client is ready. Prochaska developed a model of the developmental stages of change. These include:

◉ **Pre-contemplation:** Here the client is not even aware that there is a problem. They may be quite resistant or in denial. The homeopath can serve as a model for the possibility of change. The homeopath takes on the role of light bearer.

◉ **Contemplation:** The client faces the possibility of change, yet they're not ready to take action. Much of this is inner work. There can be much ambivalence during this phase, thus it requires patience from the homeopath.

◉ **Preparation:** The client is considering strategies, options and plans. They're actively collecting information. They often have many questions at this point. The homeopath can considerably facilitate this process by encouraging and asking useful questions in return. The homeopath takes on the role of guide.

◉ **Action:** The client is finally ready to act. Here the homeopath takes on the role of coach and cheer leader.

◉ **Maintenance:** Maintaining a change is often more difficult than the initial change itself. The homeopath helps to take on the role of monitor and historian. Assessing where a client is in the process of change is vital to determining how best to work with them.

The Special Ingredients

Every practitioner and teacher has certain skills, knowledge and qualities that are unique to them and that make them good at what they do, like a secret ingredient that a master chef uses in his signature dish. This is part of the magic and mystery that makes homeopathy work. Good clinical teachers don't focus so much on imparting this quality to their students as helping students discover their own unique gifts in order to enhance their practice.

Clinical Assessment

> *A sudden, bold, and unexpected question*
> *doth many times surprise a man and lay him open.*
> —Francis Bacon

Assessment of clinical training is generally more difficult than assessment in didactic work. Students often experience a negative clinical evaluation personally, whereas a negative didactic evaluation is more easily kept at a distance. It's important that supervision creates a safe environment within which to learn, otherwise, in order to get a better clinical evaluation, students may fear sharing their work too deeply, or distort what they do.

Many of the same rules for evaluating apply to both didactic and clinical training (see Chapter Four). However, in clinical training there is more of a need to provide assessments that are descriptive rather than evaluative. Evaluations should be both verbal and written. They should be regularly scheduled and direct. Good evaluations are understandable, flexible, and focus on what can be changed. Most important, students need to discuss the assessment with the clinical teacher.

In conducting verbal evaluations during clinical training, it is important for students to first evaluate their own strengths and weaknesses before their clinical teacher offers feedback. Peer evaluations can be helpful, although students generally are not particularly diplomatic and lack the skills and discipline required to give balanced clinical evaluations.

Students also need to learn how to assess the effectiveness of treatment and their own work. Most students are too critical of their performance. A good clinical teacher helps the student see both their strengths and weaknesses. This comes through self evaluation and the evaluation of one's practice.

Emergencies

We learn geology the morning after the earthquake.
—Emerson

Handling emergencies requires a unique set of qualities, skills, and knowledge. Role confusion often occurs during urgent situations. Any of the four members of the clinical rhombus (student, teacher, administrator or client) may experience a given situation as an emergency. There's a natural inclination for the supervisor or administrator to take over (rescue) during crises, sometimes due to pressure from students and clients. Although rescue by clinical teachers is sometimes necessary, it can prevent a student from learning. Students must learn to be comfortable in crises. However the situation is handled, it is important that role confusion be minimized.

Students may tend to only bring emergency situations to their supervisors. Some students under act and downplay urgent situations, while others treat every situation as an crisis and overreact. It's important for clinical teachers to define an emergency for their students.

Clinical teachers focus on preparing students for emergencies. This can be a challenge, as each crisis is unique. Specific areas should be explored, including medical emergencies (e.g. acute myocardial infarction, acute gastrointestinal bleeding, epiglottis or sepsis) and psychiatric emergencies (e.g. danger to self, danger to others, inability to engage in self care, child abuse or elder abuse). Content should focus on both assessment and self management during crises. Important issues include consultation and referral, personal safety, legally mandated reporting, maintaining calm, using common sense, setting appropriate limits, protecting confidentiality, mobilizing supports and creating concrete plans. Role playing can help. Teachers can also help their students develop an awareness of the importance of crises as opportunities and turning points in treatment.

Models of Clinical Training

Some say that my teaching is nonsense. Others call it lofty but impractical. But to those who have looked inside themselves, this nonsense makes perfect sense. And to those who put it into practice, this loftiness has roots that go deep.
—Lao-Tzu

A variety of models are utilized for clinical training. These can be described as four basic types: clinical observation, training clinics, supervision and consultation. Schon respectively describes the first three types as "follow me" (watching the master), "joint experimentation" (collaborative clinical training model) and "hall of mirrors" (the relationship between student and teacher mirrors the relationship between the client and the student) (Schon 1987). Each of these models has strengths and weaknesses, which include time, financial, and resource constraints. These models also represent a movement from dependency to increasing autonomy in casework. Generally, the less experience in training the student has, the more direct clinical training they'll require.

Students may be more adapted and suited to one model over another. However, a training program does best when it uses a diversity of clinical training models and approaches. By using a diversity of methods, students are ensured of having the opportunity to work with the model that fits them the best. Also, different supervisors have differing sets of skills and knowledge that they can impart to students.

A central challenge in clinical training is designing a model that gives the student maximum opportunity to participate in the clinical process, while not warping the homeopathic interview. For example, many clients feel uncomfortable with having observers in the consulting room and feel that it makes it difficult for them to give a good case. Adapting the models to giving needed support for each student while encouraging increasing autonomy and self growth is a challenge in clinical training.

Clinical Observation

> *He who hopes to learn the fine art of the game of chess from books will soon discover that only the opening and closing moves of the game admit of exhaustive systematic description, and that the endless variety of the moves which develop from the opening defies description; the gap left in the instructions can only be filled in by the zealous study of games fought out by master hands.*
> —Sigmund Freud

Clinical observation entails watching a master homeopath at work. This time-honored method of teaching a craft or vocation involves apprentices matching themselves with a master teacher and copying their methods in training. This was the predominant form of teaching before schools were formed and was traditional in homeopathy as well.

Clinical observation is based on modeling. This is an effective ways for educators to show students the artistry involved in homeopathic work. Observation is essential, but not sufficient in itself to guarantee mastery.

There are a variety of forms that observation may take. Many homeopathic schools have students watch a master teacher taking either live cases or video cases. An advantage of video cases is that it is possible to present cases of increasing complexity, even before the student sees their first live case. Another variant is having students bring in their failed cases (live or video) for teachers to observe and analyze in front of a class, although students often become bored and resistant watching other students' cases. Following the observation period, there is generally a discussion and analysis of what has been observed. This is the method around which most homeopathic seminars are currently constructed. This also is a common format for more advanced homeopathic study groups. It is important that students who observe watch not just the content of what occurs but the process as well.

The problem with this model is that it does not promote autonomy. Students whose clinical training consists of observation, often have great difficulty translating what they have observed into practice. Another central problem is that this model can create carbon copies of the master homeopath. Clinical observation interferes with the student's individual expression and style. Adult learners learn better by doing than observing. Finally, although this method is very useful in learning a craft or trade, homeopathy ultimately is more than that, as homeopaths are more than skilled experts.

Training Clinics and Problem-Based Learning Approaches

> *So far, with the single exception of the Foundation work,*
> *the teaching of homeopathy in this country is a matter of*
> *individual contacts, for while modern medical education*
> *(even in the homeopathic colleges) has sought to eliminate*
> *preceptorships, they have offered no substitute, and homeopathy, the method of prescribing for the individual, is best*
> *taught by individual attentions, in small groups.*
> —H. A. Roberts

This model focuses on creating a small, group process clinical environment, typically one teacher with 4-8 students. The work here is far more collaborative. Often one student takes the case with the clinical teacher observing and assisting the student. The other students either observe directly or by closed-circuit television. They have opportunities to provide input and ask questions during the session directly, through written questions or through an audio transceiver that the teacher/student carries. Another useful technique is to video the student who is taking the case, for later review and analysis. Following the case-taking session, the case is discussed and analyzed as a group. Training clinics typically last from one to two years.

The strength of this approach is that it provides the student more autonomy and an opportunity to put their skills directly into practice. Clinical teachers can assist the student at a variable level, depending on the student's skill level and experience. For the student, a training clinic can be an opportunity to experiment, try new things or focus in on a particular aspect of the case-taking process. They know that the clinical teacher will be there, if needed to get the case back on track. Another benefit is that the other students act like a Greek chorus. They can considerably facilitate the accuracy and depth of case taking and analysis. This model gives the clinical teacher an opportunity to observe the work of the student first hand and to see the rapport and interactions between student and client, which is not as possible with the other models. It is important that the number of students in the clinic be limited. A small group creates an intimate environment that's conducive to individualized learning and effective group process. The team-building process also creates vital skills for a homeopath's later career.

The problem with this model is that although it promotes more autonomy than clinical observation, students still have a safety net which they can overly rely on, making a difficult transition into individual practice. Another issue revolves around levels of training. For this model to work, it is critical that students are at a similar level of training. One way around this problem is to create various levels of training clinics. Logistically, this type of model is difficult to set up and maintain. It requires more administrative involvement, careful orchestration and planning. Handling follow-ups is particularly problematic. Clients may balk at this type of environment, feeling that they won't receive the individual attention they need.

Supervision

> *I studied general medicine from a homeopathic standpoint*
> *in the college; but I really learned homeopathy*
> *from Dr. Hering in the back office of his.*
> —Student of Hering

Supervision is a complex process between student and supervisor. It is one of the most effective tools in developing clinical practice (Kreisberg 2000). It is much more than transmitting skills. In the clinical work, what is deepest in the homeopathic student touches what is deepest in the supervisor. Every student will assume the roles of supervisor and supervisee on the homeopathic journey.

Although most medical professions require considerable supervision hours, in practice, students are often left to assimilate clinical work on their own or occasionally watch the master teacher. The quality of clinical training in most medical programs is quite poor. The formal supervision process is one that has predominantly descended from psychological theory and models in which the student conducts the case on their own, then brings it to their supervisor for review and analysis. This may take the form of a verbal presentation, written case notes and/or video. The supervisor takes on responsibility for the work of the supervisee. Mentorship is often an important part of homeopathic supervision (see Chapter Four).

When to Become a Supervisor

What thou has inherited from thy fathers,
earn it, to make it thine own.
—Goethe

When is the homeopath ready to take on the role of supervisor? The issue is similar to the question of "when to become a teacher," although many teachers feel more comfortable teaching in formats other than supervision. Good supervision can be one of the most difficult and challenging forms of teaching. Generally a homeopath should have many years of experience before embarking on the supervision process. Supervision skills do not develop automatically and only come through experience and careful study. Unfortunately, students are often called on to take a supervision role soon after finishing training, which can create premature expert's status.

Goals of Supervision

Clinical supervision should be designed to prepare a student for independent and autonomous practice. It creates an environment where a student can comfortably take on increasing responsibility. Supervision is also not a disguised or indirect form of doing homeopathy. The supervisor must possess the humility to allow the student to experience every supervisory suggestion as permission for experimentation rather than orders they must execute. The supervisor encourages a natural skepticism in the student. They are comfortable with their students' autonomy.

The primary task of good supervision is to enhance the knowledge and skills of the student. A secondary task is to maintain quality clinical work. Sometimes these goals conflict. Supervision is not so much concerned with finding the "right remedy." If a student brings a poorly taken case to supervision, there is little a supervisor can do in selecting a good remedy. However, supervisors can always work with students to improve their case-taking, case-analysis and case-management skills.

Role of the Supervisor

Supervisors can be tempted to blur the boundaries in clinical training, but it's critical to guard against this. Boundary issues can take a variety of forms. The supervisor may try to take over treatment and become the homeopath, especially in crises. Beginning supervisors who feel more comfortable with the role of homeopathic practioner may struggle with this. Some students want to replace supervision with treatment. In this situation the supervisee becomes more of an extension of the supervisor than a learner. Supervisors must also be free of the need to develop followers and avoid surrounding themselves with dependent admirers. This is especially a danger if the supervisor has a counseling background or is already treating the supervisee homeopathically. The supervisory relationship is prolonged and intense for both teacher and student. Supervisors must be clear about power differential in supervision and never exploit supervisees sexually, financially or emotionally (Heaton 1998).

The supervisor can also blur the boundary with homeopathic treatment in either a case-taking role or counseling role. In some students this can create patterns of dependency and stir up imitative needs. It is generally advisable for the supervisor and homeopath of the student to be separate individuals, although this can be a problem in small training programs. The focus should be on learning rather than treatment.

Setting Up Supervision

It is important when embarking on supervision that there is a contract between the student and supervisor. This is similar to establishing a mentorship relationship, although it has some differences (see Chapter Four). Much of the initial work is concerned with establishing a working relationship and developing comfort with each others styles.

When supervisors first begin, they often avoid placing many rules on their supervisees. They are overly cautious in exercising their teaching function, fear criticism and fear that the student might interpret comments as negative or hostile.

A central issue to explore is what to tell the client concerning the supervision of the student. This can create anxiety for the student. It is important that this be discussed from the outset so that the student achieves clarity about how to handle this issue.

Students generally start from previous experience in supervision. Most students have had some previous experiences with supervision and have developed a series of expectations about the supervisory process. It is very helpful for the supervisor to explore these experiences and expectations at the beginning of supervision.

There are some crucial questions that a supervisor must ask:

- Is the supervisory case appropriate?
- Does the supervisee have adequate preparation?
- Can the supervisor and supervisee work together adequately?

Other central issues include:

- Supervisor availability
- Discussion of boundaries, confidentiality issues and ethics
- Exploration of evaluations (if required)
- Creation of shared goals
- Discussion of when, if ever, to bring clients in to be seen by the supervisor
- Handling disagreements
- Handling emergencies
- Honoring each other's expertise and experience
- When and how to end supervision

The supervisor must initially assess the level of training and experience of the supervisee. There should be a discussion of what clients are appropriate for the student's current level of training. Each supervisee is unique and the supervisor will need to set up the supervision process to fit each student. Each student also represents a distinct learning opportunity for the supervisor.

Ongoing Issues

Supervisors help students plan the course of their clients' treatment. They jump start students' thinking, providing new ideas and creative solutions when they're stuck. This includes helping to clarify their students' understanding of a case's essence. They help students manage their counter transference and manage ethical dilemmas.

Good supervisors focus on the skills and successes of the supervisee, as well as pointing out mistakes in treatment. The practice of homeopathy can be a discouraging process and students need much support. Supervisors provide support in the often lonely process of becoming a homeopath. When errors are pointed out, it is crucial that the supervisor give clear descriptions of what and how it could have been done differently.

Another task in supervision is to encourage independent thinking and self reflection. The supervisor should help the student learn to give themselves feedback. The issue of disagreements is often troublesome for the student. They may either never disagree or consistently disagree with the supervisor. This is complicated because the student often knows the client much better than the supervisor, although the supervisor has more experience. The key is to learn to work collaboratively and to find ways of managing disagreements without being autocratic. It is helpful for the supervisor to acknowledge their own mistakes in practice. However, it's imperative to keep in mind who has ultimate responsibility for the case.

Students often over-focus on their new cases that they bring to supervision. A supervisor should periodically review the student's entire case load. Good supervision should be carefully balanced between new cases, practice management and mentorship.

Attention should also be paid to termination of treatment and evaluation of the students' complete practice.

It is important to not let students overly focus on a particular problem case. Beginning students often neglect much of their practice while they concentrate on problem cases. Lastly, students often attempt to cram too much into supervision, without adequate time for reflection and careful working through of case material. The supervisor must set limits in order to pace sessions.

Styles of Supervision

Most supervisors approach supervision as they do parenting. They repeat what was done to them. They draw on what they like and try to avoid what they didn't like from their own experience.

There are many differing styles of supervision, all of which are effective. It's important for each supervisor to find their own unique style. At the same time, there needs to be enough flexibility to work with and match differing styles of various supervisees. When the styles of supervisor and supervisee are too disparate, it can create ideological confusion.

A supervisor should not supervise a student if they have any doubts they can work well with that student. It's usually best to refer such a student to a different supervisor. The supervisor and supervisee must share the same basic understanding or principles of treatment for the work to be effective.

Administrative Issues

It is a supervisor's responsibility to keep track of all requirements and to see that all legal mandates have been met. Supervisors can find themselves at odds with administrators of clinical training programs. It is very helpful for supervisors (and other clinical faculty) to meet in a group setting for mutual support. Clinical faculty can struggle with feeling that they lack adequate support, have too many supervisees or lack adequate training. It's not only important for students to develop community, but also for teachers and supervisors.

Supervision as a Mirror

Supervision is a laboratory in which the characteristic problems of the student are replayed in supervision. There is a direct parallel between what goes on in the treatment room and what goes on in the supervisory room. Sometimes a bottleneck in a case can only be cleared up by a parallel process in supervision. In this way, supervision serves as a mirror for the student.

Students inevitably elicit and aggravate a supervisor's teaching issues. Ultimately, the learning problems of the student interact with the teaching problems of the supervisor, creating confusion. Much of this can come out in the dreams of both the supervisor and supervisee about the supervision process. In this way, students can serve as a mirror for their supervisor.

Students sometimes project their issues onto their supervisor. A supervisor can be seen as both a powerful ego ideal and a helper on whom they depend, or they may be seen as a punitive authoritarian. Such projection can be a stumbling block to learning.

Students who project idealizing values onto their teacher often become dependent on them and unable to establish their identity. Students who project authoritarian values onto teachers often react with anger which interferes with learning.

Supervisors need to be aware of these issues and deflect either idealization or devaluation, away from the real work of supervision. When supervision is a required part of training, supervisors need to be prepared to work with students who doubt the value of supervision. They also need to be aware of their own counter transference reactions in this process.

Another common problem for supervisees is over-identification with their clients. They may have difficulty in treating clients whom they resonate with or who seem either too similar or opposite to their nature. Good supervisors help their supervisees to perceive these needs and issues within themselves. They help their students to see their blind spots.

Notes

It is very helpful for students to provide a copy of their case notes or case videos to the supervisor before the supervisory session. This helps the supervisor review the case prior to the session and enable more effective use of supervisory time.

Supervisors should also keep some type of written record of their sessions. Not only does this serve to refresh the supervisor's memory regarding the case, but also helps to protect the supervisor from a medical/legal perspective. The file should contain the supervisory agreement or contract, dates of supervision, notes regarding the supervisory process and notes on specific clients. Records should be maintained for at least seven years.

Peer Supervision

Peer supervision can also be very effective. Students often feel more comfortable sharing their deepest fears and slip-ups with their peers. It is very important that the peer supervisor be someone at the same level of training and that there is considerable comfort between each other. In addition, the peer must be willing to view the student's work critically or learning will not occur. Another form that this can take is for each peer to see the difficult cases of the other homeopath in consultation. Peer supervision can be a very powerful experience and many students describe this experience as one of the most important aspects of their training.

Group Supervision

Group supervision is a model that some practitioners move into once they are more well established in their practices (Heaton 1998). Most often these groups are leaderless or the leadership rotates meeting by meeting. Generally the group size is kept small to encourage adequate participation. Members of the group agree on basic responsibilities of being a member, inclusion requirements, confidentiality, case or topic discussion formats, time limits and guidelines for constructive feedback. As with individual supervision, it is crucial that members have approximately the same level of experience. Group supervision is not as intimate as individual supervision, but it provides a forum for voicing a variety of opinions and reactions to presented material. A well constructed group supervision environment can be tremendously supportive and enriching for its participants.

Research Supervision

Another aspect of supervision is research supervision. This requires a different scope of knowledge than clinical supervision, but the requisite supervisory attitudes and skills are identical. Research supervision is a critical part of programmatic student theses and research projects. Provings also represent an opportunity for research supervision.

When to End Supervision

Supervision is complete when a student has learned the skill and knowledge sets necessary to practice effectively. There is always more to learn. The goal should be to become good enough and comfortable with one's professional role. The end of supervision should be a natural process. Ultimately, the student moves into the role of a professional colleague. This usually takes two years of regular supervision, though, in some instances, one year is sufficient.

Consultation

The light that a man receiveth by counsel from another is drier and purer than that which cometh from his own understanding and judgment, which is ever infused and drenched in his affections and customs.
—Francis Bacon

The last model is that of consultation. Here the roles are far more collegial. Neither participant takes on responsibility for the case material of the other individual and the process is far more informal. Consultation is a good way to run a case by another homeopath in order to get some quick feedback.

Clinical training is a vital, but much neglected aspect of homeopathic education. If well designed, it can provide and nurture skills, attitudes, and ethics necessary for effective cast taking, case analysis, and case management. It also provides a vital bridge between didactic training and eventual practice.

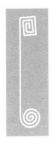

Chapter Six

Public Speaking:
Teaching from the Heart

The Importance of Public Speaking in Homeopathy

If you have knowledge, let others light their candles at it.
—Margaret Fuller

The explosion of interest in alternative medicine makes it increasingly important to present homeopathy to the world. This brings with it the potential to enter a new, golden age of homeopathy. Small things that individuals do now may have a large impact on the future of homeopathy.

This represents both a responsibility and duty for all homeopathic practitioners and teachers. Public speaking and introductory talks are often the public's first contact with the field and may either provide an opening or turn them off to the subject. Public speaking is not to be done lightly. It's common for practitioners to provide introductory talks at the beginning of their careers but neglect this service as they mature. However, even the most seasoned homeopathic practitioner can learn much from continuing to give introductory talks throughout their career.

Getting Started in Public Speaking

He who risks nothing need hope for nothing.
—Freidrich Schiller

Good public speaking differs substantially from good teaching. Different skills and talents are called upon. Speaking is addressed to a group consciousness, while teaching is more individualized. Many good speakers make poor teachers and vice versa. Educators often find speaking easier than teaching, thus public oration is a good way for the homeopathic professional to move into the teaching field. This is especially true of introductory talks.

When is someone ready to begin public speaking in homeopathy? This varies from practitioner to practitioner. Some wait until late in their careers, while others begin early in their training. One must begin public speaking and teaching from where one is. Ultimately, the key lies in having greater knowledge than one's audience and having confidence as a public speaker.

When I was first asked to give an introductory talk in homeopathy, I felt "there's no way that I'm ready." It took me some time to practice and become prepared. I had to be willing to "put myself out there," and risk making a fool of myself. I found that I felt much more alive after that first talk, and it brought me deeper into the heart of homeopathy.

Practice, Practice, Practice

Constant practice is a key to gaining confidence. Those who only speak occasionally never have opportunities to develop their skills. Although it may provoke anxiety, one must accept opportunities to speak. The greater the diversity in venues and audiences, the more helpful.

Self Assessment

Self assessment is another important aspect. The following questions should be considered:

◎ What has been my experience of homeopathic speakers and introductory talks in the past?

◎ What has been my experience of public speakers in the past?

◎ What has been the best public speech that I have heard? What made it especially good?

◎ What has been the worst public speech that I have heard? What made it especially poor?

◎ What has been my own experience in public speaking? What are my strengths and weaknesses? Where do I most need to improve?

Overcoming Anxiety

The human brain is a wonderful thing.
It operates from the moment you're born until the first time
you get up to make a speech.
—Burt Decker

Overcoming anxiety is the first task for many speakers. Stage fright is the predominant issue that participants raise in workshops on public speaking. This usually stems from heightened sensitivity, a fear of poor performance and a fear of humiliation. Some are more comfortable lecturing or mentoring as a consequence. Many speakers have had negative experiences in the past that they must overcome.

Research studies show that there is an optimal level of anxiety for performance. Levels of anxiety that are either too high or too low cause a decline in performance. The goal is not to rid oneself of all anxiety but to learn to effectively manage and channel the anxiety into the presentation. The following strategies can be helpful in coping with fear:

You Are Not Alone

The fear of public speaking is the most common fear in the world today, followed by heights, insects, financial problems, deep water, sickness, death, flying, loneliness and dogs, in that order (Wallechinsky 1977). It is helpful to a student to recognize that they're not alone. Audiences are there to hear one succeed. This is especially true of homeopathic audiences, who are often very enthusiastic about the subject and can provide much support. Having a partner, friend or someone directly supportive in the audience can be helpful.

Preparation

The most important key to overcoming anxiety is adequate preparation. It is crucial to give oneself adequate time to prepare. In particular, the first few minutes are often where the greatest anxiety occurs. Practicing and preparing the introductory segment can help to alleviate this. Breathing is another important aspect of preparation. Consciously reminding oneself to breathe can significantly reduce anxiety.

Focus on Homeopathy

Homeopathy is a "great" subject. It is much more than "who" and "what" one is. When speakers immerse themselves in homeopathy, it has a way of taking over and leading the talk. It's important to focus on the subject rather than on oneself during the delivery.

Appearing Confident

Everyone appears much more confident than they feel. It's common for a speaker to be quite nervous during a presentation, with an audience having no awareness of this anxiety. Even well known performers Johnny Carson, Carol Burnett, Merv Griffin, Joan Rivers, Liza Minnelli and Sidney Poitier admit to significant performance anxiety.

Confidence comes with experience. The more one practices public speaking, the better one becomes. Joining organizations that facilitate public speaking such as Toastmasters (http://www.toastmasters.com) can be very helpful.

Projecting confidence is also important. It's possible to shape an audience's perceptions of a speaker by the way one dresses, stands, and projects their voice. An important area to cultivate is the walk to and from the stage, in order to begin one's talk and leave one's talk with confidence. Choosing clothes carefully can help a presenter feel more confident. Those who feel young and inexperienced can be helped by dressing up. Those who want to connect intimately with an audience and meet them where they are, might find dressing down to be helpful.

It's critical to learn to project one's voice. Anxious speakers tend to begin with confidence and then trail off to a whisper. Lastly, visualizing a successful completion of the talk can assist one in feeling more confident.

Authenticity	Talking about nervousness and sharing it with others can be helpful. This creates a feeling of authenticity in a talk, although parading insecurity and lack of confidence often backfires. Speakers should own up to their mistakes in presentations. Another strategy is to turn a mistake into an advantage through humor. "Let me try that again in English."
Channeling Nervous Energy	It is vital that the anxiety have an outlet. Some speakers can successfully channel their anxiety into their talks. They have the capacity to transmute this anxiety into movement, vocalizations and dramatic gestures. Be careful not to fidget, shuffle papers or repetitively

play with the microphone or its cord during the presentation. Remembering to breathe deeply can help to cut this nervous energy and promote relaxation.

Taking a Dose of Gelsemium Some speakers routinely take a dose of Gelsemium before a major presentation. In the allopathic community this often takes the form of using the drug Inderal (Propranolol). However there are many remedies that can be effective in stage fright. It's much more effective to find a constitutional remedy that helps the individual cope with their stage fright.

As a child I played the piano and performed at recitals many times per year. I was often so paralyzed with anxiety that I forgot the piece of music that I had memorized. My hands and feet would shake so much that I had difficulty finding the right keys and keeping my feet on the pedals. Later with college performance, I found that Calcium could be quite helpful in reducing the tremors associated with anxiety, although not touching the emotional component of fear.

Preparation

Sometimes when we have to speak suddenly we come
closer to the truth than when we have time to think.
—Madeline L'Engle

Good preparation is crucial to public speaking. Those who "wing it" seldom give good presentations. Life brings requests for unexpected speeches and presentations. However, even with these, it is generally possible to prepare for a few minutes before the presentation. These moments can be crucial in developing a structure, key points and goal for the presentation (Krannich 1998). If the speaker is asked to speak often, it is helpful to have a few "canned" presentations in reserve for urgent calls to fill in.

The most critical step in planning talks is setting goals, which imbue a talk with focus and clarity. Speeches can be good (enjoyable to listen to and able to capture the hearts of an audience) or they can be effective (creating learning and change). The best speakers are able to accomplish both, although the skills required are different. Classically, three goals of public speaking have included informing (e.g. explaining what homeopathy is), convincing (e.g. convincing someone to become a homeopathic patient) and actuating (e.g. helping someone to take the next step on their homeopathic journey).

Increasingly, objectives are being required prior to presentations. Often this is a requirement for programs to offer continuing education credits. For many teachers, the writing of objectives can be intimidating. However, objectives can help to focus the talk and inform students of what they really need to know. They also help to determine visual aids. The writing of good objectives should include an action or activity, the requirements if any, the degree of accomplishment expected and the standard for which the expected activity will be accomplished. An example is the following: "The practitioner will learn how and when to effectively consult with others to reduce the risk of disciplinary complaints and demonstrate compliance with the appropriate standard of care."

A talk should be practiced. It can be gone over in one's head, although practicing aloud is more effective. Taping (audio or video) can be a powerful method to critique one's skills in delivery, including pace and inflection. Timing the speech is also important to ensure that you cover all of the main points in the allotted time. At this stage, attention must be paid to proper pronunciation. It is possible to practice too much. Room should be left for improvisation and spontaneity. It is important to anticipate problems. Everyone has experienced homeopathic speakers who were paralyzed and unprepared when they experienced a technical breakdown during their talk. It is best to have a contingency plan, especially if one is relying on equipment. If you will be introduced, it is helpful to give the master of ceremonies key points to include in their introduction.

The beginning and ending of a talk demand the most preparation. These are the points where the audience is most likely to connect with a speaker and remember what they say.

Handouts are a common challenge. Audiences often expect such materials and are critical of speakers who don't provide them. Studies have proven the optimum length for handouts is neither too detailed, nor too simplified. Good handouts usually point the way to further information rather than trying to exhaustively cover all the material themselves.

Another important step in public speaking is assessing an audience. The talk must be tailored to their needs. It is helpful to determine what is appropriate to listeners' understanding and acceptance levels. Key questions include the following:

◎ What is the relative size of the audience? This affects the intimacy level of the talk.

◉ What do they already know about homeopathy? A diverse audience is often more difficult to speak with, as the speaker must pitch the talk to all levels of the knowledge. This can require splitting of the presentation into more advanced and introductory sections.

◉ What is their attitude toward you? What do they know about you? For example, there may be negative preconceptions toward the speaker as either a physician or a non-physician.

◉ What is their attitude toward the subject? It is important to know if the audience is antagonistic so that the speaker can spend more time building bridges.

◉ What are their occupations, economic backgrounds, educational level, culture, male-female ratio, and age? This is especially important in determining case material and examples that the audience can relate to.

◉ Do listeners have a choice in attending? Are they only there to obtain credits? It is much more difficult to speak to an audience who is required to be present.

◉ What time of day will the talk occur? Whom do you follow and who comes after you? Presentations that occur at the end of the day and after lunch must be more dynamic. Speakers that start programs off often have more difficulty catching the audience's attention as participants are often tired from travel and their attention is not fully focused.

◉ What is the purpose of the meeting or conference? Is this stated or implicit? Participants can become angry when a presentation does not fit with the stated goals for the conference.

It is also important to assess the facilities where the talk will occur. This generally includes a visual check before the talk to determine if changes should be made, in time to allow for such changes. It is best not to rely on the commitment of conference or talk organizers to have such issues resolved. Conference leaders are often too busy during a conference to attend to problematical details that arise. Key questions include:

◉ What are the size and layout of the room?

◉ What equipment is available for voice projection? Is it operational?

◉ Is a lectern available that meets the presenter's needs?

◉ How is the lighting?

◎ Are there sufficient electrical outlets?

◎ Is the required audiovisual equipment operational?

◎ What is the arrangement of the seating? Is it theater style or circular? Can it be changed?

◎ How is the temperature? Is it comfortable?

Preparation can immeasurably improve the quality and success of a talk. A wise speaker takes the time to prepare.

Anatomy of Talks

> *If human beings don't keep exercising their lips, he thought, their mouths probably seize up. After a few months consideration and observation he abandoned this theory in favor of a new one. If they don't keep on exercising their lips, he thought, their brains start working.*
> —Douglas Adams

Talks are generally divided into four sections. These include the introduction (15 percent of the talk), the body or discussion (60 percent of the talk), the conclusion (10 percent) and questions and answers (15 percent of the talk). The relative percentages vary greatly on the nature of the presentation and the audience. For example, in introductory presentations, the question and answer section must be longer, as listeners often come with very specific questions in their minds.

Title

It's been said that if a talk is like a foot, then its title is like a shoe. It must be slightly larger than the talk. Creating a good title is an art. Good titles both explain the nature of the talk and convey an emotional appeal. Much of the title is about advertising. It is what draws people in. However, the title also must be authentic. Audiences can become upset when they come to a talk which they felt advertised one thing, but delivered another.

Body

Preparation should begin with the main body of the talk. The introduction and conclusion should only be added once this is complete. Generally, a speaker begins with whom they are and what they already know. If one is open, their life experiences can assist them with the talk subject.

Ideas should be organized for easy understanding, either in spatial order, sequential order, or by category. Key points must be repeated in a variety of contexts, using a variety of methods.

It is important to remember that an audience reflects a diversity of learning styles. Effective communication requires a diversity in both speaking style and presentation. For example, some learners are visually oriented, some are auditory oriented and others are kinesthetically oriented.

A variety of supporting materials are useful. These help to add interest, make what is said more memorable, clarify what one is saying, and prove the validity and credibility of the presentation.

Quotations	Quotations add authority when utilized in the body of a talk. Speakers who lecture frequently can build up a collection of stories and quotations to use.
Stories	Stories add human interest. They help the listener make a more personal connection to the material being presented.
Statistics	Statistics help to clarify and allow a presenter to communicate more creditably and precisely.
Defining Terms	Depending on an audience's level of understanding, it's important to define terminology within the body of a talk. This is especially true of introductory talks, although even more sophisticated audiences often have misconceptions about the meaning of specific homeopathic terminology. Handouts can be helpful in this regard.
Avoiding Jargon	Jargon and acronyms can be very annoying to an audience unless they've been adequately defined.
Speaking Level	Speakers who speak to the lowest common denominator end up boring their audience. Those who speak to the highest level can be so challenging that they lose or alienate much of their audience. Studies suggest that speaking at a level slightly above the median seems to work best (Krannich 1998). It can be hard at times to determine this median. It's often recommended to leave an audience wanting more.

Audiovisual Aids   These can include videos, transparencies, slides, photographs, specimens of a remedy, flip chart and writing on a marker board. The wrong visual aid can be a detriment to a talk. Audiovisual aids can be over utilized. Use these only when referring to them and make them of sufficient size to be clearly visible. Talk to your audience and not to the visual aid. Be careful about being too dependent on them, should the equipment fail.

Creation of Notes   Gather information logically. Focus on ideas and not exact phrases. Notes should be sufficient only to trigger the presenter's thinking at a glance, thus permitting them to look at the audience while speaking. Leave double spacing between the ideas so that information can be inserted at the last minute. Accentuate things in color that tend to be forgotten or need to be emphasized. Note cards are best if there's no podium, while paper materials work well with a podium. Be sure to number your pages and cards in case they get shuffled, or bind them together.

Attacking Others   Some speakers belittle or attack other practitioners, teachers and fields of healing. This can be very destructive to the homeopathic community. The audience typically reacts strongly to these comments, creating polarization. It is best to stay positive.

Proving the   As with teaching, those who speak often capture the
Subject   energy of their subjects. This is especially true of materia medica presentations where it is not uncommon for speakers to do a mini proving. In this process, they experience the energy of the remedy as they prepare for their talk. When the speaker is aware and this energy is harnessed, it can be helpful in preparing the talk and providing added material.

Assess the nature of your audience before you begin. With a potentially hostile audience, common ground must be established first and only then can the presenter build on that common understanding.

Introduction

It is critical for the speaker to believe in their message. They must be passionate. A speaker must be believed to be heard by an audience. This requires authenticity and speaking from the heart.

Credibility must be established at the outset. It has been said that "You never get a second chance to make a first impression." This can be a problem for Licensed Homeopathic Practitioners with a non-professional audience who mistrust the allopathic profession. It can also be a problem for Non-Licensed Homeopathic Practitioners with a professional audience who may perceive that the presenter lacks the knowledge and skills to become a good homeopath. A good introduction can immeasurably help in establishing credibility. A speaker can also weave in credibility enhancers without seeming too pretentious. Some speakers compliment their audiences, although this can be seen as manipulative.

A strong beginning to a presentation sets the tone, fires the imagination and captures the attention of the audience. Listeners typically only hear about 25% of what is said. The average length of attention in listening to a talk is approximately 20 minutes. What is retained the most in a speech is the introduction and conclusion. Studies also indicate that after 48 hours, most of us only remember 10% of what we heard (Decker 1991).

It is important not to open too aggressively. Audience members will often shut down if approached too strongly. There comes a certain point in a talk where one can feel the individuals hearts in the audience open to homeopathy. Much of the work initially is concerned with opening these hearts.

Once the listener's attention has been captured, then the task of the presenter is to orient the audience and build rapport. The speaker sets the goals of the speech and helps the audience understand what the payoffs are to be.

There are a variety of useful strategies that can be employed in introductions. These include:

Telling a Story   This is especially important in introductory presentations where telling one's own story about entering homeopathy can be very helpful. The story should provide a vivid illustration and fire the imaginations of listeners. It is easy to forget stories that may be pivotal during a presentation unless key words are placed in the notes to trigger the memory.

Using Humor	Humor is the most common strategy in beginning a talk. Humor can open the heart and help to make an audience more receptive. Sometimes this is overdone. Humor should only be used if it relates to the focus of the speech and is presented authentically.
Quotations	Quotations at the beginning of a speech are used for impact and inspiration. They capture listeners' attention. When used in the body of the speech, quotations are more often for clarification and increasing the depth of understanding.
Emphasis	Emphasizing the importance of the subject can help to draw listeners in and add legitimacy to what the speaker is trying to say. This can be accomplished by stating something startling that captures listeners' attention. Speakers can also emphasize the importance of the occasion on which they are speaking.
Rhetorical Questions	Asking a question is a time-honored technique to begin a talk. It is often useful to keep the listener in suspense after the question is posed. Questions can also be followed by a period of self analysis and contemplation.
Activities	Getting started with an audience participation activity can help to break the ice. It also can be a method for the speaker to quickly assess the audiences' knowledge level and skill base.
Gimmicks	There are a variety of gimmicks that are utilized in beginning talks. These are risky—they can either be quite successful or backfire. Ultimately what's most important is not a specific technique or gimmick, but speaking from the heart and being authentically oneself.

Conclusion

The end is as important as the beginning. Many speakers work hard on the body of their talk and the introduction, but end weakly. Often they don't have an ending, simply moving from the body of their talk to questions. Studies have shown that the endings are what listeners most remember from a talk.

The ending of the speech, which is often announced in some way, should be planned. It's helpful to verbally mark the move from the body of the talk to its ending. Speakers commonly summarize and repeat their main points, although this is generally insufficient. Strategies that are useful at the beginning of a talk, such as telling stories, using humor, quotations, emphasis and rhetorical questions can be useful here as well. The speaker must capture listeners' attention by striking a vivid image.

Endings are an opportunity to move deeper into the heart of the subject and touch the hearts of the audience. The conclusion is an opportunity to connect the subject to a larger perspective. The ending may also connect to the future. Good speakers always point to what's next on their listener's journey.

Lastly, the ending can be a call to action. This is a direct challenge, to not only listen and absorb the material, but to change one's actions and behavior.

Questions

What separates good speakers from average ones are their capacities to get the audience participating and involved. One of the best ways to do this is through questions that the speaker asks the audience. There are many types of questions, including rhetorical ("What is homeopathy?"), fact-based ("Why did you study homeopathy?"), opinion-based ("Why should someone study homeopathy?"), comparison-based ("How does homeopathy compare to other forms of alternative medicine?") and case-history-based ("What about this case illustrates homeopathic principles?"). Mixing up the type and style of questioning is quite helpful in keeping a talk moving and alive.

For some speakers, questions and answers can be the most challenging part of their presentation, while for others this represents an important opportunity to connect with their audience. Here again, it is useful to anticipate and be prepared to answer both common and difficult questions (examples in introductory presentations are listed below). Questions that are too complex or those that would move the discussion away from the center of the talk, can be postponed until after the presentation. These questions can also be re-framed by saying "I don't know about that, but this is what I do know..."

It is important for the presenter not to be defensive. They must have a positive attitude toward their questioners. This involves skills in dealing with vague questions. Being unsure what they want to ask, students often pose vague questions. The presenter must be able to make sense of the question and give it meaning. For irrelevant questions, presenters must find ways of honoring the questioner without taking up too much time. It is important to find value in whatever the student has to offer and to validate them. Lastly, it is vital that the presenter understand the question. It is often important to repeat the question to be sure that the speaker accurately understands the question, before trying to answer it.

The audience needs time to generate questions. The speaker should give them time to respond. There's a natural pause after a talk is complete when an audience is digesting what's been said. If the audience doesn't have any questions, it can be helpful to have a few questions prepared to stimulate the discussion, eg. "Audiences often ask me...?" Many speakers also keep a second closing or ending in reserve. The first they give after the body of their talk and the second after the questions and answers.

Style

Just as our bread, mixed and baked, packaged and sold
without benefit of accident or human frailty,
is uniformly good and uniformly tasteless,
so will our speech become one speech.
—John Steinbeck

There are three styles of speech presentation: extemporaneous, read and memorized. Extemporaneous is by far the most common style. Here the speaker may use prepared notes to jog the memory, but each presentation is unique. A read speech is appropriate for more formal presentations. It is useful when the exact wording is critically important or when a specific paper is being presented. Memorized speeches are more commonly used in the political arena.

What's most important about style is that it's uniquely yours. A speaker must be authentic. Speakers who try to copy others' styles are seldom successful. One must be authentic to be believed by their audience.

Successful speakers speak from their hearts and not just from their minds. They present all of themselves in their speeches. The speaker must make an emotional connection with their audience for listeners to change their behavior. People buy on emotion and justify with facts, and much of this is decided on unconscious levels (Becker 1991).

Good speakers are dynamic and convey enthusiasm. They convey their love and passion for homeopathy by mobilizing feelings and firing the imaginations of listeners. Students forgive almost anything in a speaker except lack of enthusiasm. Speakers convey enthusiasm by involving their audience and maintaining good eye contact with them. Charisma is more important in speaking than in teaching.

Delivery

Whether Eisenhower was speaking to ten people or two thousand people,
it always seemed to me that he was talking to one individual.
—Burt Decker

A diversity of skills are required for a good delivery of a presentation. It is of highest importance for a speaker to make a connection with everyone in their audience. By connecting with listeners, each of their listeners feels attended to. They do this by seeing an audience as individuals and talking with the audience rather than to them, which requires the capacity to work with the group consciousness.

An important step in facilitating delivery is audio taping and video-taping. Much can be learned from watching and listening to oneself speak. This can be traumatic for some—most individuals hate to watch themselves. Feedback from impartial listeners is also quite useful.

The skills involved in delivery include the following:

Quality

It is important to speak clearly and distinctly. Intonation should be varied. It's helpful to practice loosening up one's facial expression if it tends to be wooden.

Rate

Speakers who speak too quickly are hard to follow. Those who speak too slowly are often experienced as boring. Pace should be varied over time. Pausing at crucial moments in the speech can help to build the energy of the presentation. The rate of speech is about 175 words per minute, whereas the rate of hearing is about 310. Consequently, students naturally check in and out during a presentation. This inattention is often called leap frogging and can be misinterpreted by a speaker or teacher.

Volume

Do not rely on the microphone. It is not unusual for audio equipment to break down. Learn to project your voice. Remember to turn your head if you cough or sneeze. Turn off the microphone immediately after the presentation to avoid sharing private comments with the larger audience.

Pauses

Pauses should be built in to the talk. It is important to give the audience time to integrate what has been said and reflect upon it. Many speakers are afraid of silence, yet silence can be an important tool in effective presentations. Pauses are especially important for emphasis of key points, after rhetorical questionsand in the beginning and ending of a talk. It is important to avoid vocalized pauses and fillers, such as "um", "you know" and "like." The removal of these unconscious fillers can be difficult for some speakers, without discipline and practice.

Motion

Speakers must be dynamic in their presentations. One aspect of this is movement. Movement can help to gain the audience's attention and convey comfort with a subject. Any change in what the speaker does creates dramatic emphasis and focuses attention. Pay attention to gestures and be sure these come across naturally. Examine the non-verbal messages communicated to your audience. Be aware that some presentations that are videotaped may necessarily restrict your capacity to move during the presentation.

Nervous Habits

Nervous habits that distract the audience should be avoided. Some speakers fidget, especially with microphone cords and pointers while speaking. Others clench the lectern so tightly that their knuckles remain white throughout the presentation. For some speakers, it's helpful to not bring extraneous materials to the talk that might be fiddled with. Nervous energy can be channeled into more effective hand gestures and body movements.

Handling Notes

Note cards are best when a speaker is not using a lectern, whereas pages work well behind a lectern. Be sure to number your pages in case they become mixed during transit. With note cards, it can be helpful to punch a hole through the cards and attach a key ring to keep them together. With pages, sliding them can be less conspicuous than rustling of pages. Make an effort to begin and end without notes.

Eye Contact/Verbal Contact

Make as much eye contact as possible. Avoid choosing a few people to focus on during the presentation. Also avoid looking to only one side of the audience, looking at people you know, or only to the front of the audience. Using participants names, if possible, can also help to maintain connection with the audience.

Visual Aids

Approximately 75 percent of learners are visually oriented (Jolles 1993). Visual aids are an important method to capture their attention and facilitate learning. It's important to offer other methods of presentation for those who aren't visually oriented as well. It is possible to use too many visual aids. By overemphasizing everything, you emphasize nothing. When using visual aids, it is helpful not to place too much information on a slide or transparency. Generally eight to ten lines of information per visual field are recommenced (Jolles 1993).

Timing

Time your speech before you give it to be sure that it fits the time requirements. Be aware that extemporaneous speeches often become longer as you practice and continue to prepare the speech. During the speech, the speaker must be flexible enough to either expand or contract their remarks to fit the allotted time as the speech progresses. It is best to shrink the body of a talk and leave the introduction and closing intact. This requires an ability to think on one's feet.

Language

It is important to keep the level of the language in synch with the level of the audience. Good speakers and teachers develop skills in explaining complex subjects with very simplistic terms. It is best to avoid acronyms.

Breaks

Studies have shown that the average attention span of an adult learner is short. Students participate better with more frequent breaks (on the hour). It is important for the presenter to not allow the breaks to run on, while starting and ending their talk on time.

Introductory Talks

*My enthusiasm grew. I became a fanatic. I went about the
country, visited inns, where I got up on tables and benches to
harangue whoever might be present to listen to my enthusiastic
speeches on homeopathy.*
    —Constance Hering

There are two essentials to giving a good introductory talk. First, the
presenter must believe in homeopathy, feel it deeply and be able to share
their enthusiasm with others. Homeopathy is a "great subject". It is one of
the most fantastic gifts of all time. The speaker can offer others the key to
their health. They help to awaken the knowledge and love for homeopathy
that already lies in the participant's heart.

Secondly, presenters must believe in themselves. An introductory talk
must speak the truth of who one is. It is not necessary to be a great homeopath to give an introductory talk. Generally, the speaker knows more than
everyone else in the room about homeopathy. If the speaker can get out of
the way and let homeopathy take over, success is assured.

For those who give introductory presentations regularly, it is important
to keep this fresh. Varying the format, stories and emphasis help to keep the
presentation vital and alive. The presentation will also vary greatly from
audience to audience.

It is important to avoid homeopathic jargon. Most listeners have trouble relating to much of the 19th century vocabulary used in homeopathy.
Find words and language that connects with listeners.

The most difficult challenge in presenting homeopathy to the public is
prejudice (misinformation and prejudgments). Everything that the speaker
says is weighed and judged according to what the participant has been
taught before. Many people feel that they have tried homeopathy when
they really haven't. Homeopathy is also more difficult to sell than acupuncture or herbal medicine. Only those with an open mind, open heart and
open spirit can hear its message.

Length

For the most part, introductory presentations should be between one
and two hours in length. It takes time to explain homeopathy adequately.
It's crucial to leave adequate time for answering questions. Many members
of an introductory audience have come seeking an answer to a specific
question and will leave disappointed unless they have the opportunity to
ask it. Typical questions are listed in the section below.

Purpose

Most introductory homeopathic talks have four purposes. The first is introducing the public to the practice of homeopathy. They grow homeopathy and provide a service to the homeopathic community. Those who have a closed mind will not be touched, but for those who are open, these talks can be significant events in their lives, providing inspiration.

The second is an opportunity for a practitioner to share themselves. Introductory talks are the single most effective way of gathering patients for a practice. Many listeners come simply because they want the opportunity to check out the homeopath as a practitioner. The practitioner must show that they are a caring person. The goal is not to sell oneself but to come from a place of authenticity, love and humility.

The third is that introductory talks help to solidify a homeopath's knowledge. Explaining the intricacies of the homeopathic method in layman's terms helps to build a new understanding for the homeopathic practitioner.

Lastly, introductory talks help keep a practitioner connected to the public. They provide a deeper opportunity to discover what is on the public's mind, than can be discovered in one's practice.

Location

There are many effective locations for introductory talks. These include church groups, health food stores, senior centers, community organizations, public libraries, private schools, radio programs, conventional medical conferences and many others. The key is to be creative and make opportunities happen.

Format

There is no right or wrong way to give an introductory talk. Content varies greatly depending on the speaker and the audience. Introductory talks are best if they are kept simple, illustrating only a few key points. It is also best not to assume that the audience has any knowledge of homeopathy. Important elements include:

Introduction   Research shows that the speaker has about three minutes to make a connection of believability and an emotional connection with their audience before they begin to lose them. People's attention spans are much shorter in today's world than in the past. A good opening is very important. The introduction is an opportunity to share the gift of homeopathy and explain its importance in the world today. Issues such as its holistic nature, offering the possibility of true cure, its relative safety, its capacity to treat diseases that are untreatable allopathically, its nonsupressive nature and its affordability can be places to begin. Non professional audiences often resonate with the idea of the "people's medicine." Some speakers begin with a remarkable case to illustrate homeopathy's efficacy. Stories are an important method of beginning as they help to open the participants' hearts.

Telling Your Story

The speaker should describe their homeopathic journey. This includes exploring one's love of homeopathy and why homeopathy is so important to them. Most often this takes the form of telling a personal story of how the speaker discovered homeopathy. This story should be dramatic and illustrate what was missing in the speaker before homeopathy was discovered and how it has changed their life.

Story of Hahnemann

One of the most important stories to tell is that of Hahnemann. Audiences resonate with his story and wish to know the origins of homeopathy. It is useful to place this in a back drop of ancient medicine describing the split between the Rationalist and Empirical forms of healing. This is an opportunity to explore concepts such as his rejection of the medicine of his times, how he discovered homeopathy, his provings, the writing of the Organon, his relationship with Melanie (his second wife), his motto, the impact that he had on healing, and the growth of homeopathy after his death.

Basic Principles

Here the underlying philosophy of homeopathy can be explored. This is an opportunity for the speaker to distinguish homeopathy from other forms of healing. Concepts such as the Law of Similars, Hering's Law, holism and suppression can be examined. It is useful to discuss the goals of homeopathic treatment and how these goals are different from those of conventional medicine. Many audiences also wish to understand the meaning of the word "homeopathy."

What to Expect When Your Case Is Taken

Most participants want to know what they can expect when they see a homeopath. This includes how they can prepare for a homeopathic consultation and how they can be a good homeopathic patient. Concepts that can be explored include length of a homeopathic consultation, matching the symptoms to a particular homeopathic remedy, modalities, general symptoms, strange, rare and peculiar symptoms, the relative importance of mental and emotional symptoms (beyond the chief complaint), relative cost of treatment, pace of healing, antidotes (do not overwhelm them with too many details) and nature and frequency of follow-up. It is also helpful to explore the differences between first aid, acute and constitutional treatment. The safety and non-toxicity of the remedies should be stressed, while aggravations can be reframed in terms of healing crises. Another technique is to explore a typical day in the life of a homeopathic practitioner.

What Is a Homeopathic Remedy?

Generally it is best to leave this area until later in the presentation, as it is often the most controversial. What resonates with many audiences is a discussion of energy medicine. Distinguishing forms of healing based on matter vs. energy can be helpful. Depending on the audience, it is often best to avoid the subject of infinitesimal doses. They often find this confusing and become resistant at this point. What can be more helpful is to focus on finding a minimum dose sufficient to trigger a healing response in the organism. Audiences love to hear about the various homeopathic substances, especially ones that they contact in their daily lives, although it is best to avoid any discussion of nosodes. Some individuals are uncomfortable with the idea of using disease products in healing. A brief review of some key points of a particular homeopathic remedy can be quite helpful here. It is important to actually bring a homeopathic remedy for kinesthetic members of the audience to touch. Finally, the administration of homeopathic remedies can be explored.

What Can Homeo-pathy Treat? One of the most common reasons that individuals come to an introductory talk is to discover what homeopathy has to offer to them in the treatment of their own particular illness. It is useful to give a description of the breadth of illnesses that homeopathy can successfully treat. It is fine to mention that homeopathy treats people and not disease, but inevitably individuals in the audience will ask "yes, but will homeopathy treat my disease?" The speaker can explore what is and is not treatable using homeopathy. People are suspicious of any form of healing that claims universal cure rates in all disease states. This is also a good place to explore the efficacy of homeopathy in the treatment of children, pregnancy and animals. It is best to avoid complicated subjects such as the homeopathic treatment of cancer and AIDS. The key here is to convey the idea that homeopathy may be able to help them more effectively than what they are currently doing.

The Science of Homeopathy Audiences vary greatly in their interest in research. As mentioned earlier, individuals buy for emotional reasons and then justify with facts. In presentations to health care professionals, research exploring the efficacy of homeopathy is critical. The general public is often much more interested in proving research. This is also a good place to speak about current thinking concerning the mechanism of action of homeopathic remedies (Gray 2000). Skeptics generally remain unconvinced, regardless of how much research evidence is presented.

Homeopathy in the World Today Participants are interested in the practice of homeopathy locally, in their state or region, in their country and in the world today. Audiences often enjoy the mention of key political and social figures who support homeopathy. This is an opportunity to explore such issues as training, certification, scope of practice and licensure. Statistics showing the rapid growth of homeopathy and strong world-wide interest can be helpful. Discussion of how homeopathy integrates into the practice of conventional medicine in one's area can also be productive.

Conclusion and Next Steps
The conclusion is an opportunity to summarize what has been said and to connect again with the hearts of one's audience. It is vital to give participants a clear and easy path to the next step. This might include information on homeopaths in the local area, encouraging first-aid usage, providing remedies to experiment with, discussion of local study groups and training programs, books for further reading (bring these with you to show), becoming a member of local and national organizations that support homeopathy and any upcoming further events in your area. Be sure to bring plenty of business cards with you or a listing of local practitioners. The introductory study group provides a wonderful next step for those individuals who attend introductory talks and yet wish more. They also provide a safe environment for beginning teachers to practice their speaking and teaching skills.

Fielding Questions
It is very important to leave adequate time for questions and answers after the presentation. It is useful to not spend too long on any particular question, so that everyone who has a question has time to speak. Be careful to avoid letting any one participant dominate the questions. Many participants do not feel comfortable asking a question but will approach a presenter after their talk. Be sure to leave adequate time for these questions as well.

Some presenters worry about hecklers. This tends to be much less of a problem than most fear. However, occasionally this can be an issue. Generally, this arises most in the question and answer period. Be aware that if an individual's mind is closed, there is little that you can do to convince them of the efficacy and validity of homeopathy. Most important is to pause and acknowledge what they say, while avoiding getting into a debate with them. If the situation escalates, the speaker can offer to speak to the heckler later, while explaining that they want to give others a chance to speak. Last ditch efforts include inviting the heckler to come up and speak, letting the audience assume responsibility (asking if they wish to continue to let the individual speak) or ending the presentation.

It is useful to prepare for this part of the presentation. Practicing answering questions with others in a safe environment can be a good way to begin. There are two types of questions that the presenter needs to be ready to answer, common questions and difficult questions. It is also important to admit ignorance when one is beyond your skill and knowledge level. Audiences generally respect this. Some examples of each type of question are listed below:

Examples of Common Questions

◎ Can homeopathy treat my problem?

◎ Have you ever treated this problem before?

◎ What potency should I use?

◎ Can I use more than one homeopathic remedy at once?

◎ What is the difference between homeopathy and herbs?

◎ I would like to do homeopathy but I am not sure that I have what it takes to do it. What do you think?

◎ How safe is it really?

◎ How do I tell who is a good practitioner?

◎ What are these combination remedies I see at the health food store?

◎ Who can become a homeopath? What are the legalities of practice?

◎ Will X antidote remedies?

◎ What do you recommend that I read for more information?

◎ How successful are you in your practice? How successful are other practitioners?

◎ Where can I find out more? What can I do next?

Examples of Difficult Questions

◎ How effective is homeopathy in the treatment of cancer, AIDS or Alzheimer's Disease?

◎ How exactly does homeopathy work?

◎ Homeopathy is nothing more than placebo, isn't it?

◎ My doctor tells me that I am wasting my time doing homeopathy. Is he right?

◎ What exactly is Medorrhinum (or nosodes)?

◎ I heard that there are remedies like sunlight or moonbeam. What kind of craziness is this?

◎ Why isn't homeopathy more popular, if it is effective?

◎ What do you think of Treatment X (non-homeopathic)?

◎ I went to a homeopath for years and it never worked. Why should I go back?

Public speaking is one of the greatest tools that we have to help homeopathy grow. Good quality presentations can open the audience to a new vision of healing and instill hope for the future.

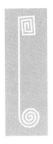

Chapter Seven
Finding the Teacher Within

Teachers are like flowers: they spread their beauty throughout the world. Their love of learning touches the hearts of their students, who then carry that sense of wonder with them wherever they may go. Teachers, with their words of wisdom, awaken the spirit within us all and lead us down the roads of life.
—Deanna Beisser

As homeopaths, the most important thing for our clients to learn about healing is that true healing comes from within. Similarly, the most important aspect of learning to teach others is contacting the "teacher within." Every teacher has two sides, the inner and the outer. Any authentic call to teach comes from the "teacher within" (Palmer 1998), and superior teachers listen to this call. It allows them to communicate from what is deepest within them to what is deepest within each student in the class. This is different from the teacher persona, which is the mask that many teachers wear when they teach. The qualities of this mask vary from teacher to teacher but all involve teaching in a superficial way that the teacher feels they should teach. In good teaching, this persona must be put aside to allow authenticity, openness, spontaneity and vulnerability.

Good teaching is a gift from one person to another. The "teacher within" represents an amalgam of teaching experiences from the past. This "inner teacher" reminds teachers of truth and asks them to reach for integrity in all that they do. In turn, students take bits and pieces of their teachers with them. In psychological terms, the student interjects the best qualities of each teacher. The kind of teaching that transforms people does not happen if either the teacher's "inner teacher" or the student's "inner teacher" is ignored.

When teachers are connected to their "inner teacher," they speak from a place of authority. It is this authority that allows one to do the impossible, to stand one's ground in the face of difficult challenges. This is quite different than speaking from a place of power (ego). To lose contact with one's "inner teacher" is to lose contact with one's authority.

The key to finding the "teacher within" is exploring the qualities, knowledge and skills central to great teaching. Qualities are ways of being in the world. They express the underlying attitudes that each teacher carries about their work, themselves and their world. Knowledge is the perception of truth. It requires awareness and a clarity of mental understanding. Skills are the ability to practice that arise from one's knowledge. They are knowledge in action. Skills require competent excellence.

What Are the Qualities of Great Teachers?

> *The bad teacher's words fall on his pupils like harsh rain;*
> *the good teacher's as gently as the dew.*
> —Talmud

Below is listed a summary of the central qualities of great teachers (Banner and Cannon 1987). Each teacher has both strengths and weaknesses in these areas. These qualities cannot be taught as much as evoked from within. Some of them are contradictory, yet great teachers somehow bring all of these qualities into their work. This is what makes teaching difficult. Ultimately, the qualities of good teachers are similar to qualities of good learners and good administrators. They also reflect the qualities inherent in good case taking.

An Ability to Teach from the Whole

> *My efforts have been spent in trying to have my fellow*
> *practitioners see the light, to goad them on to see the value of*
> *the most wonderful and most magnificent gem that was ever*
> *given to the medical world. I wanted you to see it and*
> *appreciate it; to know it as I know it.*
> —Alfred Pulford

Good teachers teach with their whole being. They teach holistically. A great teacher lives and embodies his subject at the deepest of levels. Their teaching reveals their whole selves, including both their weaknesses and strengths. They join the students, subject and self all into one rich tapestry.

Good teachers differ greatly but bad teachers are all the same. Bad teachers do not connect with their students. They are disconnected from themselves and are therefore unable to bring much of themselves into their teaching.

Good teaching is not centered on technique. Some great teachers use strictly lecture format, others engage their classes in dialectical class discussion and others focus on student-centered learning techniques. Teachers are at their best when the method that they choose is in tune with whom they are.

Great teachers also teach from the whole. With their students they embrace the intellectual, emotional and spiritual dimensions of learning. They have the capacity to give voice to the group thought of the class.

Good teaching comes from the identity and integrity of the teacher.

A classic teaching story describes a workshop leader who places a small black dot on a marker board. This individual then turns to the audience and polls them on what they see. The universal response is a "small black dot." The teacher then asks, "Doesn't anyone see the marker board?" Students tend to focus on the small details. It is a good teacher's responsibility to make them aware of the field, and place their learning in a larger context. These teachers are teaching the whole of their subject. Sitting in their classrooms, one has a sense of being connected to something "great."

A Passion for Learning

We may affirm absolutely that nothing great in the world
has ever been accomplished without passion.
—George Hegel

Great teachers not only have a love and passion for what they teach, but also for learning itself. This passion is communicated by being totally present in their work and committed to their subject. Good teachers are not just teachers in the classroom, but are teachers every moment of their lives.

This passion is often generated by appreciation of the greatness of the subject. Ultimately is not the teacher/guru that drives homeopathic education and not the students themselves, but the great subject of homeopathy itself. Homeopathy is much larger than any teacher or teaching.

Humility

Both teaching and rational inquiry at their creative and inspired best, thus lead us to the very threshold of ultimate mystery and induce in us a sense of profound humility and awe.
—Theodore Meyer Greene

Humility is the attitude that teachers hold in their hearts when doing their best work. Humility is what they feel in the face of a subject that is much larger than they are. Humility is knowing where one is and knowing one's limits. To teach effectively, teachers must be vulnerable. They must expose themselves and yet be detached enough for the student not to confuse the teacher with the message.

Compassion

A teacher is a counselor, a role model, and often a friend.
—Taylor MacKenzie

Compassion comes from Latin word meaning "suffering with." Compassion requires acting as a whole person. Great teachers remember what it was like to sit in the chair of the student and they are aware of the limitations, fears and troubles that beset their students during the learning process. The great teacher respects all states of understanding within their students. They have a capacity to teach to whatever state their students are in.

The handling of rude and angry students is the true test of compassion. Avoiding favoritism is also a challenge for every teacher. In each class there are students who want to ask the teacher for more attention but are afraid. It is the teacher's duty to find and help those students.

The teacher must achieve a balance between the personal and the impersonal. As in homeopathic practice, one must model for one's students empathy (emotional attunement) without sympathy (emotional merging).

Educators cannot teach without compassion. Banner and Cannon describe it well by stating, "Those who experience difficulty in accepting the place of compassion in the classroom, who resist the idea of sympathetic emotions, or who prefer their working lives to be exclusively intellectual should avoid teaching altogether and probably consider devoting themselves to less demanding occupations such as politics or crime" (Bannor and Cannon, 1987, p. 89).

Courage

> *Only the brave should teach. Only those who love the young*
> *should teach. Teaching is a vocation. It is as sacred as*
> *priesthood; as innate a desire, as inescapable as the genius*
> *which compels a great artist. If he has not the concern for*
> *humanity, the love of living creatures, the vision of the*
> *priest and the artist, he must not teach.*
> —Pearl S. Buck

Teaching requires courage. Teachers put themselves on the line every time they stand up in front of a class. Popular literature and movies, such as like *Mr. Holland's Opus, The Browning Version, The Pride of Miss Jean Brodie, Black Board Jungle, To Sir with Love* and *The Dead Poets' Society,* are filled with images of the heroism of teaching.

New teachers quickly learn that ambiguity and unpredictability are central aspects of teaching (Fink 1984; Eble 1988). This uncertainty is generated from the incompleteness of our homeopathic knowledge, yet also is an integral part of the dynamics of teaching. Teachers have been described as "gladiators of ambiguity" (Jackson 1986, 1990). Classrooms are full of surprises and shocks. They can be deeply emotive, generating uncomfortable feelings in student and teacher alike. Teaching is a messy and chaotic experience (Salzberger-Wittenber, Henry, and Osborne, 1983). Periods of calm are interspersed with hectic learning activity.

A teacher should have a willingness to take risks and follow the path of the class, wherever it leads. Great teachers have the capacity to stand in the face of all this ambiguity and uncertainty and not cling to lesson plans. They must be highly flexible and make a very quick series of judgments about what to do next and how to respond to unforeseen eventualities (Calderhead 1984). These decisions are primarily based on gut instinct.

A Clear Vision

> *Truth is like a ghost, seen in the misty distance for the frac-*
> *tion of a moment and even that vision is so awe inspiring*
> *that one may only imagine what it is like to see the whole*
> *of the truth all the time.*
> —Pierre Schmidt

Great teachers have a clear vision of what is to be accomplished in the class, and the ability to hold this vision always in front of the students. Homeopathic teachers must help their students maintain a clear vision of what it is to be a good homeopath. Without clarity there is a lack of sense of direction, a meandering confusion. The vision then provides a compass in the stormy seas of teaching and learning.

Vision is established by identifying a purpose in teaching or a philosophy of practice. Teachers do this by developing a critical rationale (Smyth 1986). A critical rationale is a set of values, beliefs and feelings about the fundamental purpose of teaching. Students draw strength from the passion and conviction that accompanies this vision.

It is not enough simply to have a clear vision. A great teacher must also communicate this vision to the students. The teacher must show the students where the class is going, and why it is important to go there.

Playfulness

> *The best teacher is not the one who knows most, but the one who is most capable of reducing knowledge to that simple compound of the obvious and the wonderful which slips into the infantile comprehension. A man of high intelligence, perhaps, may accomplish the thing by a conscious intellectual feat. But it is vastly easier to the man (or woman) whose habit of mind are naturally on the plane of a child's. The best teacher, in brief, is one who is essentially childlike.*
> —H.L. Mencken

Great teachers can play with their subjects and make learning fun for their students, whose childlike nature is fulfilled. They bring a sense of wonder into their classes, and convey the pleasure and joy that they have in knowing their subject.

Great teachers enjoy their students and take pleasure from witnessing the successes of their students. Their classrooms are filled with laughter and humor, true humor that does not just entertain but opens the heart. They bring humor into their work and a sense of cheerfulness.

The Ability to Inspire the Imagination

The mediocre teacher tells.
The good teacher explains.
The superior teacher demonstrates.
The great teacher inspires.
—William Arthur Ward

Great teachers have the capacity to strike or fire the imagination. Teaching homeopathically is concerned with capturing the imaginations of students, striking images that resonate with their minds and hearts. Only by bringing out the magic and mystery of homeopathy can the teacher capture the hearts of their students.

A great teacher brings their subject alive. Even if they utilize the works of the old masters, they have the capacity to apply what they teach to the world of practice today. This is what inspires students and holds their attention. In this way, teachers provide nourishment for soul.

These teachers expand their students' boundaries and open them up to new possibilities and ideas. They help their students soar past what they think is possible. They bring freedom into their teaching on all levels. In learning, imagination is more important than knowledge (Einstein 1935). William James said in *Talks to Teachers*, "In teaching, you must simply work your pupil into such a state of interest in what you are going to teach him that every other subject of attention is banished from his mind; then reveal it to him so impressively that he will remember the occasion to his dying day; and finally fill him with devouring curiosity to know what the next steps in connection with the subject are."

Imaginative teaching finds new and varied ways to reach students. Launching into uncharted territories is risky but as long as it is grounded in the great subject of homeopathy, the enthusiasm will generally carry the day. Good teachers can imagine themselves in their students' places. Imaginative teachers clarify issues before their students even reach them in their studies, anticipating their problems. There is no unimaginative teaching but there are unimaginative teachers.

Transformative Teaching

To live a single day and hear a good teaching
is better than to live a hundred years without knowing such teaching.
—Buddha

Good teachers are transformative. Teaching is the alchemical journey of transforming nothing into something. These teachers have the capacity to serve as change agents and to change their students lives. They impact them so that they are not the same when they leave. Their students may not be aware at the time and only realize in retrospect how important a figure that teacher was in their lives.

Part of what helps teachers to accomplish this is the trickster archetype (Hooks 1999). A good teacher is a chameleon and can take on many roles and shapes.

The Ability to Be Self Reflective

A teacher is one who, in his youth, admired teachers.
—H. L. Mencken

Awareness of the qualities of great teachers can take one a long way toward becoming an effective teacher. Reflection on one's own experiences can be helpful in this process. A useful exercise is to reflect on the following questions:

◎ Who were the most important teachers in your life?
◎ What qualities made them important in your learning?
◎ What made them effective?
◎ What part of them have you taken with you and is part of you?
◎ What was there about you that allowed the great teaching to happen?
◎ Who were the worst teachers that you had?
◎ What qualities made them ineffective?

This exercise can be conducted individually or in a group format as part of teacher training.

No teacher can embody fully all of these qualities. All good teachers have strengths in certain areas and weaknesses in others. It is important for good teachers to recognize and embrace their strengths while developing an awareness of and working on their weaknesses.

The Importance of Knowledge

It is probably part of the human condition that cosmologists (or shamans of any age) always think they are knocking on eternity's door, that the final secret of the universe is in reach. It may also be part of the human condition that they are always wrong. Science, inching along by trial and error and by doubt, is a graveyard of final answers.
—Dennis Overbye

A teacher must have more knowledge than his students. This knowledge is not just about the subject. The knowledge must also be about one's students, about the process of learning and about oneself. Knowledge is more than information. It is a state of individualized understanding and one comes to it through the process of trying to make sense of new information as it relates to what one already knows. It is also being aware of the limits of one's knowledge.

Thorough Knowledge of the Subject and of the Learning Process

The half known hinders knowing.
Since all of our knowing is only half,
our knowing always hinders our knowing.
—Goethe

Great teachers have a thorough knowledge of their subject. This is a challenge in homeopathy because to be a good homeopath means to be a student of life. For geologists, the rocks speak, historians are those who hear the voices of the long dead, writers hear the music of words, but homeopaths must hear the voice of all of life speaking. Great teachers must teach a love and respect for all life.

These teachers serve as guardians of knowledge and they model being a contributor to that knowledge. When teachers stop learning they become bored and cannot help but communicate this to their students. Good teachers must keep current. They must wrestle with their knowledge constantly. They are beguiled by their students' curiosity and have a willingness to be pulled into their students learning process.

These teachers have an awareness of the limits of their knowledge. They are honest and open concerning when they exceed this limit. They are not hindered by this lack of knowledge but demonstrate their constant drive to learn more.

Great teachers also have a deep knowledge of how students experience learning. They understand the problems of learning, cycles of learning and developmental stages of learning. They can work effectively with this understanding in their teaching.

Learning is highly individualized. All knowledge has a personal element to it. Some learners are acoustically focused, others are visually focused, while others are somatically focused. Some students learn best through lecture format, others through books, others through schools, others through seminars and Internet and others through independent study. Great teachers are comfortable using a variety of methods. By experiencing a variety, the majority of students will find their preferred mode of learning.

Thorough Knowledge of One's Students

> *The best teacher will be he who has at his tongue's end the explanation of what it is that is bothering the pupil. These explanations give the teacher the knowledge of the greatest possible number of methods, the ability of inventing new methods, and, above all, not a blind adherence to one method, but the conviction that all methods are one-sided, and that the best method would be the one which would answer best to all the possible difficulties incurred by a pupil, that is, not a method, but an art and talent.*
> —Leo Tolstoy

It is vital to understand one's students in order to tune into their needs. Great teachers respect their students' individual differences and honor who they are and where they are. They see them in the context of their whole lives, not just the classroom. Teachers who can see this will understand the obstacles to learning for each of their students. They can identify their needs and problems and help them to see themselves more clearly. Good teachers also know where their students are on their homeopathic journeys.

Bad teachers often utilize only one teaching method. Much like vaccinations, they feel one dose fits all. Great teachers, on the other hand, individualize their teaching, although this becomes increasingly difficult as class size increases. Then they attempt to find a method of teaching that is *similar* to the way each student best learns. It is important to remember, however, that students' learning styles change over time (Kolb 1983). Teachers must periodically reassess their teaching methods.

Thorough Self Knowledge

Know thyself.
—Plutarch

Great teachers cannot know their students until they first know themselves. They must know their strengths, skills, blind spots and weaknesses, and teach from who they are. Self knowledge is the key to the maturity of the teacher.

Teaching holds a mirror to the soul and forces one to face their inner nature. This is not always comfortable, as it can reveal the teacher's neuroses and unresolved issues, thus it's tempting to avoid what one sees. At the same time, it is easiest for teachers to avoid their weaknesses and teach to their strengths. Yet it is often the teachers' weakness that is the source of their greatest strength. Acknowledging that they are not perfect brings authenticity into their teaching. It also models to the students one's humanness and helps them have the courage to deal with their own neurosis.

One of the keys to self knowledge in teaching is to remember what it was like to be a learner and to identify with that role. Good teachers are willing to retrace the steps of their own homeopathic journey. They also continually renew themselves as learners throughout the teaching process.

What Are the Skills of the Best Teachers?

A teacher is a very special person who uses his or her creativity and loving, inquiring mind to develop the rare skills of encouraging others to think, to dream, to learn, to try, to do!
—Beverly Conklin

Although skills are important in teaching, they are less central to the role of being a good teacher than qualities and knowledge. However, many new teachers focus too much on skill development at the cost of deeper issues. Technique is said to be what one uses until the teacher arrives (Palmer 1999).

Skills represent the science of teaching. What are the skills that identify great teachers? There are many but a list of these should include at least the following:

Ability to Balance Order and Flexibility

*A man who is pleased when he receives good instruction
will sleep peacefully, because his mind is thereby cleansed.*
—Buddha

The capacity to be structured yet flexible in one's teaching approach is a fine balance. It requires the teacher to modify one's teaching style to meet the needs of the class at hand. It also demands a clear focus and a refusal to deviate from this. Teachers who have the proper sense of order create a teaching space that is bounded yet open.

Great teachers can find order in the midst of the chaos, a capacity that arises out of a teacher's leadership. Students require a certain amount of structure from which they can learn best. Without this order, students may experience the classroom as too chaotic and have difficulty imposing inner order themselves. Great teachers provide a frame in which learning takes place both internally and externally. They are responsible for protecting this frame and guarding it from disruptions. They are also fierce protectors of the truth. This order provides a sense of mental security for students.

Students also require the freedom to speak and imagine. Chaos in a classroom brings surprise and uncertainty, both elements that are critical to the learning process. Students often learn best when the greatest moments of chaos and uncertainty lead suddenly to order and understanding.

Great teachers are well prepared to teach. They have done their home-work, yet when they start class they are willing to discard their preparations and be flexible.

Ability to Balance Support and Challenge

*It is that openness and awareness and innocence of sorts that I
try to cultivate in my dancers. Although, as the Latin verb to
educate, educere, indicates, it is not a question of putting
something in but drawing it out, if it is there to begin with…
I want all of my students and all of my dancers to be aware of
the poignancy of life at that moment. I would like to feel that
I had, in some way, given them the gift of themselves.*
—Martha Graham

There is a delicate balance between support and challenge (Daloz 1986). Good teachers teach to where students are and then stretch them. With no challenge and no support there is inertia; with high challenge and low support there is retreat; with low challenge and high support there is

194

affirmation; with high challenge and high support there is growth. Great teachers create a space for learning that is hospitable and welcoming, yet charged with challenge. They do not intervene prematurely, nor do they stand back when students are becoming too comfortable with their self-defeating habits.

Good teachers constantly challenge their students. They help to overcome inertia by enthusiasm and encouragement. They have the ability to lead the class more deeply into a subject. By asking questions that deepen, they avoid shutting down the process of learning. They constantly keep moving the goal beyond their students' reach. They challenge them to think critically and with alternative perspectives.

Teachers also need to create a safe learning space for their students (Palmer 1998). This space is made up of physical, emotional and mental factors. In psychological terms, Winicott calls this a holding environment (Davis and Wallbridge 1987). It is important to have a place where students can feel safe and secure, a place where it is safe to make mistakes. Here they feel nourished and can rest. Learning can be a fearful process (see chapter five) when students are faced with the unknown and significant change. They may feel overexposed. Yet they must not feel so safe that they are bored.

There is a natural instinct in teachers to protect their students. There have been many stories throughout history of teachers sacrificing their lives for students. This is also an aspect of the mythic journey of teaching and learning. Many cultures describe such myths. Telemacheus and his student Mentor in the *Odyssey*, along with Ben Kenobi and his student Luke Skywalker in the movie *Star Wars* exemplify teachers' heroic nature.

Good teachers acknowledge the efforts that their students make. They support them when they are confused or lost and empathize with their emotional distress. They help to normalize their experience of education by supporting them through the difficult phases and transitions. Good teachers turn discouraging experiences into encouraging ones.

The word education derives from the Latin verb *educere*. This is defined not as putting something in, but drawing something out. Knowledge is already in students, it is just waiting to be revealed.

Capacity to Listen Actively and Comfort with Silence

Education is the ability to listen to almost anything
without losing your temper or your self-confidence.
—Robert Frost

The capacity to truly listen is a rare skill in our culture, even among healing practitioners. Great teachers truly listen to their students questions and perceive what is most central to what they are saying. They are able to weave this into the tapestry of the class.

Practitioners often extol the virtues of silence and active listening in their practices and yet seldom practice this in the classroom. Teachers and students view silence as something to be avoided at all costs. Typical groups can only tolerate about 15 seconds of silence.

Judicious use of silence can be an extremely valuable skill. It is a method that deepens learning. There is an important interplay between action and reflection in the classroom. It is important to keep these balanced. Students talk of information overload, feeling that they will explode from the amount of information to crammed into them. It is important to have periods of reflection where learning can be assimilated.

Encouragement of Self Learning

Any piece of knowledge which the pupil has himself acquired—
any problem which he has himself solved, becomes, by virtue of
the conquest, much more thoroughly his than it could else be.
The preliminary activity of mind which his success implies, the
concentration of thought necessary to it, and the excitement
consequent on his triumph, conspire to register the facts in his
memory in a way that no mere information heard from a
teacher, or read in a schoolbook, can be registered.
—Herbert Spencer

Just as the most important form of healing is self healing, the most important form of learning is self learning. In self-directed learning, students make the ultimate decisions and have more autonomy. Self learning is integrated more fully and completely into the mind, heart and spirit of the learner than any form of external learning. Great teachers lead students to the thresholds of their own minds. They know that much of learning is about pointing the way, without telling their students what to see.

After students graduate from training programs, much of their continuing education will come, by necessity, from self learning. It is very important that they be ready for and comfortable with self learning.

Encouragement of Critical Thinking

Goal 5. The proportion of college graduates who demonstrate an advanced ability to think critically, communicate effectively, and solve problems will increase substantially.
—*America 2000: An Educational Strategy*
(U.S. Department of Education, 1990)

Contemporary allopathic education does not encourage students to think (Wales 1993). Yet thinking skills can be learned (Resnick 1987). Critical thinking is a method of helping students to become personally empowered. It opens their minds and enables them to take control of both their own learning and their own destiny. Critical thinking brings a sense of personal control or self efficacy.

Teaching critical thinking means having students continually question their learning and themselves. In this way, critical thinking promotes the development of an inquiring mind. King has done research on critical thinking and demonstrated that it improves long-term memory retention and understanding of the material (King 1993). He says that teachers must stop lecturing, "like a sage on the stage and learn to function as a guide on the side" (King 1993). With critical thinking, students evolve from dualists, who believe that all issues have right and wrong solutions, to relativists, who realize that problems have good, better and best solutions (Perry 1970). Students who are in a dualist mind set often resent teachers who do not give them final answers.

Future Direction

I touch the future. I teach.
—Christina McAuliffe

Much of teaching is planting seeds. Sometimes there can be no visible effect, or what is planted takes years to bear fruit. Farmers often plant crops whose only purpose is to rejuvenate the soil, and it may take years for the land to be ready for a crop that can be harvested. Similarly, much of a teacher's work is concerned with preparing the soil (see Chapter Four).

Great teachers deeply affect the minds, hearts and spirits of their students. Often only in retrospect can a student see how deeply they were moved by a given teacher. Teachers also provide road maps for the futures of their students. They help prepare them for what comes next so that they are ready for practice when they leave the classroom. They serve as a potential role model for what is to come.

Patience

> *Don't despair of a student if he has one clear idea.*
> —Nathaniel Emmons

Teaching requires great patience and persistence. There must be a willingness to repeat, repeat and repeat again, while continually keeping fresh what is taught. This often challenges a teacher's equanimity. The teacher meets the student at their level and gives them the time that they need to learn. They resist the temptation to rush through material they know well, but give students time to digest. They are not annoyed with the slowness or confusion of some of their students, but use this as an opportunity to become a more effective teacher.

Great teachers also encourage patience in their students and patience with the learning process. They help their students see the stages of stagnation and growth that are intrinsic to learning. They serve as a model of patience in both the classroom and clinical settings. Ultimately teachers must be patient not only with their students, but also with themselves.

Ability to Balance Solitude and Community

> *Man is the only one that knows nothing,*
> *that can learn nothing without being taught.*
> *He can neither speak nor talk nor eat,*
> *and in short he can do nothing at the prompting*
> *of nature only, but weep.*
> —Pliny the Elder

Teachers build a space that supports solitude and yet is surrounded by community. The teacher listens carefully to the voices of their students. Each student has a unique voice that must be heard. But teachers must also listen to and express the group voice. It is similar to taking the case of the class. Teachers work with the group consciousness as well as working with each individual.

Learning demands solitude, and it is important that teachers respect this need in their students. There must be opportunities to reflect on what we have learned in order to integrate it. Many students choose not to speak in class, yet are active participants within themselves. At the same time, when facilitating discussion, teachers must ensure that each individual who wishes to speak is heard.

What helps students survive the rigors of training is a supportive community. The community helps students feel less alone, so that they are part of a shared journey and connected to a much larger whole. It is also helpful for students to know that the homeopathic community extends much further than the classroom. They are part of a community of great homeopaths who have traveled the same path before.

Community provides a place where one's ignorance and prejudice can be aired and worked through. The politics and personalities of the classroom serve as a model for the politics and personalities that the student will eventually face in the practitioner's office (Shor 1986).

Teachers often feel exposed and self conscious when their work is scrutinized. Many teachers describe the difficulty they have teaching while being observed by another teacher. Teaching can be a deeply personal process that is not easily shared. Yet receiving feedback from both administrators and peers is a vital part of facilitating teaching skills.

Teachers must find a balance between being part of a community of educators and finding their own voices in their work. Teaching can be a lonely and isolating experience(see Chapter Three) and support from a community of teachers can be essential to survive in the teaching profession.

Ethics

First the patient, second the patient,
third the patient, fourth the patient, fifth the patient,
and then maybe comes science.
—Bela Schick

Ethics can be summarized in two simple statements: Do all that you have agreed to do and do not encroach on others or their property (Mayburry 1993). In teaching ethically, the teacher makes the welfare of their students their primary concern. They build a sacred place that honors their students. Good ethics in the teaching environment are student centered.

In doing all that they agree to do, teachers honor their commitment and contract with their students. For example, this means starting and ending on time. When they make changes in what they intend to do, they carefully explain why to their students. Some teachers never get through half of their lesson plans and lack the capacity to create a coherent whole.

In not encroaching on others or their property, teachers keep clear boundaries in class. They never threaten or harm their students. They realize that it is unethical for a teacher to engage in sexual relations with one of their students. They never take advantage of their position of greater power.

Ability to Provide Valuable Feedback

They have a right to censure that have a heart to help.
—William Penn

Good teachers have excellent communication skills and rapport with their students, both very important when providing feedback to their students. The teacher's challenge is to make sure that the evaluation promotes learning (see Chapter Five). Good feedback is both usable and realistic, offering concrete practical steps for improvement. Good teachers maintain a tone of respect and support the homeopathic learners' self esteem. They can help them see the feedback as a movement forward rather than backward.

The teacher's struggle to be honest while at the same time supporting the student can be heart wrenching. Often what affects the teacher's own ability to give feedback is their difficulty in receiving it. It is useful for teachers to examine their own experiences with feedback in learning and in teacher evaluations.

When Does a Teacher Become a Leader or Administrator?

We cannot all be masters,
nor all masters cannot be truly followed.
—William Shakespeare

Usually teachers become leaders and administrators because they are called upon to serve. There is a growing idea in the teaching literature of "lead teachers" (Devaney 1987). They also have been called master teachers, mentors and teacher advisers. These are teachers who choose to work into leadership roles. They often assume an assisting role with other teachers, while continuing to teach and improve their own teaching. This can be a challenge, as teachers are often resistant to advising and supporting each other. These lead teachers also organize and lead peer reviews of school practices and participate productively in school decision making. They help to organize and lead in service education. They work into a core faculty role and take on a supervisory capacity.

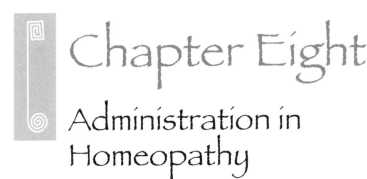

Chapter Eight

Administration in Homeopathy

The heart of leadership lies in the hearts of leaders.
—Bolman and Deal

There are two parts to administration: leadership and management. Leadership is the process of persuasion or modeling by which an individual or leadership team induces a group to pursue objectives held by the leader or shared by the organization. Management is the process in which individuals hold directive posts in an organization, presiding over the processes by which the organization functions. Both are critical to effective administration, but, although there's some overlap, leaders and managers can be distinguished in the following ways:

- ◎ **Time:** Leaders think longer term. Managers have a short-term focus.

- ◎ **Scope:** Leaders grasp connections to larger realities. Managers focus on their immediate organization.

- ◎ **Vision:** Leaders emphasize vision, ethics and motivations. Managers focus on day-to-day problems and structure.

- ◎ **Politics:** Leaders have political skill in dealing with multiple constituencies. Managers have skills in working with human resources within their organization.

- ◎ **Growth Versus Maintenance:** Leaders think in terms of continual growth and renewal. Managers focus on maintaining what exists and ensuring the smooth operation of the organization.

◎ **Experimentation:** Leaders must be willing to experiment and embrace change. Managers try to copy and imitate what exists. Joel Barker says that "you manage within a paradigm, you lead between paradigms" (Barker 1992, p. 164).

◎ **Meaning and Purpose:** Leaders focus on infusing an organization with meaning and purpose. Managers are involved with stewardship, accountability for resources and ensure that the rules and structure of an organization are closely followed.

◎ **Strategy:** Leaders are strategic in their work. Managers are tactical.

Administrators who identify more with a managerial role may initially focus on the rational and technical features of their work, such as analysis, planning and restructuring. They only grow into the more visionary and emotional aspects over time. Administrators who identify more with the leadership aspects of their work may struggle with the more "mundane" managerial aspects of what they do.

Some administrative situations call for more management, while others require leadership (Yukl 1989). The skilled administrator can function in both roles interchangeably.

This chapter focuses on leadership, while Chapter Nine deals with management. Chapter Ten explores the qualities, knowledge and skills necessary to being a good administrator.

The Importance of Good Homeopathic Leadership

Great necessity calls forth great leaders.
—Abigail Adams

Good leadership is central to the success of a school (Miller 1995). The more complex the school system, the greater the need for leadership (Fullan 2000). Good leadership helps to provide an education that liberates the mind from prejudice and opens the door for a lifelong journey of learning.

Good leaders stay focused on homeopathy. They maintain equal distance from students, teachers and community without over-identifying with any one role (see Appendix A). When a teacher comes to an administrator for advice about problems with a particular student, it is often easy to blame the student for the problem. The administrator must maintain objectivity. Leaders who also teach may have difficulty with blurred boundaries.

Why Become a Leader?

You can't make being a leader your principle goal,
any more than you can make being happy your goal.
In both cases, it has to be the result, not the cause.
—Gloria Anderson

Leaders do not generally set out to become leaders. They set out to become themselves and express themselves fully. Each individual has the capacity to transform himself into a leader. Some have the false belief that leaders are born not made. Yet the opposite is true; leaders are made. In fact, leadership training, when it is done well, can be a very effective tool in facilitating leadership.

Leaders are often called forth by the times they live in. Leadership always occurs within a historical context, and homeopathy is currently at a crossroads. As a homeopathic community, we face the decision of remaining fixed in our current position or growing into a leading health care movement. Now is a time when there is a strong need for homeopathic leadership. We cannot sit around waiting for someone to take the reins.

Leadership requires full deployment of oneself. Individuals become leaders when that expression becomes of service to their communities. Individuals lead because they must and because they are needed. There is a great joy in helping and nourishing something. This is certainly true of teaching, but even more of leadership. Leaders can touch many more individuals than teachers.

Leaders can make a difference. Even small positive changes that they affect can have rippling effects throughout the entire homeopathic movement. At the same time, the seeds that a leader plants may take considerable time to grow.

Whom does the leader serve? Ultimately it is not the students, nor the teachers, nor the community. Leaders must serve the "great subject" that is homeopathy. It is this that gives them the courage to go on amid the chaos, confusion and attacks that leadership attracts.

Leading from Within

At bottom, becoming a leader is synonymous with becoming yourself.
It's precisely that simple, and it's also that difficult.
—Warren Bennis

Leadership begins from within. It is a journey of inward discovery and rediscovery of one's spiritual and ethical center (Palmer 1999). There is no map on this part of the journey; each leader must find his own way.

One leads from one's center, from what is deepest within oneself. Kent describes this as "government from the center to the circumference" (Kent 1979). It has been said that good leaders are self directed and that they invent themselves. Once this inward journey is completed, they can then return to help transform the kingdom.

Neither good leaders nor good schools are made by copying others. The desire to replicate success destroys local initiative.

Good leaders build their leadership outward from their core commitments and vision (Bolman and Deal 1995). It is a path that leads from where they are to where they dream of being. Leadership is a gift of oneself. It is the ability to express oneself fully. A leader must find what gifts he can offer others, gifts of the heart and spirit. This necessitates openness of spirit, heart and mind.

Good leaders constantly listen to their inner voice. They have learned to trust their inner guidance and vision and have found that this is where they are most effective in their work. They have found what is truest in themselves and both nurture this and give it expression. They do not simply lead from rationality but also include their heart and their spirit in their work. In this sense they lead holistically.

It is this quality that gives leaders "character" in the true sense. People around them see them as authentic. Who they are is congruent with what they do and have become. This authenticity allows others to trust them and share their vision and purpose.

Stages of Leadership Development

With the insights we have gained into health and disease in the last decades we have come to the point where we can connect these miasms with the different phases of the individual process of mankind. When we do this we can see how each miasm corresponds to a different phase of the life process.
—Van Der Zee

Leaders go through developmental stages, as do learners and teachers. Leadership is a constantly evolving journey. Leaders never fully arrive. They may lead in very different ways at various points in their careers, as they themselves grow and develop. There are many guideposts along the way that can assist leaders in seeing where they are. Unless these guideposts are consciously sought, they are seldom recognized.

As with learning and teaching, leadership development can be viewed miasmatically. Miasms are part of the growth process and necessary to become who we truly are (Van Der Zee 2000). From this viewpoint, leadership becomes a developmental stage of what it is to be human and to fully individuate. Leaders go through stages of development associated with pre-miasmatic(contemplating leadership), psora (beginning stages of leadership), sycosis (middle stages of leadership) and syphilis (end stages of leadership).

Leadership and administration represent more the syphilitic aspects of the homeopathic journey. This is the stage where the archetypes of the king, queen, anima, animus, wise old woman and wise old man are explored. Issues that arise during this stage include death and rebirth, egotism, hope and despair, creativity, courage, responsibility, love, altruism, service, self assertion, isolation, vision, transcendence, freedom, wisdom, enlightenment, fulfillment and transformation (Van Der Zee 2000). It is in this phase that homeopaths unite the divisive forces inside of them, beginning to truly create, connecting to their spiritual nature and taking responsibility in the world for the benefit of all life.

Styles of Leadership

We need a vision of leadership rooted in the enduring sense
of human wisdom, courage and compassion.
—Bolman and Deal

Style is the total of how a leader presents themselves to their followers. Each leader is unique and has their own style. They must develop the style that is right for them through time. Leadership styles are also called forth from the differing homeopathic communities and homeopathic organizations. There should be a good fit between the homeopathic community and the leader's style (Fiedler 1967). The best administrators are ones who can be flexible in their style to meet the demands of each new situation (Hersey and Blanchard 1982).

A key condition that influences leadership style is the maturity level of the followers. Immature followers need more structure, which decreases as their maturity level grows. Power issues also play a role. High power and control positions call for more task-oriented styles. Similarly, low power and control positions require task-oriented leaders, whereas moderate power and control positions call for human-relationship-oriented styles (Fiedler and Garcia 1987). Attitudes on change and the use of authority also have a significant impact on style.

Leadership style strongly influences the behavior of subordinates within the homeopathic community. Typically this occurs in such a way that the subordinates' behavior supports the use of the leaders preferred style and mirrors their needs. This creates challenges for new subordinates who are accustomed to a different leadership style.

Some administrators over-identify with their administrative role and feel that they can do administration anywhere and with any program. They may down play the importance of homeopathic knowledge or specialized homeopathic skills in their work. However, homeopathic programs offer a unique set of problems and issues that are not present in any other form of administrative work. It is critical that the homeopathic administrators have a basic knowledge of homeopathic practice, homeopathic learning and homeopathic teaching to be effective in their roles as administrators.

McGregor (1960) described two distinct types of leadership beliefs that he calls "Theory X" and "Theory Y." Leaders' styles are adapted around these beliefs. Leaders who adopt "Theory X" have underlying beliefs that people dislike and avoid work if they can, shirk responsibility, are inherently lazy, desire security, resist change and require external direction and rigid structuring. These leaders are typically rigid, inflexible, inconsistent in their decision making and arbitrary. They often treat students as children who have to be taken care of and teachers as somewhat older children. They have trouble delegating authority. They break problems down into the component parts, yet lose any sense of connection to the whole. "Theory X" is allopathic leadership. Allopathic schools close down more minds than they open.

Leaders who adopt "Theory Y" feel that work should be as natural as play, that students and teachers are capable of self direction, that they seek and accept greater self direction and can be trusted with authority and responsibility. These types of leaders are flexible, dynamic, embrace change, give their constituents autonomy and are comfortable with ambiguity. These leaders do not cover up secrets and are open with their constituents. Theory Y is homeopathic leadership.

It is helpful for leaders to recognize their natural leadership style and the styles of those around them. This helps to give these leaders a vision of how they are perceived by others, a road map for growth and an awareness of the pitfalls that they will face in their work.

Terrence Deal and Kent Peterson (1998) describe various types of leadership roles that determine how leaders interact with their constituents, colleagues and community. Blanke and McCanse (1991) also describe a variety of leadership styles: control and dominate; yield and support; balance and compromise; evade and elude; prescribe and guide; exploit and manipulate; and contribute and commit.

Control and Dominate

This is a dictatorial style that focuses on results and not people. Relationships are seen as issues that slow the achievement of results. This style is often experienced by others as militaristic.

Yield and Support

This is an accommodating style in which the leaders have little concern for results and great concern for others. These leaders are warm and friendly but lack purpose. They focus on nurturing others and keeping everyone happy, while downplaying any consequences for poor performance.

Balance and Compromise

Here there is a medium level of concern for both results and people. The leaders often focus on mediation and arbitration of conflicting forces. The objective is not excellence but risk-free conformity. Information is used to reduce controversy.

Evade and Elude

This style stems from indifference. The leaders often seem to be just going through the motions. There is a low level concern for both results and people. The leaders strive to be invisible and neutral in all situations, to blend in without attracting attention. Often the leaders do not want to be disturbed and like to work independently so as not to be observed.

Prescribe and Guide

This is a paternalistic style of leadership parallel to that of a parent to a child. The style is less controlling and dominating than above, because the leaders also seek approval and admiration from others. They hold themselves to high standards of performance, and expect others to maintain the same high standards. They do provide more support, guidance, encouragement and help than leaders who adopt other leadership styles. These leaders have trouble delegating and must intervene if a task is not done just the way they want.

Exploit and Manipulate

This is an opportunistic style of leadership. The leaders use the position to advance their own goals and always determine what is in it for them. They show little concern either for others or the school. They use and deceive others to gain trust and support. They prefer short-term relationships where exposure is less likely or situations of unilateral authority where it does not matter what others think.

Contribute and Commit

This is said to be the most effective style of leadership. Here there is high concern for both results and people. These leaders are effective at encouraging teamwork, and they rise above politics and fears to evaluate effectiveness against standards of excellence. They are not afraid to take risks and test the limits of their creativity. They utilize feedback and criticism well. They have the capacity to learn from experience. They know how to encourage others without a fear of retaliation. They come from a place of openness.

Whatever the leadership style, it is important that it be authentic. This style must be congruent with that needed for the particular homeopathic community.

The Hero Archetype

*We in the United States, dearly love noise and show and
are given to hysterical fervor and exuberance, almost on a
par with the old-time Methodist camp meeting; we are
fond of fooling ourselves and of being fooled and thus
exhibit a naiveté which for the foreigner at least, is
difficult to understand.*
—Rudolph Rabe, M.D.

The inner psychological dimensions of leadership have been historically tied to the image of the hero. This champion typically is masculine,
aloof, all-powerful, mysterious, charismatic, lives on the edge of society and
stands for rugged individualism. Typically these individuals do not need
anyone else and perform on their own. Characters such as the Lone Ranger,
Dirty Harry and Rambo all reflect this image. Many great homeopaths of
the past also fit this archetypal role.

The heroic leader has a vision that is personal and guides his organization toward that vision. He must be extremely knowledgeable, possess
strength, display initiative, be courageous and have tenacity. He communi-
cates forcefully, aims to amass power and uses it for organizational improvement. He has a take-charge attitude and enjoys solving difficult problems.
A heroic leader is a lion who patrols the borders of the organization. He
absorbs and manages all the uncertainty that comes from the outside and
serves as a buffer so that others can remain undisturbed.

Although heroic leadership may have been sufficient in the past, this is
no longer productive for leadership in today's world. With the increasing
complexity and rapid change in today's world, problems can no longer be
solved by a single leader. Typically these savior/heroes are few and hard to
find. Because their contributions depend on who they are and their charisma, they typically are not lasting. Heroic leadership fosters dependency
on the part of its constituents.

There is likewise a shortage of leaders in homeopathy today and without
solid leadership, homeopathy cannot move forward as a dominant form of
healing. This is also true in school leadership roles in other professions.
Schools and organizations suffer when they demand too much of their leaders and too little of themselves. There is much role confusion for educational
leaders and it has been described as a time of transition (Cunningham 2000).

The types of leaders that are important to start a movement are very
different from the kinds of leaders who are needed to continue and grow

that movement. (Cronin, 1989). Homeopaths are typically very independent individuals. This has been a necessary characteristic in the leader who helps to break away from allopathic medicine and create the strong identity needed to survive in the face of the allopathic attacks and criticism. However, there comes a time when homeopaths must move beyond this, not for themselves but for homeopathy. Only in this way can homeopaths come together and form a unified profession.

Narcissism and Leadership

> *Are you one who carries a chip on his shoulder for those who do not see the homeopathic truth as you see it? Knock it off yourself immediately and forget it. Concentrate your thoughts on the truth of homeopathy as you have found it. Make it so vivid that all the world must get a vision but even then don't expect all to register it alike. When a ray of light is thrown upon a diamond it flashes back red or blue or gold, but the diamond remains steadfastly clear.*
> —F. E. Gladwin

The shadow of leadership is narcissism. Everyone knows an authority figure who abuses their power and control. These pseudo leaders are often more focused on themselves and their own needs than those of their constituents. They are filled with arrogance and greed for power and lack vision beyond themselves. These individuals typically tell rather than show and are unwilling to give up control. They put together teams that only reflect themselves and their ideas. Likewise, faculty and students must mirror them to survive. They must adapt to their leaders, rather than be themselves. Homeopathy is no different from any other profession in this way.

Narcissistic individuals become over identified with their own ideas and theories. They rigidly and fixedly follow their own belief system. They believe that they have the only correct way of perceiving truth and that all others are deluded and foolish. Students who learn from these paternalistic teachers and leaders end up feeling that their teacher is the greatest homeopath in the world and that there are no other teachers worth learning from. The intense prolonged nature of training lends itself to this type of experience.

The outgrowth of this is polarization, division, isolation and alienation for the homeopathic community. Some homeopathic schools have their own allegiances with too little trust and respect for each other. Homeopaths become unable to work together to build a homeopathic community.

There is little dialogue between homeopathic schools or their leaders. They may criticize each others work in unprofessional ways. Ultimately they recreate the situation in America around the turn of the century where political infighting among the various homeopathic factions helped lead to the decline of the homeopathic movement. NANHE is working actively within the educational community to address this situation (see Appendix D).

Towards a Homeopathic Vision of Leadership

Leadership is a relation rooted in community...
—Bolman and Deal

What is leadership that is homeopathic in nature? Homeopathic leadership is holistic, institutionalized and dispersed throughout an organization. There is a need for high performance shared leadership at every level of an organization, not just at the top levels. Single leaders become replaced by a leadership community where higher echelon leaders work to strengthen the community. Their ability to lead comes from the strength and sustenance of those around them.

Contemporary thinking is that leadership is no longer simply a quality of individuals, but also a quality of organizations and schools. Thompson sees leadership as something that flows through organizations, spanning levels of hierarchies (Thompson 1967). Rather than waiting for a heroic leader to come along and guide us to our homeopathic destiny, each of us must embrace leadership as part of our homeopathic journey.

With such leadership, the leader engages his constituents (students, teachers, staff and community) in a discussion of the quality of the training and makes a constant effort to help the organization grow through this process. The leader also models what needs to be done and the qualities of good leadership. He encourages constituents to evaluate his own work for quality, rather than evaluating it himself. The leaders helps to create an environment in which good leading, teaching and learning can flower. Finally he serves as facilitator for the constituents' homeopathic journeys.

This change in leadership philosophy implies moving from directing and controlling to facilitating, supporting and coordinating. It is also useful to focus on the unheroic side of leadership (Murphy 1999). Unheroic qualities such as acknowledging weakness, depending on others, surrendering or letting go and developing a shared vision are critical factors in becoming a good leader today.

The homeopathic challenge is ensuring that homeopaths individualize themselves while remaining a community. This requires the skills of good leadership.

Transformation and Meaning

There is no exercise better for the heart
than reaching down and lifting people up.
—John Andrew Holmes

Leaders are transformative agents (Murphy and Lewis 1999; Fullan 1993). In an alchemical way, they help to transmute that which is material and base (lead) into that which is energetic and profound (gold). They assist in realizing the inner potential and creative energies of that which is around them.

Leadership is not simply about doing. Leaders also must help provide meaning and understanding to those around them, as well as help others to find their own meaning. They work to keep others conscious and aware of where they are on their respective homeopathic journeys. They put organizations and individuals in touch with that which gives them passion and purpose.

This necessitates reaching out and connecting what is deepest inside the leader with what is deepest in each individual. Only in this way can there be a raising of consciousness and establishment of meaning. This requires courage, spirit and hope (Bolman and Deal 1995).

Resistance to Leadership

"Continue to work as we have done for such a long time, carry
on my mission; you know Homeopathy and you know how to
cure as well as I do." I replied: "But I am a woman, my body
has grown tired, my hair has become white under the strain of
this difficult work, I have well earned a little rest." "Rest!"
said Hahnemann and raised himself up in his bed, "Have I
ever rested? Forward, ever forward against the wind, struggle
against the strain, always cure and everywhere, and by con-
stantly curing you will compel justice to be done to you; cur-
rent opinion will support you respectfully after having opposed
you on your path."
—Melanie Hahnemann

Everyone has had negative experiences with leaders and administrators. This is particularly true of homeopaths who often have dealt with allopathic persecution and resistance from conventional organizations. Frequently these experiences become generalized to a point of distrust of all administration and leadership. There is a desire for rugged individualism, with the feeling, "let me just do it on my own with no interference."

Individuals often project their underlying unconscious feelings and attitudes onto their leaders. These are feelings that they cannot accept in themselves and must be seen outside in the world. The experience of leaders as "other" and "alien" to oneself encourages individuals to do this. These projections are often parental in nature. They seek a powerful figure to guide them and on whom they can lean. And yet they resent their dependency when they have given their power away.

Leaders are frequently initially idealized and then, once they cannot meet the high expectations of their constituents, they are devalued. There is a social prejudice that administration and leadership are for incompetents, someone who could not make it as a practitioner or teacher. This often causes behaviors where individuals will try to pull leaders down, trip them up or make them fail. These behaviors can be either conscious or unconscious. Some leaders react to this by hardening their hearts from the repeated attacks they experience. Others avoid leadership altogether because they fear these experiences.

The foregoing sections have focused on the philosophical aspects of educational leadership. The remainder of the chapter will examine more practical leadership issues.

Getting Started as a School Leader

A leader is a follower is a leader.
—Gertrude Stein

Not all good homeopathic leaders are practitioners or teachers. What is far more important is that they are homeopathic learners. They need to have a life-long commitment to learning.

Whether they recognize it or not, every school leader has some experience in leadership for every person gains leadership experience from life experience. To understand one's own leadership experience, begin with a review of one's life experience. Writing a one page statement of one's philosophy of leadership can be helpful. It often involves a process of careful self reflection. Important questions to ask include the following:

◎ What are the qualities of good leadership?

◎ What has been my experience as a follower? What makes a good follower?

◎ Are there leaders in my life that I particularly admire or dislike?

◎ What experiences were vital in my own development and were turning points in my life?

◎ How do organizations stifle or encourage their leaders?

◎ What are the values and ethics that have guided me as a leader?

This leadership review also requires self knowledge about one's strengths and weaknesses as a leader. Inevitably there are well-ingrained habits (obstacles to leading) that hold individuals back from leadership. These must be examined and resolved before the educational leadership journey can begin.

Another important step is the creation of an educational platform (Sergiovanni and Starratt 1998). This should be a one-page statement of one's philosophy of education comprising fundamental values and beliefs about educational development, the nature of learning and teaching and the purpose of education. Ideas that should be considered include the following:

◎ The goals of education
◎ The image of the teacher(s)
◎ The image of the learner(s)
◎ The image of the administrator(s)
◎ The preferred kind of pedagogy (teaching philosophy)
◎ The preferred school climate
◎ The preferred student, teacher, administrative interactions
◎ The value of the curriculum
◎ The significance of quality homeopathic education to homeopathy
◎ The ethics of oneself and one's community

The platform should then be compared to one's own behavior to determine how authentic their actions and philosophy are. Areas of disagreement should be explored and examined. This educational platform should be in general agreement with the mission, philosophy and goals of the school system in which they work.

A new concept in contemporary education is that of teacher-leaders (Lieberman, Saxl and Miles 2000). This represents an intermediate step between teaching and leadership. These individuals play leadership roles as teachers, supervisors and mentors. They work gradually into these leadership roles.

Mentorship can be a crucial aspect of leadership. Leaders are often isolated and alone. Pairing with a good mentor can be vital to assist in providing good feedback and fostering self reflection. Formal training programs in educational administration, reading on the subject of education and administration, attending conferences and attending school board meetings can also be helpful.

Ultimately there is no substitute for experience. This is the best teacher and the best method to become a leader.

Leading a Homeopathic Learning Organization

I took a good deal o' pains with his education sir;
let him run the streets when he was very young,
and shift for his-self. It's the only way to make a boy sharp, sir.
—Charles Dickens

A central task of the homeopathic educational leader is to build and manage a homeopathic learning organization (Senge 1990). This is a holding environment, a safe place where quality teaching and learning can occur. It is both a physical and a psychological environment. A leader helps to nurture this space, thereby allowing those within it to flourish and grow. A leader accomplishes this through being an example and facilitating the formation of a living culture in the organization (see the following). They create opportunities that allow energy (dynamis), information and the human spirit to flow within and through the system.

In learning, it is critical to have a safe place with minimal stress. In this environment, the student is comfortable with self discovery, which includes making mistakes, experimenting and creating. A leader helps to define the limits and boundaries to this space. They also assist the organization in reinventing itself over time.

The physical space is important, although less so than the psychological space. Successful schools have been held in very small, cramped spaces. The physical space should reflect the school's history and identity. Pictures of homeopaths, remedies, graduation, awards and certificates all can help to create an environment that solidifies this homeopathic identity.

The psychological space must feel safe and orderly. Effective school leaders are fierce protectors of a fragile psychological ecosystem. This is especially true of beginning, fledgling schools. There is an intricate web of interdependent relationships that the leader maintains (Lambert et al, 1995). These relationships include those with students, faculty, the homeopathic community, state political and governing agencies and other educational institutions. As the community grows, it becomes self renewing and takes on a life of its own, permitting the leader to gradually step back.

It's helpful to have the homeopathic community design and create the space. This gives it a feeling of ownership by the community and the space provides a bridge to the homeopathic community.

Characteristics of a Learning Environment

It is difficult to effectively lead a learning organization unless one is aware of the learning organization's unique characteristics.

Learning organizations are organic in nature. They are founded on the following principles:

◎ **Self Awareness**: One of the primary tasks of being the leader in a learning organization is to ensure that the organization knows itself. The leader helps the members of the organization stay in continuous dialogue about what it is and what it is becoming. This dialogue centers on leading, teaching and learning. The leader does this by helping others to challenge their assumptions and holding up mirrors to assist others in seeing themselves. The leader looks for patterns to explicitly identify and name the group process. The leader also does this by modeling self reflection on leadership, teaching and learning.

◎ **A Strong Homeopathic Community**: Central to building a learning organization is the presence of a strong homeopathic community that supports it (see below). There must be a commitment to nurturing both internal and external community. The leader helps to build a bridge between the external and internal homeopathic communities. This requires the establishment of a common language.

◎ **Systems Thinking**: It is vital that all members of the learning organization have skills in working together, as well as expertise in teaching and learning. Systems thinking helps individuals feel connected to a larger community and the world. It helps them to see how they create their reality and the effects of their actions. It also encourages meta-level learning where there is learning concerning how to learn together and teaching about teaching.

◎ **Encouraging Growth as Learners**: The leader in a learning organization encourages learning at all levels, from students and teachers to staff or other administrators (Beck and Murphy, 1996). It is important to move beyond the concept of learning only for the students. The leader serves as a model through constant self learning and self reflection. In this way, the leader can then help others to live their lives in the service of their aspirations. They also do this through personalizing learning and creating a diversity of learning opportunities. Good leaders instill in students, teachers and staff the self confidence that together they can learn whatever needs to be learned to accomplish the collective vision. It is a spirit of collaborative inquiry.

◎ **Encouraging Growth as Teachers and Leaders**: The leader focuses on resources aimed at building the capacity of people within the community to teach and lead. The leader encourages teachers to solve their own problems, rather than solving problems for the teachers. The leader encourages continuous, incremental and systemic improvement.

◎ **Building a Shared Vision**: A good leader does not dictate a vision to others, but works with others to develop a common shared ideal. This involves surrender and allowing the collective aspiration to be set free.

◎ **Team Learning**: Teams are the fundamental units in learning organizations. In many educational institutions, individuals may be quite intelligent whereas groups work at a very primitive level of understanding. Not only does individual growth and learning need to occur, but also team learning. The leader helps to ensure this by facilitating the growth of new knowledge throughout the organization and through the promotion of collegial feelings.

◎ **Humanism**: Leadership of a learning organization is by necessity humanistic. High priority is placed on initiative, valuing autonomy and freeing everyone to do their best and most creative work. This is a community of reciprocal care and shared responsibility, where each person's welfare and dignity is respected and supported (Kellogg Leadership Project Report entitled "Leadership in the Twenty First Century," 1997).

◎ **Self Management:** Leadership of a learning organization requires the promotion of self management and self organization. The process of self organization is a natural one that occurs in life from the smallest microbes to the evolution of the galaxy. In a learning organization, students, teachers and staff are encouraged to manage their own work. Research has shown that this markedly increases productivity.

Creation of a Culture

Like night dreams, stories often use symbolic language, therefore bypassing the ego and persona and traveling straight to the spirit and soul, who listen for the ancient and universal instructions embedded there. Because of this process, stories can teach, correct errors, lighten the heart and the darkness, assist transformation and heal wounds…The tales people tell one another weave a strong fabric that can warm the coldest emotional or spiritual nights. So the stories that rise up out of the group become, over time, both extremely personal and quite eternal, for they take on a life of their own when told over and over again.
—C. P. Estes

One of the central tasks of a school leader is assisting in the formation of a school culture (Schein 1985). This culture is based on facilitation, growth and mutual support. It embodies the accumulated wisdom of the community, including beliefs, assumptions and patterns. According to Bennis (1989), this culture can give an organization transformative powers to continuously improve itself.

School leaders help culture formation by facilitating shared stories, dreams and myths that carry the identity of the organization. Myth is a public dream, whereas a dream is a private myth. Without shared dreams, organizations falter and perish (Bolman and Deal 1995). Stories and myths help individuals to learn from their experiences by placing them in a shared context. Learning organizations need their own stories.

Leaders also identify and embrace the secret symbols of daily activities and rituals. Many of these are unconscious and taken for granted. They must be aware of the power of these elements.

Every class has its own personality and its own organic identity. Good administrators celebrate and honor each class's uniqueness.

Ceremonies and Celebrations

You have seen the fires of passion and hell,
My son, and now you arrive
Where I myself can see no further
I have brought you here by wit and by art.
You take as your guide your heart's true pleasure.
You have passed through the steep and narrow places
And now the sun shines bright upon your brow.
See around you the flowers and young grasses
which the soil of paradise grows.
Your eyes, whose weeping once brought me to you,
now shine far and full of bliss. I can go no further.
Expect from me no further word or sign
Your feel is right, and sound, and free.
To disobey it would be a fault.
Therefore, I give you yourself
Crowned and mitered, you are yours
                              —Danté

The beginnings and endings of the school year help school leaders to nurture the community and embrace and honor the participants. The ceremonies make transitions a collective experience and connect everyone to their common roots (Deal and Key 1998). Ceremonies weave together the past, present and future. They are how people summon and celebrate the power of the human spirit (Bolman and Deal, 1995). They help each participant to have courage in taking the next step on their homeopathic journey. Learning must be celebrated.

To engender enthusiasm and passion, celebrations and ceremonies must be authentic. They should be an integral, carefully planned part of the school community. It is not enough for a school to only celebrate at the time of graduation. Celebrations should be a part of every important milestone along the homeopathic journey. In this way, these celebrations become rites of passage. Milestones must be acknowledged not just for students, but also for faculty and staff (award banquets, retirement parties, holiday gatherings, etc.).

The journey is seldom embarked on alone. It is also important to honor students and faculty's loved ones who become a vital part of their educational process. These individuals support both the students and educators. Graduations and ceremonies provide opportunities to acknowledge this and express gratitude.

Every academic cycle begins with initiation. There are three parts to the initiation process (Gennep 1989). The first is separation. Here the student moves from the familiar into the unfamiliar. This involves embracing not knowing as a developmental step. The second phase is the threshold experience. This is the transformative part of the curriculum, which is often chaotic and timeless. This is a state of feeling betwixt and between. Students can bear witness to their experience through myth and ritual. Every homeopathic class develops its own myths and rituals over time. Retreats can be a powerful way of celebrating this stage (see below). The last phase is the incorporation stage. This is a time of healing and movement back into the everyday world.

It is also important to celebrate endings. Endings are particularly emotional, and include feelings of grief, fear, joy, excitement, relief and disappointment. It is important to draw people together at these times to mourn loss and renew hope. This is also one of the most important times to build community.

Retreats

Nothing gives rest but the sincere search for truth.
—Pascal

For several reasons, I have found that retreats are essential in a homeopathic training program. First, they provide an opportunity for students to pull back from the day-to-day grind of their studies and see where they are, where they have been and where they are going on their homeopathic journey. Second, retreats build community by bringing administration, students and faculty into one unified whole. Students have the chance to give feedback to the administrator(s) and the faculty in a more relaxed setting than the classroom. Third, retreats provide an opportunity to work on group process. They enhance students capacity to work in group environments, a skill that is quite important when they get into practice. Group process also facilitates a deepening of students' experience through listening and sharing with others. The sharing of group dreams (dreams about the group or about the educational process) can be a powerful technique. Group process is often emotional, yet can be a very rewarding experience for students. Fourth, retreats provide an opportunity to give feedback to the administrator(s) and the faculty in a more relaxed setting than the classroom.

Retreats can be optional or required, although they are more productive when the entire class attends. Typically these last for one day and occur once or twice per year. They are best held in a setting away from school or where classes normally meet in a more relaxed and intimate atmosphere. As a rule, co-led retreats are more successful than those with only one leader, as this more greatly facilitates group process. The leaders should establish a basic structure and generic guidelines, but otherwise the format can be loose. Most important is that the students should feel safe and comfortable in self expression. The preparation and sharing of meals together can also be an important aspect of retreats.

Critical incident review (Brookfield 1990) can be a powerful technique at retreats. It can help students understand and take control of their learning process. Important issues to explore include:

◎ The most rewarding and the least valuable educational moments in training

◎ Characteristics of good teachers and good students

◎ Students' new insights about effective teaching and learning

◎ The most painful and pleasurable aspects of training

◎ Moments when students desired to give up their training and what kept them going

◎ Moments when students first had the confidence to disagree with conventional wisdom

◎ Group-shared experiences, including myths, rituals and shared dreams

On Building a Strong Homeopathic Community

Community is a place where conflict can be resolved
without physical or emotional bloodshed and with wisdom
as well as grace. A community is a group that fights gracefully.
—M. Scott Peck

What is a homeopathic community? The word "community" is derived from the Latin word *communis*, which means "shared." A community is a group of people who get together to share a common interest. That interest, such as homeopathy, is larger than the individual. This sharing also includes a similar geography, shared set of rules, a common set of beliefs, values and customs, emotional bonds, a sense of obligation to fellow members and a shared sense of belonging.

We live in a global village. By coming together, a homeopathic community can flower and grow. The community can provide the structure that will allow expression of the spirit (dynamis) of homeopathy. It keeps alive the creative spark that is homeopathy.

What is the importance of a strong homeopathic community? Its presence will ensure that homeopathy will not falter for the future. It provides a resource and a place to renew one's inspiration and love for homeopathy. It keeps homeopathy vital and fluid in the community. It helps people remain fresh, current and inspired. Homeopathy has always been the "people's" medicine. It does not belong to any one group or faction of practitioners but to the entire world community.

Homeopathic study groups, clinics and schools often falter because they lack a strong community base. One of the problems with contemporary homeopathy is that too much attention has been focused on the later stages of development of the homeopathic community (e.g., schools) without creating the solid foundation and underpinnings of a strong homeopathic community. This would involve moving from a practitioner-centered growth model to a community-centered one. One of the reasons homeopathy is not growing as fast as other forms of alternative medicine is its lack of a strong homeopathic community.

The homeopathic community gives back to the practitioners through referring patients and providing support. It is this mutual give and take that allows each to grow. The practice of homeopathy can be an isolating experience. The community can help the practitioner stay connected. It also helps in the various stages of development in becoming a homeopath.

Homeopathic educational programs and leaders should work to develop and grow community (Kreisberg 1999). This requires school leaders to nurture cooperation between school and community and to promote face-to-face involvement within that community.

The Developmental Stages of a Homeopathic Community

Good company in a journey makes the way seem shorter.
—Italian Proverb

When is a community ready to open a school or to create a study group or to create conferences? It is important to only introduce a school into a community when the community is ready to sustain it. Otherwise the school will falter and fail.

What follows is a description of the stages of growth of a homeopathic community. It is an example of one model and certainly not all-inclusive. This model may be effective in certain areas of the world, but not in others. It represents a community- rather than practice-based model. There is a progression in this model, with each stage building on the last, although the order of some of the stages can be transposed (Rowe and Hesselmann 2001).

Stage 1: Introductory Talks

The most central step in the growth of homeopathic communities is the establishment of introductory talks (see Chapter Six). These can be held at various locations throughout the community. They are also one of the most important ways to help beginning practitioners establish a practice. The main task at this stage is to get the word "homeopathy" out to the public and to connect newcomers with practitioners.

Stage 2: Introductory Classes

One way to teach the beginner is to organize an introductory class, which deals with the basics of homeopathy. Newcomers often have trouble integrating into a beginning or intermediate study group. They need a basic foundation and language with which to understand what is being taught. The introductory classes can provide just such a grounding. There are two main objectives. The first is to provide a place where new homeopathic patients can immerse themselves in homeopathy, even if they are not interested in attending a study group. An understanding of homeopathy will help them to become better homeopathy patients. Happy patients will tell their friends, and the word will spread. The second objective is to bring the newcomers to a level where they can understand and participate in a beginning study group without feeling lost in terminology or immediately being too far behind. A benefit of the introductory class is that it provides a place for beginning-level practitioners to teach and practice their teaching.

Stage 3: Formation of a Beginning Study Group

Once a group of people have shown interest, they can hold a meeting with the goal of forming a study group. The leader should be someone who is knowledgeable about homeopathy and a good teacher. The leader must be willing to commit a fair amount of time to the teaching. A new group probably needs a minimum of six to twelve months of regular meetings to establish a foundation, both of the knowledge of homeopathy and for the group.

The leader develops a curriculum to keep the study group members interested and moving forward. Such a beginning program can repeat every one to two years, as required and as new members 'graduate' from the introductory sessions into more advanced stages. The beginning study group can provide a place where new practitioners teach. It can also become a resource center for the community.

Stage 4: Formation of a Newsletter and Website

A newsletter helps to keep study groups together by providing a common communication center. It provides a vehicle to let everyone know what is going on in the community. The newsletter should not be the sole responsibility of the editor. An interesting newsletter is best created by a team.

A website can also be a useful way for study group participants to work together. Newsletters can be published on the website, as well as calendars of local and national activities. Links can also be created to national websites.

Stage 5: Formation of an Intermediate Study Group

The next step is the formation of an Intermediate Study Group. The leader of the group can give deeper level lectures or enlist others who can. Intermediate programs can be ongoing and do not have to be repeated periodically, like the introductory and beginning material. Many study group members feel that they can move on to homeopathic schools after this step. Others chose to pursue more formal medical training such as a medical school, naturopathic school or nurse practitioner school. As they become students themselves, they also become candidates for teaching their homeopathic study groups. The intermediate study group also provides an opportunity for practitioners to hone their homeopathic teaching skills. It is important to have enough teachers to share the load to prevent teacher burnout.

It is also useful at this stage to have externally-based conferences with nationally or internationally known speakers. These conferences generate enthusiasm and inspire and encourage students to go to further stages. Students of homeopathy are exposed to more well-known speakers and new ideas. These conferences also generate income, which helps the community grow. Hosting conferences before this stage may be less successful.

Stage 6: Formation of an Advanced Study Group

The advanced study group is a place for practitioners and serious students to meet. Here, the level of instruction is turned up a notch. This is where difficult cases can be discussed and practitioners learn from each other's experience. The advanced study group provides a forum to notify the community of upcoming homeopathic events. Here also, community-wide planning of homeopathic activities can be done on a somewhat higher level.

This group can be the foundation for a speakers/teachers bureau that is available to teach community wide. A speakers bureau can be advertised to local community organizations, schools and hospitals. This is also an ideal stage for medical students, naturopathic students and medical residents to interface with homeopathy. Here they can see and hear cases in a supportive setting that is more tailored to their medical needs than the typical beginning or intermediate study group.

Stage 7: Community-Based Seminars and Conferences

A community-based seminar is quite different from an externally based (from outside the immediate homeopathic community) national or international speaker conducting a seminar. A community-based seminar does far more for building the homeopathic community. With the presence of a solid homeopathic community that becomes a base from which to draw attendees, it should be possible to launch a successful regional conference.

Community-based seminars offer a good opportunity for intermediate-level and advanced-level practitioners to teach. It is useful to have three components to these seminars: a newcomer program, a beginning-level program and an intermediate to advanced-level program. It is advisable to have a foundation of knowledge developed through work in the previous stages, before bringing in speakers or organizing expensive conferences.

This is also a good stage to introduce provings into the community. Provings offer an important way to bring a community together. They can demonstrate the heart of the homeopathic process and allow participants to experience homeopathy on a more visceral level.

Lastly, there are opportunities at this stage for connecting more to the regional level, and extending homeopathy to the far reaches of the region. Traveling introductory homeopathic programs can be created extending into various rural areas and undeveloped urban communities. From these programs, seed groups can be started which can then connect back to the central group.

Stage 8: The Homeopathic Center

At this stage, a physical structure is needed that is dedicated solely to homeopathy. It is important to have a central location. This also provides the study group a larger space in which to work and expand. This center can become the place where newcomers discover homeopathy, where classes are held, and where introductory/intermediate training programs are held. It can also house a homeopathic library and a homeopathic pharmacy.

Another important facet of this stage is supervision by experienced homeopaths, to meet the needs of the growing number of practitioners. This is an opportunity for students to present their case material and have the undivided attention of the experienced homeopath. The center also makes more easily possible clinical supervision, videotaping and video viewing by the supervisor, as well as informal curbside consultation with other practitioners and peers. The homeopath can ensure that nothing was overlooked and the student has the benefit of someone knowledgeable with whom to discuss the case.

At this stage, history becomes increasingly important. A common history has the powerful effect of bringing together a homeopathic community. The center can also house a homeopathic archive that contains the recorded history of the homeopathic community.

Stage 9: Clinical Training Program

Once a solid didactic program has been established, homeopathic clinic(s) become possible. These clinics provide more serious students with the opportunity to practice homeopathy under close supervision. They bridge the gap between didactic training and practice. The development of a clinical training program is a critical piece in the development of the homeopathic community.

The clinic environment provides an ideal place for medical students, residents and other practitioners in training to experience homeopathy first hand. There are more and more opportunities for homeopathic practitioners to work with allopathic practitioners, through allopathic hospitals, training programs and medical centers. Alternative medical centers and schools provide further community-building opportunities. Students at alternative schools are prime candidates for study group activities, either as students or teachers. Study group activities can also be held at the schools/centers as a way of supporting the organizations.

Conventional research in proving the validity of homeopathy becomes more possible at this stage. Clinics can be utilized as centers for research grants and centers for affiliation to universities.

Stage 10: Homeopathic Schools

This stage focuses on the establishment of a homeopathic school. The school can use the homeopathic clinic(s) as a base for homeopathic clinical teaching. Schools can affiliate with local teaching institutions, thereby further supporting the community.

A homeopathic foundation becomes important at this stage. Funding through donations can support the school with scholarships and can help to promote homeopathic research.

Creating a school broadens the connection to homeopathy to a national level, and provides a place for advanced-level practitioners to teach. Again, it is important that there be sufficient community support before undertaking a school or it will falter over time. Many new homeopathic schools are springing up and it is no longer as feasible to draw students from distant locations. Increasingly students are selected from within the local, homeopathic community.

Stage 11: Certification/Licensure

Once the homeopathic community is strong enough, political action becomes possible. At this point there can be movements toward homeopathic licensure and the creation of homeopathic boards. Homeopathic certification becomes increasingly important as it helps the public differentiate the quality of the practitioner's practice (see Appendix J). Licensure is available in some states and confers the legal right to practice.

At this stage, it is important to recognize achievement in the homeopathic community through honors and awards. This is a way for the homeopathic community to give something back to its members.

Homeopaths can also begin to serve in the worldwide community through international organizations such as Homeopaths Without Borders. Here there are increasing opportunities to interface with the media through television and radio. This can seed the earlier stages of community development. Ideally, a full-time marketing person is enlisted at this stage.

Stage 12: Formation of Homeopathic Hospitals/ Nursing Homes

At this stage, it is possible to form homeopathic hospitals and nursing homes. There are increasing international connections with opportunities for teaching and mutual collaboration, such as international symposiums. It is also at this stage that homeopathy can take a more proactive approach towards public-health policy, including public-health clinics and free clinics.

Creation of Partnerships

It takes an entire village to raise a child.
—African Proverb

A critical step in school success is the creation of alliances and partnerships (Cordero and Loup 1996; Gardner 1983; Jehl and Kirst 1992). These partnerships connect the school to the homeopathic community, as well as to the larger community. They allow pooling of resources and mutual growth. Important to the success of partnerships are leadership, trust, stability, good communication and a common agenda (Cordeiro and Monroe-Kolek 1996).

Partnerships are either school-linked or school-based. They can be between people or organizations or agencies. These include partnerships with the homeopathic community, alternative medicine community, allopathic community, governmental agencies, nonprofit agencies, higher-education institutions, education-related organizations, the virtual community, social/ ethnic organizations, media, business, industry and social-service agencies.

Good leaders must find ways of balancing the inner and outer community work. They are the living link between the school community, the professional community and the community at large. The danger is that administrators can find themselves so overwhelmed with outer tasks, that they lose touch with the school community.

Ethics

Out beyond ideas of right-doing and wrong-doing
there is a field. I'll meet you there.
—Rumi

Ethical leadership is critical to the formation of an ethical learning community. It is also essential in the formation of successful leaders (Badaracco and Ellsworth). The skills of ethical leadership can be developed (Mertz 1997; Shapiro and Stefkovich 1997; Duke and Grogan 1997; Craig 1999). The two basic principles of ethics, "Do all you have agreed to do and do not encroach on other persons or their property," are especially important in leadership positions (Mayburry 1993, p. 31). A school that goes back on its promises to its students or creates an environment that is not respectful of its students' space will soon find itself closing its doors.

Most important, to build an ethical community leaders must be ethical themselves (Fullan, 1993). They must come from a place of authenticity. They must attend to their own moral development and have the courage to be honest and the humility to change. This involves self-reflection, awareness, dialogue amongst the community members and modeling of good ethical behavior. Another aspect of this is that relations between teachers and between teachers and administration must be collegial and reflect the values of the school and learning community.

One model of ethical leadership involves three ethics that must be followed. These are the ethic of caring, the ethic of justice and the ethic of critique (Staratt 1986 and 1994).

Ethic of Caring

This is concerned with the confirming of others and is focused on relationships. These relationships include connections to each other, to patients, to the community, to the environment and to the world. Effective leaders must develop the attitudes and skills necessary to sustain caring relationships. Ultimately this leads to transcendence in connecting to something greater than themselves. Important aspects include:

◉ **Working for the Good of All**: Ethical school leaders make the well being of students the fundamental consideration of their decisions and actions. They avoid using their position for personal gain through political, social, religious or economic influence.

◉ **Fostering Learning Together**: Ethical leaders help the community to move away from competitive learning to shared learning.

◉ **Community Service**: Ethical leaders understand the importance of learning and teaching through service. Service learning requires that students serve their communities as a fundamental part of their education.

Ethic of Justice

This ethic focuses on equity and fairness in relation to individual and community. Administrators must serve as advocates for their students, teachers and staff. Important aspects include:

◉ **Respect**: These leaders see the interrelationship of everyone in the school community and treat them with respect and dignity. They fulfill their professional responsibilities with honesty and integrity. They honor diversity and majority/minority interests.

◎ **Ownership**: Ethical leaders are personably accountable. They encourage students and teachers to feel that they have a stake in their program. Ethical leaders are also loyal to their community and stand by them through the problems and conflicts that arise.

◎ **Obeying Laws**: Ethical leaders obey local and state laws, while working to correct those laws and policies that are not consistent with good educational goals.

◎ **Due Process**: Ethical leaders support the principle of due process and protect the civil and human rights of all individuals.

◎ **Honoring Contracts**: Ethical leaders honor all contracts until fulfillment. They keep their promises.

Ethic of Critique

The ethic of critique fosters critical thinking, which questions the basic assumptions and the framework of the way one thinks and organizes one's life. This allows students, teachers and administrators to open their hearts, minds and spirit. Important aspects include:

◎ **Encouraging Diverse Perspectives**: An ethical leader helps communities explore issues from diverse perspectives, such as feminism, post-modernism and critical theory.

◎ **Self-Reflection**: Self-reflection is critical to self-awareness. Self-reflection entails the writing of an ethical platform or including this as part of the leader's educational platform. Comparing and contrasting ethical codes of conduct from a variety of sources is an important part of this process.

◎ **Strong Goals**: Without clear and consistent goals, schools founder. Leaders must not just do things right, they must do the right thing. They must pursue excellence in all its forms.

When Does a Leader Become a Student?

The true leader is always led.
—Carl Jung

The educational journey moves full circle as the leader becomes the student once again. The leader lets go of their creations to make room for new learning. This helps the leader to renew oneself and the organization.

Leaders must become committed lifelong learners. This requires a certain degree of humility. Good leaders experience, model, display and celebrate what is expected from their teachers and pupils. This is especially true in learning from those one would like to silence. It is important for a school leader to surround himself with individuals who do not just espouse the leader's views but who question and challenge those views.

Leadership Renewal

Success is a journey, not a destination.
—Ben Sweetland

There is very little available in the homeopathic community that helps to support its leaders. There is a need for leadership for leaders, creating the conditions where leaders can flourish. This process begins with an awareness of the importance of homeopathic leadership and mutual support. Mentorship is a critical part in nurturing the growth of new leaders. Ultimately this will require the establishment of conferences and leading centers where leaders can go for inspiration and renewal (Covey 1997).

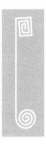

Chapter Nine

Stewardship of a Homeopathic Training Program

O, it is excellent to have a giant's strength,
but is tyrannous to use it like a giant.
—William Shakespeare

Stewardship is management at its best. Stewardship means holding something in trust. Block describes it as "the willingness to be accountable for the well being of the large organization by operating in service, rather than in control of those around us…Its underlying value is about deepening our commitment to service." (Block, 1993)

Great administrators are stewards of their organizations. These administrators have an underlying ownership and responsibility to their organization. They are chosen by the people with whom they work. This has been described as servant leadership (Greenleaf 1970).

Before discussing the intricacies of stewardship, it is important to understand the current trends in homeopathic education.

Overview of Homeopathic Schools in North America

He who thinketh he leadeth but hath no one following him
is only taking a walk.
—Anonymous

In May 1998, Kreisberg and Phelps did an extensive survey of North American homeopathic schools, called *Trends in Homeopathic Education: A Survey of Homeopathic Schools in Northern America*. They distributed their questionnaire to 36 schools, with 23 responding (64 percent). At the time of the survey the schools had graduated a collective 650 students. Kreisberg and Phelps obtained the following additional results:

◎ 17 percent of the schools had graduated between 1-20 students;
22 percent between 20-50 graduates;
13 percent between 50-100 graduates;
10 percent more than 100 graduates

◎ 61 percent of the schools had been established in the last ten years

◎ There was virtually no alumni follow-up by any of the schools

◎ 78 percent only focused on homeopathy

◎ 60 percent had some type of governmental recognition (i.e. licensure)

◎ 60 percent were non-profit

◎ 30 percent were identified as postgraduate programs only for licensed health professionals; of the remaining programs, typically there was a ratio of five to one unlicensed to medical personnel

◎ 61 percent required at least one research project

◎ Library facilities were available at 56.5 percent of facilities

◎ 13 percent had only one professor;
56.5 percent had between 2-5 faculty;
22 percent had 6-9 instructors;
8.5 percent had 10 or more teachers

◎ 52 percent have advisory or governing boards

◎ Nearly all the programs were weekend-seminar based, averaging one weekend per month: 8 percent were less than two years in length; 22 percent trained students for two years; 35 percent were three year programs; 35 per cent took four years to complete training

◎ Total Hours: 22 percent of programs had 200-400 hours; 22 percent had 400-600 hours; 22 percent had 600-800 hours

◎ Student Body: 56.5 percent had less than 50 students enrolled; 17 percent had between 50-100 students; 13 percent had between 100-150 students; 13 percent had more than 150 students

◎ 70 percent of programs spent 75 percent of curriculum time in lecture; 25 percent spent 50 percent of curriculum time in lecture

◎ 25 percent offered no clinical supervision

Homeopathic programs are well known for having short lives before they fold. What was not included in the survey were the many programs that had started and stopped in the preceding decades. The above survey gives an indication of the current state of training. There is much that needs to be done to improve the quality of training programs in North America. The remainder of this chapter examines some of the critical issues that are necessary to improving this quality.

Certification and Licensure

> *To begin with, the highest and strictest standard of home-*
> *opathy must be established and tested thoroughly in the*
> *arena of actual clinical results. To this end, teachers must*
> *be trained thoroughly to the highest standards. These teach-*
> *ers, with the help of the finances and talents of an inter-*
> *ested public, can then establish full time schools for the*
> *training of homeopathic prescribers. The very professional-*
> *ism and clinical successes of these schools should be able to*
> *overcome the inevitable political and legal resistance to the*
> *emergence of a new profession...*
> —George Vithoulkas

A critical factor in the growth of homeopathic education is the certification and licensure of homeopathic schools. Certification is an indicator of quality of practice, whereas licensure confers the legal right to practice.

Currently in North America, licensure is only on the state level and only 50 percent of training programs are licensed (see previous section). Certification in North America is through the Council for Homeopathic Education (see Appendix B). Only a few schools are currently certified in North America. The certification process, however, is a vital step in the establishment of a homeopathic profession. Only through national certification can homeopathic education begin to be recognized as legitimate.

Creating a Faculty

> *A man who knows a subject thoroughly, a man so soaked in it that he eats it, sleeps it and dreams it-this man can always teach it with success, no matter how little he knows of technical pedagogy.*
>
> —H. L. Mencken

Creating a faculty requires careful planning. In hiring faculty, one of the central questions is whether the school offers one teacher or many. A disadvantage of a single-faculty program is that this encourages dependency and discipleship and prevents diversity. It also makes critical thinking for students more difficult.

The disadvantage of multiple-faculty programs is that coordination in teaching can be difficult, causing unnecessary repetition. Diversity can also create cognitive dissonance in students that stems from multiple perspectives. This can result in confusion.

The challenge in assembling a diverse faculty is to allow differing styles of teaching (see Chapter Three) while preserving the same core philosophical tenets. School directors seeking diversity encourage students and faculty to find their own style, rather than creating carbon copies. It is also important to have a balance between male and female faculty. This balance helps to prevent polarization between students and faculty and provides a more rich tapestry of experience.

A distinction can be made between core faculty and adjunct faculty. Core faculty must be more available to the students and provide both mentorship and supervision. Adjunct faculty simply come to teach and have little responsibilities outside of this. Often they come from further away.

Clinical faculty are particularly difficult for institutions to find. It is difficult for schools to adequately reimburse faculty for clinical training. Clinical training is often volunteer based, and it is difficult for volunteers to sustain a commitment over time.

Faculty and Staff Management

*I find the three major administrative problems
on a campus are sex for the students, athletics for the alumni,
and parking for the faculty.*
—Clarke Kerr

Faculty and staff need strong leadership from the school director and administration. Administrators need to provide clear and consistent feedback to the students, staff and teachers. Student evaluations, classroom visits, review of videotapes of classroom activities and the expectation of faculty development are all important in this regard. Regular faculty meetings can be very helpful. These meetings can utilize teaching consultants or be based on a series of focused facilitated exercises.

Handling problematic faculty can be a challenge. It is important to clearly document any problems before taking remedial action. Teacher problems are sometimes better handled by other teachers than by heavy-handed administrative action. It is best to avoid quick fixes, but provide support as the faculty work it out among themselves, when possible.

Palmer describes a useful model where four individuals (usually faculty) focus on one teacher's problem, creating a clearness committee (Palmer 1998). The teacher first writes a few pages about the problem, including a clear statement of the nature of the problem, its relevant background and foreground. The committee meets for two to three consecutive hours, giving undivided attention to the teacher. Participating members are forbidden to speak to the person in any way except through open-ended questions. This helps to strip away the layers and allow the teacher to listen to the teacher within. The participants may not speak about the meeting afterwards. This model can be tremendously productive in focusing, clarifying and resolving faculty issues.

Faculty and Staff Development

*Was putting a man on the moon actually easier
than improving teachers and education in our public schools?*
—B. F. Skinner

Administrators think constantly about teacher and staff development. They work to identify with the needs of each member of the school community. Staff development can take many forms including individualized development plans, in service training, workshops, independent study, college-level courses, networking or conferences. The creation of homeopathic learning centers, teaching centers and leading centers (virtual or reality based) is part of this process. These centers provide a source for renewal and inspiration.

Good administrators, like good mentors, not only help members of the community develop within their current roles, but also assist them in moving from one role to the next. This includes assisting students in moving into teacher roles and teachers in moving into leadership roles.

It is important for the administrator to support not only individual learning and growth but also team learning and organizational learning (Cunningham 2000). Teams learn in different ways and at different rates than individuals. Good team building requires periodic group activities to be effective.

Choosing a Program Structure

There never were, in the world, two opinions alike,
no more than two hairs, or two grains;
the most universal quality is diversity.
—Montaigne

Currently, a variety of program designs and educational models exist, ranging from short, introductory programs to extensive, four year, full-time schools. Ultimately all programs must embrace three principles: training for practice, personal growth and development of community. In North America, nearly all programs are currently structured as one weekend a month for two to four years (Kreisberg and Phelps 1998). The advantage of this approach is that students have the time to study independently during the month and can adequately prepare for class. In addition, this model allows an individual to support themselves financially during their training.

It is also important that schools train their students to effectively sit for national certification exams. Minimum standards for nearly all North America certification boards include a minimum requirement of 500 hours of training (see Appendix J).

Schools must be individualized. School certification boards should honor the individuality of schools. It is difficult to bring a school from one location to another and expect to duplicate the school structure. Each school needs to make allowances for locale, culture and community.

Choosing a Learning Approach

Men must be taught as if you taught them not,
And things unknown proposed as things forgot.
—Alexander Pope

Before a school can even approach the issue of curriculum design they must develop a basic learning approach. This is also called learning transfer (Detterman 1993 and Sternberg and Frensch 1993). A learning approach attempts to create the optimum learning conditions for learning transfer to occur. It should also create the optimum conditions for good teaching.

New schools are often expected to provide more learning options for their students. They are required to be creative and willing to experiment with new ideas in teaching and learning. Many new programs are arising where students teach each other—creatively and interactively. For more information see: www.aasa.org/reform.approach.htm. Some examples of learning approaches include constructivism, apprenticeship, thematic learning, accelerated schools, essential schools, success-focused schools and critical teaching.

Constructivism: The constructivist view of learning is that individuals learn best when they actively acquire knowledge through exploration. Learning is an active process, where individuals construct knowledge rather than receiving it. New knowledge is acquired when an interaction occurs between one's existing knowledge and new situations that the individual encounters.

Apprenticeship: Traditionally homeopathy has been taught primarily through an apprenticeship model. This is one of the oldest models of learning and requires situational learning in context. Key factors include witnessing, attuning, imitating, helping, collaboration, interacting, experimenting, transmitting and investigating (Moffett 1994). Apprenticeship at its best is mentorship.

Thematic Learning: Thematic learning requires integration of many disciplines brought to bear on a central problem, theme, issue, topic or experience (Cunningham 2000). Here, learning is not by course, such as materia medica, history or repertory, but is woven together into one bright tapestry that is interdisciplinary and synthetic.

Accelerated Schools: Accelerated schools (Brandt 1992) give their students a great deal of autonomy and responsibility in learning. The students are actively involved through open-ended problem solving and hands-on activities. Students work in teams and receive constant feedback from other students. Fundamental principles include unity of purpose, empowerment, responsibility and capacity building.

Essential Schools: Essential schools feel that curriculum should be much simpler. Homeopathic schools that utilize this approach may teach fewer remedies, but in much greater depth. Teaching emphasizes problem solving over rote learning. The curriculum helps students connect with the community and is future focused (Sizer 1996).

Success-Focused Schools: Success-focused schools center on the success of every student (Slavin 1996). Success can be measured in many ways including effectiveness on national certification and licensure examinations. Each school must weigh its relative focus on preparing students for these exams versus teaching students what they need to know to effectively practice as a homeopath. Successful schools can accomplish both.

Critical Teaching: Critical teaching arises from critical theory. This refers to "a deliberate attempt to construct an environment through which educators and students can think critically about how knowledge is produced and transformed in relation to the construction of experience informed by a particular relationship between the self, other, and the larger world" (Giroux 1992). Here the focus is more on learning how to learn.

Liberal Learning

> *I believe a liberal education is an education in the root meaning of liberal—liber, "free"—the liberty of the mind free to explore itself to draw itself out, to connect with other minds and spirits in the quest for truth. Its goal is to train the whole person to be at once intellectually discerning and humanly flexible, tough minded and open hearted, to be responsive to the new and responsible for values that make us civilized. It is to teach us to meet what is new and different with reasoned judgment and humanity. A liberal education is an education for freedom, the freedom to assert the liberty of the mind to make itself new for the other minds it cherishes.*
> —Giamatti

Liberal learning is study that fosters openness and self reflection in the search for truth. Liberal learning helps students grow not just as homeopaths, but also as individuals. It fosters critical thinking skills, provides students with an emotional, intellectual and social context, helps students to question themselves and their values, encourages students to adapt to a changing world and assists them to communicate effectively with others.

Liberal learning capitalizes on a liberal education, although it is not a collection of required courses or prerequisites.

Traditionally liberal learning and professional studies have been taught in different kinds of institutions (Bratchell and Heald 1966). Yet liberal learning is the responsibility of all who teach. Increasingly, professional organizations have agreed on the importance of liberal learning for those entering their professions (Armour and Furhmann 1993). They also have agreed on the importance of liberal learning within their professions in developing the capacity to analyze, problem solve, communicate, synthesize and integrate knowledge from various disciplines (National Institute of Education Report 1984).

Problem-Based Learning

Never believe on faith, see for yourself!
What you yourself don't learn, you don't know.
—Bertolt Brecht

Students ultimately practice in problem-oriented environments but generally learn in subject- or discipline-oriented environments. Problem-based learning (PBL) is loosely centered on the concept of cooperative learning (Slavin 1990 and Steven and Slavin 1995). Here, the focus is on collaboration. Students serve as teachers for each other and typically work in teams of four to five individuals.

Problem-based learning is an instructional approach used increasingly in medical education (Bridges and Hallinger 1995). It also has expanded into many other forms of education (Bridges and Hallinger 1995; Boud and Feletti 1998). It uses a tutorial format and begins with a practical problem that the student is likely to encounter in the "real" world of practice. Problems are chosen to illustrate core concepts in the school curriculum and typically are open ended. Often these are written cases, live cases or simulated patient presentations. Students must identify the problems in the case, formulate tentative hypotheses, identify learning needs, access resources, pursue the implications of their hypotheses, reformulate the problem and come up with a plan of action.

Students are given considerable responsibility and autonomy for directing their learning. Learning is done in dyads or small teams of ideally six to seven students. Students demonstrate their learning through a project or direct evaluation of their performance. Through this process, students gain skills in self direction, reasoning, problem solving and collaboration. Ultimately, they gain a feeling of what it is like to be a practitioner.

The key points for problem-based learning are as follows:

◎ The starting point for learning is a problem.

◎ The problem is one that students are likely to experience as a professional.

◎ The knowledge that students are expected to acquire during their professional training is organized around problems rather than subjects.

◎ Students assume a major responsibility for their own instruction and learning.

◎ Most of the learning occurs within the context of small groups, and lectures are seen as supplemental.

The teacher has a different role in PBL. They serve more as a facilitator, a cross between a mentor and a teacher. They challenge their students through questioning designed to stimulate their thinking and their assumptions. These teachers support their students by helping to foster a feeling of collegiality and creating a nurturing and supportive environment. They work to build each student's capacity for learning.

Teachers who use problem-based learning methods encourage diversity and self reflection. They model effective listening techniques, group process skills and communication skills, while ensuring that the group stays focused on the task. They encourage individuals to take ownership in the process by knowing when to keep quiet and when to intervene. The teachers demonstrate learning alongside their students. Lastly, they direct group members to resources both within and outside the group.

Groups typically take on roles of recorder, process observer and manager. They create ground rules before beginning to work together and agree on a process to use. This helps to teach students how to effectively collaborate, a skill that will be vital once they begin practicing. Students typically rush to solve the problem without fully understanding it or try to incorporate a solution into their initial understanding of the problem. The teacher must refocus them on the larger task.

Homeopathic Curriculum:
A United States Historical Perspective

> *The ebbing vitality of homeopathic schools is a striking dem-*
> *onstration of the...incompatibility of science and dogma...It*
> *will be clear, then, why, when outlining a system of schools*
> *for the training of physicians on scientific lines, no specific*
> *provision is made for homeopathy. For everything of proved*
> *value in homeopathy belongs of right to scientific medicine*
> *and is at this moment incorporated in it...*
> —*The Flexner Report*, 1910

Once the optimal learning conditions are created and the basic teaching and learning approaches are identified, the school can turn toward the curriculum. It is valuable to first have some understanding of the history of curriculum development in American medical schools.

Curriculum reform in medical education demonstrates a pendulum swing from a linear, technical rationality (Dinham and Stritter 1986) to reflective practice models, also called deliberative curriculum theory (Harris 1986). By the turn of the century there were approximately 22 homeopathic colleges in the United States. In 1909 the Carnegie Foundation commissioned Abraham Flexner to visit all the medical schools in the country. He prepared an 850-page report entitled *Medical Education in the United States and Canada*, which lambasted the status of homeopathic - education in the United States (see Appendix H). He criticized their inadequate facilities and lack of quality clinical training. The status of homeopathic schools was already in disarray at that time and the report only worsened this process (Cooke). More important, he recommended a specific program for medical schools to follow based on the Johns Hopkin's model, which focused on a basic science format for the first two years of training. He also helped to create state board licensure and competency evaluations.

Ironically, what came to be known as the Flexner Report did far less damage to homeopathy than it did to allopathic medicine. What followed was nearly a full century of medical training that was academic in orientation and prepared students poorly for practice. The Flexner Report de-emphasized practice and focused on technical research. It promoted schools where teaching was divorced from practice. Schools of medicine began to be moved into the research universities and the scientific component of medical education was greatly increased (Jencks and Riesman 1977). This movement inspired other professions to follow suit, with Reed's report on legal education in 1921 and Gies's report on dental education in 1926.

These movements have had lasting affect across professional education and the structure of the professions (Rice and Richlin 2000). The keystone of a professionally oriented society became the modern university (Parsons 1968). The task of the academic professional is the pursuit of cognitive truth. Pursuit of knowledge became organized by discipline and ultimately specialization and sub specialization. Scholarship increasingly became independent and prior to practice. Training focused on the mind, leading to increasing intellectualization, reductionism, loss of spirit and loss of heart. Palmer describes this as the "death-dealing energies of contemporary education" (Palmer 1998).

There have been occasional signs of this changing. In the 1950s, Case Western Reserve University organized its pre clinical curriculum around organ systems through interdisciplinary presentations (Williams 1980). In the mid- 1960s McMaster University Medical School in Canada and Michigan State University went to a problem-based curriculum (Barrows and Tamblyn 1980; Barrows 1985). Other medical schools have begun to follow suit, most notably Harvard Medical School. Overall, however, there has been little change.

Creating Curriculum

First we shape our institutions,
and afterwards they shape us.
—Winston Churchill

Curriculum design is one of the most controversial areas of homeopathic education. What makes it problematic is the diversity of approaches with respect to curriculum content. Ultimately, each school must choose its own content, which is in part determined by local, national and international standards. In addition it is critical that the school and the homeopathic community pinpoint its basic philosophy. Without this, the curriculum is not grounded and floats without direction. Each school must determine how focused they will be on meeting standards versus their core philosophical approach, which often contradict one another. What is essential is that what is most important to the homeopathic community drive the curriculum design.

Another challenge in designing curriculum is the varying levels of students. Many programs have students with varying levels of knowledge at the outset of the training. By the end of the program, students generally catch up to each other. For the more advanced students, it is helpful to design the beginning of programs to offer something that is both interesting and challenging.

In creating a curriculum, it is useful to have a team (Harris 1991). This should include faculty, as it is critical for faculty to be enthusiastic about the content they teach. It is also important to have participants from the homeopathic community.

Curriculum design is a complex task and it is easy to miss critical steps if there's not considerable feedback from students, faculty and the homeopathic community. The challenge is to create a certain uniformity of basic concepts and requirements without destroying curiosity and creativity. Reviewing curricula from other schools can be helpful, but ultimately each school must determine its own curriculum.

Not all homeopathic education is designed to train homeopaths. There are some students that choose to serve homeopathy in other ways (e.g. research, writing, public speaking). Good leaders need to communicate that it is possible to serve homeopathy without being a practitioner. Schools also have a responsibility to train their students to become good homeopathic learners, teachers and leaders. Curriculum needs to reflect this.

There is also a difference between being a successful homeopathic prescriber and a successful homeopath. Brilliant prescribers can be poor healers and good healers can be poor prescribers. Good homeopaths are complete healers, considering all aspects of a case and utilizing all available tools (Sankaran 1996). Homeopathic students must be trained to be not only homeopaths but effective healers as well.

Tanner

According to Tanner, there are five types of content for curricula design (Tanner and Tanner 1995):

- ◉ **Specific Education:** Designed toward training someone to become a homeopath.

- ◉ **General Education:** Geared toward connecting specific education with other fields of endeavor.

- ◉ **Enrichment Education:** Avocational, but enriches and broadens one's life. Much of mentorship falls into this category.

- ◉ **Exploratory Education:** Education that pushes the student to explore beyond the known and their limits.

◎ **Special-Interest Education:** Provides an intense learning experience beyond the needs of vocational and avocational pursuits. Research projects and theses often fall into this category.

Doll

Doll (1986) also describes five types of curriculum design:

◎ **Subject Design:** Stresses content

◎ **Interest Design:** Based on needs and interests of students (PBL)

◎ **Process Design:** Emphasizes learning how to learn and thinking skills

◎ **Social Activity Design:** Highlights social and community issues

◎ **Competency Design:** Represented by behavioral objectives and descriptions; this is a curriculum based on standards and meeting specific behavioral objectives.

Eisner

Eisner describes three types of curricula (Eisner 1991):

◎ **Explicit:** Curriculum in the conventional sense

◎ **Implicit:** What is taught at the school but never overt. It is "what it teaches because it is the kind of school it is" (Eisner, 1994 p. 97).

◎ **Null:** What is not taught. This can be just as important as what is taught. It is similar to the Japanese concept of the "ma." In Japanese gardens, the ma is that part of the garden that is empty and formless, yet has a critical role in defining and creating the garden.

Issues of Curriculum

There are many important decisions to be made in curriculum design. These can be summarized through the following issues: level; integration; breadth; organization; development; balance; intensity; mentorship; clinical training; preparation for practice; flexibility; options; medical training; research; and pauses.

◎ **Level:** At what level of training is the curriculum targeted (see Chapter Three)? For example, how much of the curriculum focuses on acute versus constitutional prescribing?

◎ **Integration:** How integrated should the curriculum be? Should home-opathy be taught through different subjects in a lecture format or through more interactive learning, such as a problem-based approach?

◎ **Breadth:** Is the curriculum designed to cover the entire materia medica or a few remedies in great depth? What is the process by which remedies are chosen (i.e. based on philosophy or certification and standards)? How diverse should the training be? Should the teacher teach the overall gestalt or focus on all the details? Is the program balanced between essential knowledge and special interests?

◎ **Organization:** How is the curriculum organized? Is the order of remedies presented randomly, alphabetically, miasmatically, patho-logically, by families or using another concept?

◎ **Development:** Are there certain concepts that must be taught first? Are there certain ideas that should be left for last? Are there any topics that must have foundational grounding before being taught? Are there cer-tain topics that must be taught inductively versus deductively?

◎ **Balance:** Is everything around a particular concept taught at once, or is this spread out over time? For example, is ethics taught at only one point during the curriculum or is it integrated into the curriculum?

◎ **Intensity:** How do you fit everything in that needs to be taught? Is there enough time for everything without making the program too intense? How long should the program be?

◎ **Mentorship:** What type of mentorship experience has been designed into the curriculum? Is adequate time designated for these experiences?

◎ **Clinical Training:** What part of the curriculum is clinical training? How much time is devoted? How is the clinical training designed (i.e. supervision, observation and clinical teaching environments)? How is clinical training integrated with didactic training?

◎ **Preparation for Practice:** Does the curriculum help prepare stu-dents for practice? How much of the curriculum is theoretical versus experientially based? What is missing in this preparation?

◎ **Flexibility:** Is there any room in the curriculum for flexibility? Is there room to teach special areas at the request of the students?

◎ **Options:** Are there program options available to the students? Is the curriculum responsive to the special needs of the students, such as gender issues or multi-culturalism?

- ◎ **Medical Training:** What part of the curriculum is reserved for medical training or review? Is this part of the curriculum, a prerequisite or a concurrent requirement to be obtained elsewhere?

- ◎ **Research:** Will research projects or theses be a required part of the curriculum? Are there any provisions for community research projects? What opportunities are there for students to participate in ongoing research at the school? How are faculty and administrators modeling research practices and research involvement?

- ◎ **Pauses:** Self reflection and pauses are critical to the learning process. What types of pauses and rhythms are designed into the curriculum? Are there retreats scheduled? Are there celebrations and ceremonies that are part of the curriculum, other than graduation?

Curriculum Improvements

If you want to truly understand something, try to change it.
—Kurt Lewin

Curriculum design is a complex and multi-faceted process. Ultimately, a series of compromises must be made to meet all the varying needs. Once the curriculum has been settled, then curriculum improvement begins. This is a constant and never-ending process of renewal. Many schools put considerable attention and energy into curriculum design, but fail to reevaluate the curriculum over time. Curriculum should be reviewed periodically, as well as in response to issues that arise during the program. It is important that curriculum be regularly compared to current educational standards and to any change in the fundamental philosophy and orientation of the program.

Surveys show that more than two-thirds of organizational changes fail (Wheatley 1992). The most frequent reason for failure is lack of communication within the organization (Sizer 1996). Ultimately the most effective improvements in schools come from people improvements (staff development). Factors that are crucial to the success of school improvements include (Fullan 1993):

- ◎ **Goal Focus:** Everyone must share the same goals and mission.

- ◎ **Effective Communication:** This needs to occur at all levels of the organization.

- ◎ **Resource Utilization:** Resources must be obtained and used effectively.

◎ **Cohesiveness**: Members of the organization should work together and be part of the team.

◎ **Morale**: There is a positive morale and a wish to grow together.

◎ **Innovative**: There is an excitement and willingness to change.

◎ **Autonomy**: This reflects how the organization maintains its internal structure when faced with outer stress and pressures.

◎ **Adaptation**: There is a flexible ability to handle stress and to adapt to change.

School Governance

In the first place God made idiots.
This was for practice.
Then he made school boards.
—Mark Twain

Many homeopathic schools currently do not have a governing board or advisory board (see *Trends in Homeopathic Education* above). In a homeopathic learning organization, the creation of such a body becomes critical.

Part of the job of the school board is to assess the overall school performance. Typically the board serves as a policy-making body, while the school director executes the policy. One of the central tasks of the board is to create a mission or covenant about teaching and learning. This covenant helps to capture the beliefs of the community about quality homeopathic leadership, teaching and learning. This covenant must reflect the voices of everyone in the school.

In a learning organization, the school board is made up of students, faculty, administration and members of the homeopathic community. Shared governance becomes a way for the homeopathic community to impact and help shape the school. It is a method to keep the control of the school close to its people. Shared governance gives ownership to the students and faculty in the school. It also assists individuals to grow by encouraging them to move into leadership roles.

Entrance Requirements

The births of all things are weak and tender,
and therefore we should have our eyes intent on beginnings.
—Montaigne

One issue that each school must resolve is entrance requirements. The most central aspect of this question consists in deciding whether the school will only accept medically licensed students or be open to a broader base. This will be determined by both state and local laws as well as by the central philosophy of the institution. For those institutions accepting non-medically licensed students, it is important to decide the medical prerequisites prior to entrance, or whether these medical requirements are to be concurrent with the program.

Another important area is knowledge of the natural world. It is becoming increasingly important for homeopaths to have knowledge of the natural world including biology, anatomy, physiology, pharmacology, chemistry, physics, botany, zoology and mineralogy. These courses can either be required as prerequisites, as concurrent survey courses or integrated into the curriculum.

Special Needs Students

Schools are places where pebbles are polished and diamonds are dimmed.
—Robert Ingersoll

Schools must be aware of the special needs of each of their students. The goal is to help each student succeed, regardless of their life situation. Disaffected students can have a significant negative impact on the program. Studies have shown that disappointed students tell nine to 15 people about their bad experience, while satisfied students tell only two to five people (Cunningham 2000).

Programs must be in place to help individualize the teaching program. This can take a variety of forms including language issues (e.g. when the primary language of a student is not the primary language in the classroom), cultural issues (e.g. when students are not familiar with the cultural norms of their fellow students and patients), physical disabilities (e.g. hearing-impaired or vision-impaired students), cognitive disabilities (e.g. learning-disabled students), slow students and gifted students. Each of these groups may require a specialized learning plan to help them adapt the program to their needs.

The challenge is to ensure that the specialized needs of the individual student do not interfere with the flow of the normal class process.

The school must also have programs in place to help resolve these issues and problems as they arise. Interventions include counseling, remedial education, peer tutoring, mentoring and student advising (Schwartz 1995).

Post-Graduate Programs

Every individual with whom you can converse
has his own ideas and theories.
When he questions you about Homeopathy,
you hesitate because he has not the beginnings.
—James Tyler Kent

Many homeopathic schools end their connection to their students upon graduation. However, a growing number of schools are creating post-graduate programs that offer continuing education to their students and the homeopathic community. This most often occurs in the form of periodic seminars or conferences. There is a strong need for modeling of continuous learning after graduation.

Most continuing professional education in homeopathy is self directed. It is important that post graduate teachers and administrators find ways to support these efforts, rather than simply placing homeopathic practitioners back in a student role. To accomplish this, new models of post-graduate education will be required, which will include a much greater equality between learner and teacher.

Post-graduate programs should be limited to graduates of homeopathic training programs. A problem with some contemporary post-graduate programs is that they accept all comers into their trainings. When this occurs, the program often moves to the lowest common denominator in learning (Kreisberg 1996).

There are two types of post-graduate conferences: community-based and externally-based (see Chapter Eight). Training programs should perform long-term follow up of their graduates, to ensure adequate training. They need to assess how many of their graduates go on to practice, become certified or licensed. This is often done through the form of surveys and alumni organizations.

Human Resource Management

*Theories and goals of education don't matter a whit
if you don't consider your students to be human beings.*
—Lou Ann Walker

A critical factor in the success of a school is the ability of the administration to care for the staff, teachers and students. The quality of education in large part depends upon the quality of the human resources within the school system. Why do students leave their training programs? The answers vary but reflect the same reasons patients drop out of practice. The most common reasons are financial and time (Gaines 1994). Other important factors include underestimating the difficulties of training, disagreements with administration and teachers and lack of determination or perseverance (Kaplan 1997).

For many schools, staff are chosen as volunteers from the homeopathic community. Many schools utilize work study positions to assist in administrative efforts. The board of governance is also typically composed of volunteers. What attracts these volunteers is the reputation, image and vision of the school and the opportunity to serve homeopathy. It's also an opportunity for alumni to give something back to their school. The administration has a responsibility to create a climate in which volunteerism can flourish.

Human-resource management focuses on helping each member of the staff to reach their highest possible level of achievement and performance. The administrator helps them to link to the organization's vision and purpose, works to motivate them and maximizes career development (Webb and Norton 1999). Administrators must realize that the needs of each staff person vary greatly and should be treated in an individualized manner. The needs of staff members when first starting are quite different from that of seasoned employees. It is also important for administration to find employees who do not share their own personality traits. These individuals are more likely to challenge them to grow and they must be willing to listen to them.

Key factors in human resources management include:

◎ **Utilization**: This includes staff planning, recruitment, selection, orientation, assignment and staffing, compensation, security, benefits and employee records.

◎ **Environment**: This includes organizational design, job analysis, job specifications, job descriptions, job enrichment, employee wellness, Employee Assistance Programs (EAP) and the creation of an organizational chart.

◉ **Development**: This includes performance appraisal, staff development, induction into the staff and organizational development.

Assessment

Examinations are formidable even to the best prepared,
for the greatest fool may ask more than the wisest man can answer.
—Charles Caleb Dolton

Assessment involves evaluation of students, faculty, supervisors and mentors, administration, staff and overall school performance. This must be both internal (comparison to internal standards) and external (comparison to community, state, national and international standards).

Assessment is continuous (especially self assessment) as well as periodic (i.e. audits). Assessment is more than recitation of information. It must be authentic and grounded in a wide repertoire of knowledge and skills that mirror life. This knowledge and skill must be demonstrated in solving complex, multi-step problems. Good assessment is more than an auditing tool. It improves performance.

Traditional schools assess more by external standards, which students meet to move on in their training. Typically this is in the form of standardized tests. Learning organizations additionally utilize performance assessment (also called alternative assessment) and self assessment. Performance assessment occurs when students are asked to perform work that illustrates higher-level thinking and problem-solving skills.

When a student becomes a practitioner, self assessment becomes increasingly critical. Unless students have been trained to utilize self assessment, they may be unable to incorporate this into their practice.

Assessment of faculty should be both from students and from administration. It is vital that faculty review their evaluations from students and that they receive feedback from administration. Administrators may need to assist faculty in integrating this feedback, without overreacting or denying its significance.

Administrators must also be open to feedback themselves. There are seldom formalized methods to achieve this. Good administrators seek this out from members of their organization, community and peers.

Financial Concerns

People spend what's in the budget, whether they need it or not.
—George W. Sztykiel

It is very difficult for a homeopathic school to survive on a long-term basis utilizing tuition as its only funding source. Schools must be flexible, using non-traditional revenue sources and exploring a variety of funding strategies. One of the most important initial decisions is whether to incorporate the school as a for-profit or non-profit entity. This decision is based on legal issues and the community's needs as well as the fundamental school philosophy. For-profit corporations permit greater control and independence, while non-profits often better meet the needs of the community.

Establishing a foundation is helpful in moving the school forward financially. This foundation creates a vehicle for obtaining gifts from individuals and corporations that can be targeted at special projects, scholarships and awards. This foundation also helps to foster partnerships and secure donors.

Alumni are a strong resource and are often among the largest sources of gifting. Three key sources of non-tuition funding can be explored (Meno 1984):

1. **Donors:** Donations include cash gifts, real property from individuals, private-foundation grants, corporate gifts, non-profit gifts, fund raisers, donated services, donated supplies and donated equipment.

2. **Enterprise:** Enterprise includes services leased to other schools, lease of facilities, community education, sale of school access and distance-learning projects. Distance learning is popular currently and is an easy target for attracting grant funding.

3. **Cooperative:** Cooperation includes shared programs with other homeopathic schools, cooperative programs with universities, cooperative programs with other alternative medicine organizations, programs sponsored by other organizations (i.e. corporations), and work-study programs.

Grant-writing skills are becoming increasingly important for administrators (Ruskin and Achilles 1995). These minimally include:

◉ Identifying a philanthropist or foundation

◉ Developing a comprehensive and individualized plan.

◉ Designing a short-term strategy and long-range plan for support

◉ Making personal contacts with the funder

◉ Devising a plan to enlist support of other key people

◉ Sending a letter of inquiry and interest

◉ Submitting the proposal: A calendar for grant follow-up should be provided.

◉ Establishing ongoing dialog with the funder

◉ Stewarding the funder through various phases of the project

Hidden Costs

There are many hidden costs in designing a homeopathic training program, and actual costs often far exceed initial projections. Costs for the establishment and maintenance of a homeopathic program typically include the following:

◉ Salaries: Faculty, supervisors, mentors, clinical and administration
◉ Instructional supplies: includes books and photocopying
◉ Instructional equipment
◉ Operation of the physical plant or facilities
◉ Library costs
◉ Food services
◉ Maintenance and repairs
◉ Licensure and certification costs
◉ Partnership costs
◉ Insurance
◉ Marketing and publicity
◉ Accounting
◉ Legal services
◉ Parties and celebrations
◉ Contingency costs

Of particular note are the contingency costs. Planning for the unexpected becomes critical in the uncertain world of education. Programs also must plan in their budgets for recidivism of the student body. Most programs lose 25 to 50 percent of their students from the start of a program to its completion (much of this is determined by program length). Unless this recidivism is planned for, programs can find themselves in financial trouble as the program progresses.

Legal Issues

We must all hang together or assuredly we shall all hang separately.
—Benjamin Franklin

School administrators are often uneasy about their knowledge of the law. Yet they must keep abreast of legal issues within their communities. Private-school associations can be quite helpful in charting current legislation so that changes in law are reported to school administrators. They also frequently have lobbyists who can work to make positive changes in school legislation. Homeopathic education is still in its early developmental stages. Because of this, it is imperative that schools proceed in a legal manner. Small legal mistakes that one school makes can have a large impact on other schools and training programs.

It is important that all school personnel, faculty and administration act reasonably regarding the rights of others. In-service trainings can be helpful in this regard. Schools may only regulate free speech when it is necessary to achieve a compelling purpose, such as when it disrupts the school's educational purpose or invades the rights of others. Student suspension and expulsions are significantly guided by state boards and state law. Students must be given an opportunity for a fair and impartial hearing before exclusion from school. Students with disabilities must be afforded an education from which they may reasonably be expected to benefit. Guidelines regarding access and confidentiality of student records should be established.

Creation of Clinical Training, Supervision and Mentoring Programs

A single conversation across a table with a wise man
is better than ten years' mere study of books.
—Longfellow

Clinical training, supervision and mentoring are vital parts of the training program. These should not be included as after thoughts. These programs are often difficult to develop and take more energy and commitment from staff. They also require considerable involvement from the homeopathic community. The establishment of these programs often takes much time and requires patience and persistence by the school administration.

Clinical training and mentorship should be set up with an eye to diversity. Students should be exposed to as rich a client population as possible, so that they will be prepared to deal with diverse situations once they arrive in practice. Careful attention should also be placed on what types of clients students initially see. In the allopathic model of medical training, students generally see the most difficult cases at the beginning of their training (i.e. hospital-based tertiary-care settings). Often these are patients that no one else will care for and are extremely complex and challenging. These types of cases do not always represent the best learning cases for the beginning homeopath.

There are many factors to be explored in the designing of these programs. Key issues to examine include the following:

◎ **Define the Vision**: What purpose does the program serve? What are its goals? Whom does it serve? What programs already exist?

◎ **Identify the Name**: What is the name of the program? How are participants designated?

◎ **Finding Students**: Do the students come only from within the school? Who is eligible and after what level of training? Is the program open to students from within the community?

◎ **Find Faculty**: Is there sufficient faculty from within the school or is outside faculty needed?

◎ **Identify Roles**: What are the roles and responsibilities of students, faculty and administration for the program?

◎ **Develop Pairing Protocols**: How are the individual students matched with the faculty? What role does personal preference play?

◎ **Develop a Training Program for Faculty**: What type of training and education is needed? What knowledge base and skills are required? What type of orientation is needed? What type of ongoing support will the faculty need?

◎ **Create Celebrations**: How does the program celebrate success?

◎ **Define Administrative Needs**: How will the program be administrated? How will it be coordinated? What personnel needs are required? Who is the contact person? How will confidentiality be handled?

◎ **Establish Evaluation**: What methods and procedures are necessary for tracking progress and providing for continuous improvement? How is feedback obtained and monitored?

◎ **Anticipate Problems**: What types of obstacles and road blocks can be anticipated? Where will be the greatest resistance to implementing the program?

These programs require considerable resources and participation from many individuals. At their best, they serve as a vehicle to knit the students, faculty, administrators and outside homeopathic practitioners into a vital homeopathic community.

Creation of a Learning Center

The true university of these days is a collection of books.
—Thomas Carlyle

The creation of a homeopathic library and archive is an important element of a training program. This library is more than a collection of books. If well designed, it can become both a learning and teaching center. Most students have trouble affording books beyond the required texts and need a comfortable location where they can peruse the homeopathic literature and journals. The library provides a resource for homeopathic research. Libraries also serve as gathering places for students, which in turn facilitates collaboration.

In summary, homeopathic education has far to go. In many ways, it is still in its infancy. Yet there's a strong quality of stewardship in many leaders of homeopathic institutions today. If this can be nurtured and permitted to flower, homeopathic education will have a bright future indeed.

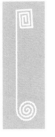

Chapter Ten
The Art of Homeopathic Leadership

Quality homeopathic education will be critical to homeopathy's growth in the twenty-first century. The future of homeopathy depends on the establishment of good leaders and managers (administrators). This administration must be homeopathic in nature, and as the healing marketplace becomes increasingly complex, this becomes challenging. What it means to practice homeopathic administration must be defined and methods to enable homeopaths to practice good quality leadership must be established.

Defining Good Administration

We govern for the benefit of the governed.
—Plato

Individuals can only learn to become administrators by administrating. However, a careful study of what it is to be a good administrator can help on one's leadership journey. Useful self-reflective questions to ask in evaluating yourself as an administrator include the following (Neushcel 1998):

- Do I have a mission as an administrator? How closely have I lived this mission?

- How good have I been as an administrator? How effective? What improvements have I made in my leadership and management skills in the last few years? What are my attitudes about change?

- How do I continuously evaluate myself as an administrator? Am I improving? What are my goals in improvement?

◎ How has my organization improved under my administration?

◎ Have I thought deeply and in an organized way about learning, teaching and administration?

◎ How well do I know how the students, faculty and staff are performing under my administration?

◎ How am I perceived by the students, faculty, staff and community? To what extent am I viewed as a leader?

◎ How well am I preparing my successor? Have I helped to train other leaders in my organization?

◎ To what extent do I feel comfortable making difficult decisions? What have been my most important decisions as a leader? How well did I handle these? How stressful is decision making for me?

◎ How high are the demands that I place on others and on myself? How much do I hold myself and others to those demands?

◎ What is my level of stamina and endurance? How do I handle leadership stress?

◎ To what extent can I delegate and let go of control?

◎ How much character and integrity do I possess as a leader? How do I handle power?

The Qualities of Homeopathic Leadership

The moment one gives close attention to anything,
even a blade of grass, it becomes a mysterious,
awesome, indescribably magnificent world in itself.
—Henry Miller

The concept of leadership is elusive. It is said to be like beauty, hard to define and inexact. Possessing good leadership traits does not guarantee success as an administrator. Yet, awareness of the qualities of homeopathic leadership can take one forward on the journey toward becoming an effective homeopathic leader.

The question arises, "Are good administrators born or made?" The answer is both, although they're more often made (Cunningham 2000). Good leadership qualities can be nurtured. Even an individual with good leadership potential may never realize this potential unless life throws them into an opportunity to lead.

Being of Service

He who has never learned to obey, cannot be a good commander.
—Aristotle

One of the most central keys is the idea of a servant administrator or servant leader. This is the antithesis of narcissistic leadership. Servant leaders share their power, rather than trying to accumulate it for themselves.

Leaders and followers represent a continuum. The leader's own style of following provides a model for those within their organizations. All leaders are also followers (Neuschel 1998). Administrators must first serve in order to better lead. It is their privilege to serve. Through service they help others grow. In this way they have the capacity to unleash the power of their community.

A good administrator will help a student leave a program if this is what is right and best for them. The interests of the students come before the needs of the program.

Having Vision/Essence

The vision of things to be done may come a long time before the way of doing them becomes clear, but woe to him who mistrusts the vision.
—Jenkin Lloyd Jones

Vision provides a sense of purpose and inspiration. Leaders clarify the mission and values of their communities and help to hold a vision. They work to develop formal structures to enhance the vision and goals. This vision is of a positive future for their organization and community. Leaders have the capacity to not only see the world as it is, but as it could be. Albert Schweitzer talked about a sleeping sickness of the soul. He described this as a malaise, loss of enthusiasm and lack of zest for life that comes from a lack of goals and vision. Vision helps one come alive to realize their potential and their dreams.

The vision must be mutually shared. It belongs to the whole community and comes from all levels. It is held in trust by the leader. The leader celebrates others contributions to this vision. The vision is a change agent that helps to bring about transformation. It has been described as the "grain of sand in the oyster, not the pearl" (Heifetz, Ronald and Sinder, Riley 1987). It is the impetus to cause the organization to grow beyond itself. This vision is often a general direction rather than a clear specific focus. It contains a description of the limits of the program and its boundaries. It also identifies the barriers to its implementation, within the organization and community.

Vision requires the capacity to grasp what is most important. This is the capacity to see the essence or heart of one's community and organization.

This vision must include a belief in everyone's ability to be educated. It focuses on maintaining high standards of learning and teaching, self learning and continuous school improvement. It focuses on ensuring that students have the knowledge, skills, qualities and identity necessary to become effective homeopaths.

Attention to the mundane balances this grand vision. Good leaders can translate a grand vision into very concrete terms for their community, students, faculty and staff. This requires attention to the keynotes of the organization, to the strange, rare and peculiar things that make each organization and community unique and individualized.

Embracing Challenges and Change

*It's self evident that if we can't take the risk of saying
or doing something wrong, our creativity goes right out the
window...the essence of creativity is not the possession of
some special talent, it is much more the ability to play.*
—John Cleese

Good leaders embrace challenge and change. They use conflict as a resource and are willing to learn from their mistakes. This requires great resilience. Babe Ruth set both a home run record and a strikeout record. Most educators are paralyzed by their mistakes. Studies show that successful schools are ones that embrace problems rather than avoiding them (Cunningham 2000). Successful school leaders reframe problems so that they can be seen from a wider and more holistic perspective.

Students, teachers and patients have a natural tendency to avoid the challenge to grow. They utilize both conscious and unconscious efforts to seduce the leader out of the change role. They may avoid this through fighting or projecting their problems onto the leader. A leader must gently confront avoidance of the difficult work of change. Schools should build in the capacity to change and to grow.

For change to be effective, there must be a realistic sense of what can be achieved. There also must be a fundamental shift in mind set to a "change mentality" and change oriented leadership (Neuschel 1998).

Bringing Order to Chaos and Chaos to Order

In order to survive, we must break tradition.
—Walter E. Goddard

An organization's order and tradition help it to build community and culture. Chaos in a system creates a lack of equilibrium, yet a lack of equilibrium creates change and growth. Chaos can become a source of energy and momentum. Administrators must be comfortable with ambiguity.

Successful organizations adapt and change through confusion, debate, conflict and chaos. Schools and organizations go through stages of chaos as they evolve. This requires leaders to have comfort with ambiguity, mystery and uncertainty (Neuschel 1998).

Some leaders adopt a "circle the wagons" mentality, in which they attempt to prohibit change and uncertainty. Their need to control can inhibit learning. Wheatley suggests a shift in thinking in which leaders look for order and chaos rather than control in their organizations (Wheatley 1992).

Leaders must be willing to take risks and face the perils of the path through chaos that leads to order, and from order into chaos. It's often their own inner peace and calmness that brings stability in chaotic situations.

Modeling

Each man is a hero and an oracle to somebody.
—Ralph Waldo Emerson

Leadership is more about how to be than how to do. Leaders must serve as an example before they can ask others to make changes. This is especially important for leaders because of their high visibility. Most importantly the leader models authenticity and living of the group's core beliefs qualities, and values. This modeling also includes life long learning, community service, an ethical stance, embracing change and ambiguity, challenging assumptions, diversity, building bridges and serving others.

With this comes great responsibility. The actions, thoughts and feelings of leaders can have profound effects on those who look to them for leadership.

Seeing the Totality

*It is interesting that the words "whole" and "health" come
from the same root. So it should come as no surprise that the
unhealthiness of our world today is in direct proportion to our
inability to see it as a whole.*
　　　　　　　　　　　—Peter Senge

Great administrators have a capacity to grasp the totality, and thus, to see
and work from the whole. Historically, these leaders have often been travelers
because it gives them a capacity to see the world from new perspectives
(Neuschel 1998). They can see both sides of opposing views and possess the
gift of being able to move toward "both/and" or "win/win" resolutions to conflicts and problems. In conflict resolution, they often widen the gaps between
the opposing viewpoints until the middle ground can be clearly seen.

They are only able to do this by leading from their whole selves. This
means utilizing their mind, heart and spirit in all of their work.

Promoting Diversity

*The key to community is the acceptance—in fact,
celebration of our individual and cultural differences.*
　　　　　　　　—M. Scott Peck

The key to individualization in leadership is diversity. Good administrators promote diversity of all kinds. Administrators who embrace diversity
encourage dissent and encourage differing viewpoints. They design effective
learning environments for a wide range of learning and teaching styles. They
encourage a culture that is multi-generational, ethnically diverse and has balanced gender perspectives. This requires interpersonal sensitivity.

Good administrators prevent any one school of thought from dominating their organizations. Single schools of thought in training programs
lead to master/apprentice models of learning. This is the foundation of
prejudice. Homeopathy is one of a very few vocational programs of study
that requires one to have a very broad base of knowledge and education.
The more life experience one has, the better the homeopath they become.

Projecting Dynamis/Energy

Fortune favors the bold.
—Machiavelli

Good administrators must be dynamic. They energize those around them. They have the capacity to free themselves and their communities from the danger of stagnation and identification with the status quo. This requires that they can learn from their own experiences.

They are oriented toward growth, development, exploration and experimentation. Not only do they embrace this themselves, they also encourage the learning culture to innovate and to leave its comfort zone. These administrators support risk taking and curiosity. In embodying this themselves, they encourage the fundamental attitudes necessary for good quality research to take place within their communities.

Living with Integrity

The shortest and surest way to live with honor in the world is to be in reality what we would appear to be; all human virtues increase and strengthen themselves by the practice and experience of them.
—Socrates

Integrity is a consistency between one's values, goals and actions. This is what inspires trust. It requires personal maturity, self knowledge, character and candor. Good administrators have high flash points and the ability to draw on deep reserves of energy.

Leaders must honor their commitments and "walk their talk." They provide an anchor in their organizations through their integrity. They ensure that everyone is treated with fairness, dignity and respect.

Showing Humility

Everyone who is seriously involved in the pursuit of science becomes convinced that a Spirit is manifest in the Laws of the Universe-a spirit vastly superior to that of man and one in the face of which we, with our modest powers must feel humble.
—Albert Einstein

Good administrators know their limits and aren't afraid to admit to them. They realize that they are there to serve and that they're no more important than anyone else in their organization. Although they have the final authority, they use it sparingly. In Japan, top executives clean toilets in their organizations as a way of remaining humble and connected to the small things.

Being Accountable

> *The buck stops here.*
> —Harry Truman

Good administrators do not pass the buck. They carry final responsibility and authority for their programs. These administrators accept responsibility and refuse to blame others. They hold themselves accountable for student learning, faculty teaching and staff performance. Through their modeling, they help others accept responsibility for themselves.

Being Steadfast Yet Flexible

> *We must adjust to changing times and still hold to unchanging principles.*
> —Jimmy Carter

Good administrators must be tenacious and hold to their convictions. This requires sheer grit, self discipline and the ability to pace oneself. They are reliable and steadfast through adversity. It also means being available to others. Many changes sought by administrators take time, sometimes well beyond the tenure of a particular administrator. Good administrators plant seeds which they patiently nurture. Through their steadfastness they set the pace for their organization. This also requires accessibility.

Conversely, it is important for administrators to be flexible. The spirit of the law in leadership becomes much more important than a rigid adherence to the letter of the law. Good school administrators foster a climate in which there is dedication to the school values and traditions but openness to innovation (Peters and Waterman 1982).

Appreciating and Motivating Others

> *You will always need the favor of the inhabitants...*
> *It is necessary for a prince to possess the friendship of the people.*
> —Machiavelli

Great administrators expect the best of people around them. This arises from a deep desire to grow and see others grow. They work to establish the highest of standards of training and clinical services possible. They hold to the belief that they and their communities can be greater than they are. It is also critical that the administrator provide sufficient resources (ideas, finances, direction and manpower) to accomplish the task at hand. They bring out the best in others and help them to realize their creative potential. This requires the intuition to know what makes other people motivated and enthusiastic, as well as modeling passion about one's work. For people to change, they must be moved and inspired. This requires not just an idea, but a leader who advocates.

Good administrators have a way of generating loyalty. Their followers become caught up in their vision and inspiration. Their self confidence helps to create such loyalty. They also accomplish this by appreciating each student, faculty and employee. In this way they build bridges between people. It isn't possible to force participants in a learning community to do things they don't want to do. It is only this appreciation that helps to empower students and staff to experiment and innovate.

Having a Future Focus

> *Change is the law of life. And those who look only*
> *to the past or present are certain to miss the future.*
> —John F. Kennedy

Hockey star Wayne Gretsky once said: "You always skate to where the puck is going, not to where it's been." Good administrators are proactive and take the long view. Administrators look to sustainability of their programs over time. This requires a careful knowledge of school history and homeopathic educational history. A leader cannot look to the future without a knowledge of where they've been.

A school program only has meaning to students if it can endure over time. This necessitates providing for systematic, continuous improvement. A school must create a vision of what holds the greatest promise for improving education for the future. Part of what sustains this focus is an attitude of hopefulness.

Being Courageous

> *Furthermore, I am convinced, and have history to prove it,*
> *that the meek shall not inherit the medical world of our gener-*
> *ation. With frankness, that legacy, in its state of therapeutic*
> *chaos, is not for us homeopaths. We must build anew, like a*
> *homeopathic prescription, a structure composed of a minimum*
> *of material substance but a wealth of energy. It is only through*
> *our honest sincerity that we can will this. Any effort short of*
> *idealism is doomed. Without the will we shall find no way.*
> —Anthony Shupis

Good administrators have the courage of their convictions. They move from thought to action, to live their dreams. They know when it's time to move forward and make decisions. The difference between those who gain mastery and those who simply dream is their commitment to action (Bennis 1989). Courage is, in part, what makes leaders worth following.

Knowledge Areas in Homeopathic Leadership

Not knowing, that is, being willing to admit that we don't know, is one of the keys that opens the door to creative intelligence. It takes humility to open that door. Our ego, doesn't like not knowing and would prefer to go over and over what we already think and believe, rather than trust in a subtle, unknown process like creative intelligence.
—Richard Carlson and Joseph Bailey

Post-modernist thought encourages diversity of knowledge. It teaches that all forms of knowing have equal legitimacy, that there are no hierarchies of wisdom. It encourages multi-frame thinking and reframing of problems in larger contexts (Glickman 1998). Post modernist thought is homeopathic in nature and serves as an antidote to allopathic thinking. Effective leaders also model continuous learning and self improvement.

The latest techniques in management and leadership are seldom helpful in becoming a good administrator. Knowledge can be accumulated through careful study, but more importantly, a leader learns how to lead through leading. This education must include knowledge about education, politics, communities, systems theory, organizations and self knowledge.

Organizational Knowledge

A valuable executive must possess a willingness and ability to assume responsibility, a fair knowledge of his particular branch of business, and a nice understanding of business principles in general, also to be able to read and understand human nature. There is no phase of knowledge which anyone can safely dismiss as valueless.
—Charles Cheney

Educators must create a culture that parallels that which students find outside their schools. This requires a variety of types of knowledge.

268

Knowledge that's important to effective administration of a school includes all of the following (AASA 1993, NAESP 1991):

◎ **Leadership**: facilitating the development of a shared vision for the school and a shared strategic plan to accomplish that vision; identifying and accomplishing school mission; encouraging and helping to develop leadership in others; recognizing both individual needs and the needs of the entire school; providing a sense of purpose and direction; setting priorities and goals; understanding leadership and organizational theory; planning, organizing, actuating and directing; coordinating and controlling; developing an awareness of the change process for schools and organizations

◎ **Problem Analysis and Synthesis**: analyzing and synthesizing disparate information; identifying the important elements of a problem by gathering and analyzing data, facts and possible causes; seeking additional needed information and bringing it together into a meaningful whole; creative problem solving strategies; conflict management techniques; systems theory

◎ **Decision Making**: making decisions that are well informed and represent the best interests of the school and individuals; reaching logical conclusions founded on ethical and moral standards; making timely decisions; analyzing alternative approaches; knowledge in gathering, analyzing and using data for decision making; the capacity to reframe problems; formulating solutions to problems; quality management; strategic plan development and implementation

◎ **Planning**: planning and scheduling one's own and others' work; setting short and long term priorities and goals; managing change; establishing time lines and scheduling projects

◎ **Implementation**: realizing the dream; putting programs and change efforts into action; coordination and collaboration of tasks; nurturing and monitoring those responsible for carrying out projects and plans; consensus building; establishing negotiation skills

◎ **Delegation**: assigning projects, tasks and responsibility; providing lines of clear authority; carefully following up on delegated activities

◎ **Supervising and Motivating Others**: encouraging participation of students, faculty and staff; facilitating teamwork and collegiality; supervising and treating staff as professionals; providing feedback on performance; providing measured growth challenges; serving as a role model; setting high expectations and goals; honoring diverse styles; designing staff and faculty development programs; developing supervision and mentorship programs

◉ **Interpersonal Sensitivity**: perceiving the needs and concerns of others; embracing diversity; recognizing multi-cultural cultural, generational and gender differences; dealing tactfully with others; obtaining feedback on one's interpersonal style

◉ **Oral Communication**: encouraging reflective feedback at all levels of the organization; making clear, easily understood oral presentations; being persuasive; utilizing appropriate communicative aids; adapting to audiences; using effective counseling skills with staff and students; articulating and defending decisions; utilizing research, facts and data to communicate more effectively; applying current technologies; using mass media; developing the capacity to actively listen; promoting higher level thinking skills

◉ **Written Communication**: expressing ideas clearly in writing; writing appropriately for different audiences; preparing brief memoranda, letters, reports and other specific documents

◉ **Group Process**: developing knowledge of group process and ability to work with diverse groups; facilitating group cohesion; involving staff, faculty, students and community; developing the capacity to listen actively

◉ **Program Design**: creating instructional programs for the improvement of teaching and learning; recognizing developmental stages and needs of both students and faculty; ensuring appropriate instructional methods; encouraging diversity of styles and approaches of faculty; accommodating differences in learning styles and achievement for students

◉ **Curriculum**: understanding major curriculum design models; curriculum planning and development; applying community needs and values; encouraging faculty input; initiating needs analyses; aligning curriculum with anticipated outcomes; monitoring social and technological developments as they affect curriculum; utilizing resources and current technologies to maximize student achievement; understanding and usage of research findings on learning and teaching

◎ **Student Guidance and Development**: understanding and accommodating student development; providing for guidance, counseling and special needs; planning student activities; celebration and honoring of developmental milestones; creating effective channels of communication for student support

◎ **Faculty and Staff Development**: working to identify and assess professional needs; planning, organizing and facilitating programs that improve faculty and staff effectiveness and growth; arranging for remedial assistance and development activities; initiating self awareness and development; modeling development; inspiring faculty and students; resolving conflict and developing consensus

◎ **Evaluation**: assessing performance, progress and effectiveness; encouraging input; fostering continuous improvement; determining what information is needed about students, faculty, staff and the school environment; conducting needs assessments; making reasonable conclusions from the available data; interpreting evaluations for others; designing, conducting, and evaluating research and evaluation studies; designing accountability mechanisms

◎ **Resource Allocation and Management**: coordinating resources; managing all fiscal responsibilities; procuring, apportioning, monitoring, accounting for, and evaluating fiscal, human, material and time resources; planning and developing the budget process; developing and maintaining the physical plant; providing a safe climate to learn and teach; conducting human resource management; developing and implementing staff procedures; selecting, assigning and organizing staff; managing time; developing and maintaining a library; finding and maintaining suitable equipment and technological resources

◎ **Ethics and Values**: identifying and modeling accepted ethical standards; establishing professional codes of ethics; recognizing philosophical influences and values in education; understanding the values of the school in its community; shaping school culture and climate; multi-cultural, generational, gender and ethnic understanding; shaping a school culture; using influence and power to enhance homeopathy rather than for personal gain

◎ **Technology**: keeping abreast of technological developments; using technology as curriculum and instructional tool; promoting appropriate technology usage among faculty and staff; use and application of technology to accelerate learning

◎ **Personnel Development**: encouraging personnel leadership and management skills; practicing and modeling self reflection; creating and attending workshops, conferences; belonging to professional organizations

◎ **Policy and Governance**: formation and development of boards of governance; procedures for working with the board; formulating policy, standards and regulations

◎ **Educational Knowledge**: philosophy and history of education, knowledge of student growth and development; learning theory; adult-learning models; the role of technology in promoting student learning, principles of development of organizations; women's issues in education

Community Knowledge

He traveled much and far in his attendance upon the meetings of societies and colleges. He spared neither time, money nor strength when called upon to lend the influence of his gracious presence and facile speech for the strengthening or building up of his beloved Homeopathy. As organizer, missionary, exhorter and peacemaker-in-general, he was well nigh ubiquitous. Wherever there was a society to be formed or reorganized, a fraternal 'breach of the peace' to be healed, backsliders and weak kneed brethren to be stirred up and strengthened, there was Dr. Allen to be found. And wherever he went he took with him that genial spirit, that charming presence, that suave address which made him always a welcome and honored guest. He was tactful and diplomatic in his dealing with man and measures.
—Excerpt from the obituary of H. C. Allen,
IHA Transactions, 1909

Besides organizational knowledge, effective administrators must have knowledge of the community and the world they live in. Good leaders engage the world. This includes knowledge of politics, community relations, legal status, partnerships, marketing and public relations.

All organizations have internal and external politics. It is difficult for a school to exist in the current climate without some political presence. To survive, a school must work within the political forces. Much of the images of politics are negative and this is often an area of homeopathic leadership that is avoided or neglected. What is needed are more positive images of becoming a constructive politician. Important political skills include agenda setting, networking and forming coalitions, and bargaining and negotiating (Kotter 1988). In the political arena, it's vital to have friends and allies to accomplish anything. This requires political savvy.

Administrators must respond to diverse groups and pressures as they work to improve their schools. This requires good community relations and skill in articulating the organization's vision and purpose to the larger community. Good administrators have the capacity to respond to community feedback and build consensus. They collaborate both locally and globally.

Schools must act according to federal and state rules, procedures and directives. This requires a knowledge of confidentiality and privacy of school documents. In many states, it is illegal for a school to operate without a state license. It is critical for a potential school to become familiar with state and federal statutes before embarking on the formation of a school program. They also should familiarize themselves with national and international standards of learning, teaching and school management. Effective administrators join professional associations, national and international organizations, to influence homeopathic policy and homeopathic standards formation.

Administrators must have a knowledge of media and public relations. They know how to respond to electronic and printed news media. This includes an awareness of local, national and international issues that affect education. They have a knowledge of community resources and can effectively manage their school's reputation. These administrators enlist public participation and support. They have a knowledge of collaborative relationships within the community to promote school programs (media, private business, teachers, researchers, business, professional associations, industry, government and special interest groups). They also know how to attract volunteers and coordinate community services.

Self Knowledge and Capacity to Change

The more you know yourself, the more clarity there is.
Self knowledge has no end—you don't come to an achievement,
you don't come to a conclusion. It is an endless river.
—Krishnamurti

Administrators must know themselves. They are aware of their strengths and their weaknesses as managers and leaders. They have learned to compensate for their shortcomings, draw on their weaknesses and others strengths, and match their talents and personalities. The more a leader accepts and acknowledges their weaknesses, the more effective they become. It is difficult for a leader who doesn't accept any weakness to ask for help.

To be an instrument for change in an organization means that administrators must be willing to change themselves. Effective administrators who lead an organization through change often say that the most important change that occurred in the process was in themselves. In this way they model growth and the spirit of research and experimentation for their organizations and communities.

Skills of Homeopathic Leadership

Try? There is no try. There is only do or not do.
—Yoda in *The Empire Strikes Back*

Good leadership skills can be learned (Yukl 1989, Drucker 1992). Some feel that homeopathy is more a skill or vocation than a body of knowledge and should be taught accordingly (Kreisberg 1999). Self study, programmatic instruction, courses, trainings and conferences can all be productive in this process.

Self Care

While I am only 61 years old, I am worn out. I have been lecturing to classes on homeopathy and materia medica since 1883, and it has been a bitter fight continuously. Though I have enjoyed it, it has worn me out.
—James Tyler Kent

Administration is quite challenging. Leaders are often attacked, both personally and in their ideology. This can create great stress, yet leaders are supposed to be strong and never get sick.

It becomes critical for leaders to find ways to replenish themselves. They must minister to their own physical, emotional, mental and spiritual needs. Good leaders are psychologically hardy (Evans 1996). They have solid inner resources to draw upon in their work and know how to cultivate those resources. Relaxation, physical fitness, humor, play, stamina, teaming with supportive peers and reconnecting to a higher purpose can all be vital in the work.

Two central skills in this process are time management and priority setting. Time must be allocated and managed wisely. Priority setting helps an administrator focus on what's important and helps avoid getting lost in the minutia of daily stress. Good administrators have skills in setting priorities and triaging what's at hand. This requires an instinct for knowing what's essential. Current surveys suggest that most educational administrators waste 2-4 hours per day on unnecessary trivia (Cunningham 2000).

Ultimately, the goal is not worth having unless the journey itself is enjoyed. Good administrators take time to smell the flowers on their journey. They also model these self-help techniques for their students, faculty and staff.

Empowering Others

There are very few so foolish that they had not rather
govern themselves than be governed by others.
—Thomas Hobbes

Administrators must create conditions that promote self empowerment and authorship. This comes through helping others realize their importance and significance and their capacity to change the world around them. Only through empowerment can students, teachers and staff learn to lead and effectively manage themselves. They begin to feel personally accountable and responsible for their actions.

This issue is particularly important in schools and organizations that rely on volunteers. Keys to this process include building unity and cohesiveness, delegation of responsibility, developing a feeling of organizational pride, giving others credit, usage of rituals, telling of community stories, symbols and music. This cannot be done through disempowering themselves as leaders. Self empowerment must be modeled on all levels.

Surrender and Delegation

The surest way for an executive to kill himself
is to refuse to learn how and when,
and to whom to delegate work.
—James Cash Penney

Delegation is not only one of the most important forms of administrative self care, but also a vital means of self empowerment for students, faculty and staff. Many administrators fear that, through delegation, they will lose control, that things won't get done correctly, that they as administrators will appear weak or that they will become too dependent on others. Delegation requires a tolerance for imperfection in others. There is also a very strong temptation for administrators to micro manage others, to ask others to do a task, but deny them the power or the tools with which to do it. Heroic leaders feel that they must do it all and protect others from both internal and external attacks. Not only must administrators effectively delegate responsibility, they must also learn to listen effectively to others.

The creation of a learning community necessitates surrender and trust by its leaders. This means letting problems and issues go, so that others can take care of them and then to support others through this process. Good administrators work hard to make others successful. Ultimately the organization becomes much larger than any of its constituents.

Communication

> *If you want to be heard you must speak in a language*
> *the listener can understand and on a level*
> *at which the listener is capable of operating.*
> —M. Scott Peck

Communication skills are an essential building block for good administration. These skills help to build connections between members of the community. The administrator must ensure that the vision and goals of the school are effectively communicated to the community, students, faculty and staff. In part, this is communicated through stories, symbols and ceremonies. The administrator also ensures that lines of communication stay open throughout their organization.

Communication skills are founded on good listening skills and the ability to acknowledge others. They require the capacity to be persuasive, provide continuous feedback, ask good questions, to gather useful information and to admit to ignorance. A skillful administrator must not only understand the facts, but also the underlying feelings, meanings and perceptions of those within their communities. This requires the capacity to communicate strategically (practically) and tactically (conceptually). This also necessitates good group process skills and an awareness of the unconscious elements that play large parts in communication.

Effective communication requires the establishment of a community-wide resource network, not just within the organization. This helps to foster connections throughout the community.

Diplomacy

> *In case of dissension, never dare to judge*
> *until you have heard the other side.*
> —Euripides

Effective administrators learn the fine art of diplomacy. They are skilled at helping others feel valued and important. Diplomacy includes skills in sociability, high visibility, maintaining an open dialog, relationship development with community leaders, the capacity to negotiate effectively, public relations, problem analysis, interpersonal sensitivity, multi-culturalism, conflict mediation and assertiveness training. They have the capacity to open the school to public scrutiny. Effective administrators can forgive and forget; they let something go and move on. This is vital in a homeopathic community that's historically been torn by dissension.

Leadership Renewal

> *It takes a long time to become young.*
> —Pablo Picasso

One of the most important skills and responsibilities of a leader is leadership renewal. Good leaders continuously develop the leadership capacity of others in their organizations. They find that there's many more individuals with leadership potential than might be assumed. Good leaders seek them out and help to develop their leadership capacities. In seeking them out, they set high expectations, provide resources and ideas, mentor, and help to set up self-improvement programs. This also takes the form of continuously preparing and grooming a replacement for what they do. Only in this way can the continuity of the organization be ensured over time.

Standards of Homeopathic Leadership

> *State a case to a ploughman and a professor.*
> *The former will decide it as well and often better than the latter,*
> *because he has not been led astray by artificial rules.*
> —Thomas Jefferson

Standards describe what we should know and be able to accomplish. In the United States, the Interstate School Leaders Licensure Consortium (ISLLC) met to establish common standards for school leaders. This was a consortium consisting of 24 states and nine associations. These standards reflect the centrality of student learning, quality teaching and school improvement. They focus on what the committee called "the heart and soul of effective school leadership." The framework is standards (norms for quality control) followed by knowledge competencies, dispositions (qualities) and performances (skills). The standards are summarized below, but in more detail in appendix H.

Standard One

A school administrator is an educational leader who promotes the success of all students by facilitating the development, articulation, implementation, and stewardship of a vision of learning that is shared and supported by the school community.

Standard Two

A school administrator is an education leader who promotes the success of all students by advocating, nurturing, and sustaining a school culture and instructional program conductive to student learning and staff professional growth.

Standard Three

A school administrator is an educational leader who promotes the success of all students by ensuring management of the organization, operations, and resources for a safe, efficient, and effective learning environment.

Standard Four

A school administrator is an educational leader who promotes the success of all students by collaborating with families and community members, responding to diverse community interests and needs, and mobilizing community resources.

Standard Five

A school administrator is an educational leader who promotes the success of all students by acting with integrity, fairness and in an ethical manner.

Standard Six

A school administrator is an educational leader who promotes the success of all students by understanding, responding to, and influencing the larger political, social, economic, legal, and cultural context.

A Look to the Future

Any one can hold the helm when the sea is calm.
—Publilius Syrus

Homeopathy's star is rising. It is said to be the fastest growing form of alternative medicine in the world today. Promoting quality homeopathic education will be a vital part of its growth, yet there are many challenges on the road ahead. The journey that we take together as educators will be fraught with peril and debate. There is much to be done. It remains to be seen whether homeopathic educators can come together as a community. It is the purpose of this book, and my fervent hope that we can join together to create a common educational vision that will move homeopathy further on its journey.

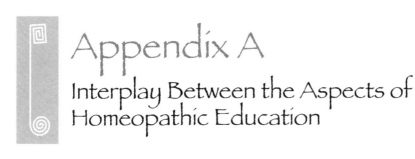

Appendix A
Interplay Between the Aspects of Homeopathic Education

Didactic Triad

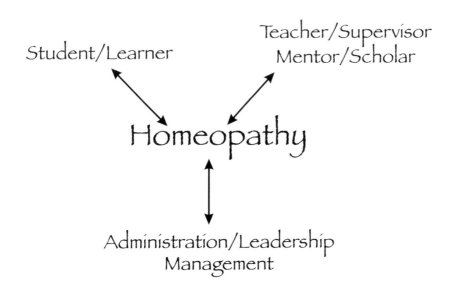

Student/Learner

Teacher/Supervisor
Mentor/Scholar

Homeopathy

Administration/Leadership
Management

Clinical Rhombus

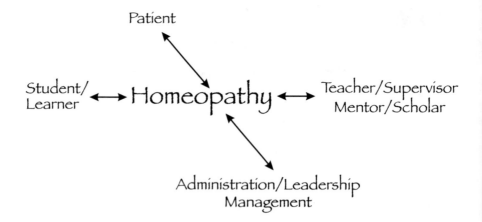

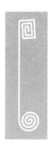

Appendix B
The Council on Homeopathic Education

The Council on Homeopathic Education (CHE) was founded in 1982 as an independent and autonomous agency. Its goals are:

- To establish, maintain, insure, and improve the quality of education in the science and discipline of homeopathy in the United States and Canada.

- To act as a resource center for questions regarding the content and presentation of lectures, seminars, academic programs, and institutions dealing with the art and science of homeopathy.

- To establish standards for the above presentations and to evaluate for approval, endorsement, or otherwise certify such presentations or institutions.

The Council has been active in evaluating educational training in the United States since 1982. Participating organizations include: the American Institute of Homeopathy; the Homeopathic Academy of Naturopathic Physicians; the National Center for Homeopathy, and the North American Society of Homeopaths. The board consists of representatives from member organizations, endorsed schools, and the public at large.

Beginning, advanced, and clinical programs are evaluated at graduate and postgraduate levels. Episodic programs for continuing education units (CEU) are endorsed as well.

The CHE can be reached at:

801 North Fairfax Street, Suite 306
Alexandria, VA 22314
(703) 548-7790

Appendix C
The National Center for Homeopathy Affiliated Study Groups Program

The National Center for Homeopathy Affiliated Study Groups (ASGs) helps to spread the knowledge and use of homeopathy and to further classical homeopathic education. This program links individual study groups into a regional and national network. It provides a structure for consumers who wish to integrate homeopathy into self and family health care. Informed consumers, in turn, promote an increased awareness of homeopathy throughout the health-care community. The program provides educational resources and training for ASG members and information that is shared throughout the ASG network.

The program was developed in 1987 by the National Center for Homeopathy in response to the renewed interest in homeopathy by individuals and groups in North America. There is a rich, 125-year history of non-professional societies in the United States. They focused on how to be a good homeopathic patient, provided interesting lectures for their members and the general public, and served as auxiliaries to the numerous homeopathic hospitals.

Homeopathic study groups have evolved a great deal since that time. The philosophical underpinnings of the study group movement are based on self-care, freedom, the formation of a grass-roots community and empowerment (Lillard 1992). As the groups grow, they are creating an increasing political presence. They can quickly mount letter-writing campaigns, trigger telephone trees, raise funds, and contact their legislators. They also encourage local communities to grow their own homeopathic practitioners to better fit the communities' needs.

For further information contact:

National Center for Homeopathy
Affiliated Study Group Program
801 N. Fairfax St., #306
Alexandria, VA 22314
(703) 548-7790
www.homeopathic.org

Appendix D
The North American Network of Homeopathic Educators

The North American Network of Homeopathic Educators (NANHE) was founded in 1995 by the Homeopathic Community Council (HCC). The Council for Homeopathic Education assumed responsibility for this group in 1997. Its meetings are open to anyone interested in homeopathic pedagogy. NANHE holds annual meetings to support homeopathic educators in North America. For more information, contact:

Council for Homeopathic Education
801 North Fairfax Street, Suite 306
Alexandria, VA 22314
(703) 548-7790

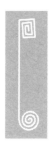

Appendix E

Standards and Competencies for the Professional Practice of Homeopathy in North America

A Report of a Summit Meeting Sponsored by The Council for Homeopathic Education

January 28-30, 2000, Mountain Lakes, NJ

Supported by the a grant from The Homeopathic Community Council

Introduction

The Council for Homeopathic Education (CHE), with the support of the Homeopathic Community Council (HCC), held a summit meeting of invited representatives of key homeopathic organizations on January 28-30, 2000. The intention of this summit was to achieve consensus on the homeopathic and medical competencies and standards necessary for the practice of homeopathy in North America. Following review by the North American Homeopathic Community, this document represents the final version of these competencies and standards.

The Council for Homeopathic Education was founded in 1982 with the mission to accredit homeopathic schools and educational programs. In 1999, the CHE identified the establishment of consensus on standards and competencies as a priority necessary to achieve its mission. Accreditation of educational institutions is a function vital to the development and recognition of homeopathy as a health-care profession.

Homeopathy is currently utilized by a wide variety of health-care practitioners in the United States and Canada. The political-legal environment in which homeopathy is practiced is in a state of evolution. These complexities make the job of the CHE in identifying the competencies and standards to which schools must prepare students a complicated task. It is a task that must be undertaken with sensitivity to many perspectives and an awareness that health care in the North America is heading rapidly toward new potentials.

While the summit group has outlined homeopathic and medical standards and competencies, we emphasize that the means of acquiring these competencies may vary from formal instruction to self-study to clinical supervision. Ideally, the training process will include all three of these elements. The important thing is that the instruction be based on definable standards and that homeopaths must be capable of demonstrating these competencies and proficiencies by the standardized measurements utilized by certification boards.

This document was distributed to the North American homeopathic community for public comment in the winter of 2000. It has been through a series of revisions and reflects commentary from many organizations, schools and individuals within the homeopathic community. We wish to thank all of the individuals and organizations who participated in the public commentary.

One of the positive outcomes of the Summit process was the high degree of consensus among participants from diverse segments of the homeopathic community, including practitioners with and without medical licenses. We believe this heartening outcome is a good omen for the future, and for harmony within the homeopathic profession. Unless otherwise indicated, statements in these documents represent consensus. For those points on which we were unable to agree, we have set forth the arguments for and against so that the larger homeopathic community can make its decision. In fact there were only two such points.

One area where opinions diverged was on whether or not it was necessary to outline potential models under which homeopaths would practice. While some felt it contributed context and substance to the discussion of standards, others felt it unnecessary and ill advised at this time. Also, there was debate about the models themselves. Ultimately, it was determined to adopt a model that reflected the practice of the great majority of homeopathic practitioners in North America.

We realize that many practitioners have a strong preference for either the word "client" or the word "patient." In drafting this document, we had to choose one, for the sake of simplicity. We have used "client" in most contexts, but we mean it as a neutral word to refer to anyone who seeks homeopathic care.

The summit process was assisted immeasurably by the monumental efforts of our professional colleagues, national and international, who have spent many hours considering, deliberating and publishing their thoughts on these issues. The documents to which we referred regularly are listed in the Selected Bibliography.

Consensus on standards for classical homeopathic practice will have important implications and benefits for the interdependent components of the homeopathic community — schools, accreditation organizations, certification boards and professional organizations. Indeed, these standards can lay the groundwork for the recognition of an independent profession of classical homeopathy in the United States.

Summit participants felt that formalizing the homeopathic and medical requirements for the professional practice of homeopathy will lead to greater unity in the profession. This has already proved to be the case within the diverse summit group, who were able to agree not only on homeopathic competencies, but on medical competencies as well. While this unity may help propel homeopathy into the mainstream, it can only happen if homeopathic principles are honored.

We submit these documents to the North American homeopathic community in the hope that they will become a powerful tool in the strengthening of the homeopathic profession. These standards represent a beginning. We fully recognize the need for growth and change. It is our hope for the CHE to hold another summit meeting to review these documents in seven to ten years.

Invited Organizations

American Association of Homeopathic Pharmacies (AAHP)
American Board of Homeotherapeutics (ABHT)
American Institute of Homeopathy (AIH)
Council for Homeopathic Certification (CHC)
Council for Homeopathic Education (CHE)
Homeopathic Association of Naturopathic Physicians (HANP)
Homeopathic Community Council (HCC)
Homeopathic Nurses Association (HNA)
Homeopathic Pharmaceutical Association (HPhA)
National Board of Homeopathic Examiners (NBHE)
National Center for Homeopathy (NCH)
North American Society of Homeopaths (NASH)

Attendees

- ◎ Summit Chair: EDWARD CHAPMAN, MD, DHt President, CHE; Treasurer, HCC; Trustee, AIH; Primary Care Coordinator, ABHT

- ◎ PEGGY CHIPKIN, FNP, CCH Board, CHC; Board, HCC; Member, HNA

- ◎ JANE CICCHETTI, RSHom (NA) Member, NASH Schools Committee; Board, CHE (representing NASH) (Resigned prior to draft of final documents)

- ◎ JOYCE FRYE, DO, MBA President, NCH; First Vice President, AIH

- ◎ KATHY LUKAS Secretary, CHE

- ◎ CHRISTOPHER PHILLIPS, CCH Board, CHE (representing CHC)

- ◎ RICHARD PITT, RSHom, CCH President, CHC

- ◎ JOSETTE POLZELLA, Treasurer, CHE

- ◎ IRIS HAGEN RATOWSKY, RSHom (NA), CCH Registrar, NASH; Board, CCH

- ◎ CAROLINE RIDER, JD Associate Professor of Management and Chair of the Department of Management, School of Management, Marist College, Poughkeepsie, N.Y.

- ◎ TODD ROWE, MD, MD(H), CCH, DHt Vice President, NCH; Board, CHC; Board, CHE

Selected Bibliography

Commission on Accreditation of Allied Health Education Programs, "Standards and Guidelines for an Accredited Program for the Physician Assistant," revised, 1997.

European and International Councils for Homeopathy, "Guidelines for Homeopathic Education"; first edition (January 1993) and second edition (March 1999).

European Council on Homeopathy and *Liga Medicorum Homeopathica Internationalis*, "Programme for the Teaching of Homeopathy," Appendix I.

Hahnemann, Samuel, *The Organon of the Medical Art*, Wenda Brewster O'Reilly, PhD, ed.; Redmond, WA: Birdcage Books, 1996.

Kent, James Tyler, *Lectures on Homeopathic Materia Medica*, Philadelphia: Boericke & Tafel; fourth edition 1956.

Kent, James Tyler, *Lectures on Homeopathic Philosophy*, Chicago: Ehrhart & Karl; memorial edition, 1929.

National Guideline Clearinghouse, an online source for nationally agreed upon guidelines for the treatment of more than 600 medical conditions.

North American Society of Homeopaths, *Record-Keeping Guidelines*, Appendix C.

Sherr Jeremy, *The Dynamics and Methodology of Homeopathic Provings*, Malvern, England: Dynamis Books; second edition, 1994. Society of Homeopaths, *Core Assessment Criteria*, 1998.

Society of Homeopaths, *Critique of Consultation Document Developing National Occupational Standards for Homeopathy*, 1998.

United Kingdom, *National Occupational Standards for Homeopathy*, Draft 25, August 1998.

Uphold, C.R., Graham, M.V., *Clinical Guidelines in Family Practice*, Gainesville, FL: Barmarrae Books; third edition, 1998. [This text is designed to help clinicians quickly access up-to-date information regarding health maintenance and commonly occurring primary care problems.]

List of Appendices

Commission on Accreditation of Allied Health Education Programs, "Standards and Guidelines for an Accredited Program for the Physician Assistant," revised, 1997.

European and International Councils for Homeopathy, "Guidelines for Homeopathic Education"; second edition, March 1999.

European Council on Homeopathy and *Liga Medicorum Homeopathica Internationalis*, "Programme for the Teaching of Homeopathy," Appendix I.

North American Society of Homeopaths, *Record-Keeping Guidelines*, Appendix C.

Olsen, Steve, CCH, ND, DHANP, *The Homeopathic Code of Professional Ethics and Ethical Standards of Practice*; January 15, 2000, version 1.3b.

Society of Homeopaths, *Core Assessment Criteria*, 1998.

Society of Homeopaths, *Critique of Consultation Document Developing National Occupational Standards for Homeopathy*.

United Kingdom, *National Occupational Standards for Homeopathy*, Draft 25, August 1998.

Council For Homeopathic Education January 2000 Summit

Part II: Statement Of Homeopathic Standards and Competencies

Homeopathic competencies are the knowledge, skills and attitudes that any practicing homeopath needs in order to prescribe homeopathic remedies and to manage the responses to those prescriptions. The means of acquiring these competencies vary from formal instruction and self-study to clinical supervision, and ideally will include all three. The homeopath must be capable of demonstrating these competencies by the standardized measurements utilized by certification boards.

These competencies are not intended to be a comprehensive outline for the structure of a curriculum or of an assessment tool, but rather guidelines to assist those who are developing them. They are meant to be an expression of what the community holds as the minimum skills, attitudes and knowledge required to practice homeopathy at a board certified level.

The following competencies are synthesized from a number of sources, the most important of which are listed in the Selected Bibliography. The competencies are grouped into the headings that make logical sense for assessment and curriculum development.

I. History of Healing

The practitioner must be familiar with the development of homeopathy and the social forces that have influenced its practice over its 200-year history. The practitioner should be cognizant of the philosophers and authors who have had major influences on homeopathic thought and be able to place them in context.

    A. History of Western Medicine: Hypocrites to Galen and Paracelsus

B. History of Vitalism: Paracelsus to Hahnemann
C. History of Homeopathy
    1. Hahnemann and his contemporaries
    2. Homeopathy in North America
    3. The Organon 1st to 6th editions

II. Homeopathic Philosophy: The Principles Of Homeopathy

The practitioner must have a thorough understanding of the principles of homeopathy that guide its theories and implementation in clinical practice.

A. The practitioner must demonstrate a thorough understanding of the principles, dynamics and nature of health and disease from a homeopathic perspective and be aware of how the homeopathic view differs from the allopathic, antipathic and other views of health and disease, both current and historical. Topics include:

    1. Requirements of the homeopathic practitioner, as enumerated in Aphorism No. 3 of *The Organon*
    2. Recognition of the spirit-like dynamic Life Force energy
    3. Causes of disease
    4. Definitions of health, disease and cure
    5. The power of homeopathic medicines to cure
    6. Concepts of similar, dissimilar and opposite symptoms
    7. Why medicines are better at curing than natural diseases
    8. Differences among homeopathic, allopathic and antipathic treatment
    9. Primary and secondary actions of homeopathic and antipathic medicines
    10. Homeopathic definitions of acute, chronic and other protracted diseases
    11. Understanding of genus epidemicus, susceptibility and miasmatic disease
    12. How homeopathy treats disease
    13. The action of potentized medicines
    14. The importance of mental/emotional symptoms
    15. Intermittent diseases
    16. Preparation of homeopathic remedies
    17. Administration of homeopathic remedies
    18. Possible reactions to remedies, including models put forward by Kent and others

19. Recognition and understanding of fundamental homeopathic laws including the Law of Similars, the Law of the Minimum Dose and the Law of Cure

III. Homeopathic Provings

A. The necessity of provings
B. The history of provings (Hahnemann through modern methodologies)
C. Types of provings (informal/partial through Hahnemanian)
D. Guidelines for conducting provings
E. Provings in relation to allopathic drug trials
F. Ethical issues related to provings
   1. The nature of the substance
   2. Informed consent and blind studies
G. Protocol of thorough provings
   1. The substance
      a) Gathering information on the history, behavior and toxicology of the substance to be proven
      b) Preparation of substance to be proven
   2. The structure of a proving group
   3. Dose and posology
   4. Record keeping
   5. Supervisor/prover contact and frequency
   6. Data management
      a) Extraction of data, including primary and secondary distinctions
      b) Collation of data
      c) Statistical evaluation of data
      d) Converting data into old and new repertory language and *materia medica*
   e) Publishing the results

IV. Materia Medica

The practitioner must have a thorough appreciation of homeopathic *materia medica*. The study of remedies is greatly enhanced by knowledge of botany, zoology, chemistry, geology and plant and animal taxonomy.

A. Knowledge of the major writers and books: from Hahnemann to the present day
B. How to evaluate materia medica sources (thoroughly proven, partially proven, and unproven data; data collection, editing, short cuts, etc.)

C. Remedy-by-remedy study of materia medica determining the characteristic symptoms, disturbances and themes in mental, emotional, physical spheres of remedies. Remedies must be understood in terms of:
1. The history, culture and behavior of the substance in the natural world
2. Toxicological history
3. Proving symptoms
4. Sensation and function
5. Mental/Emotional symptoms (including dreams and delusions)
6. Characteristic symptoms
7. Strange, rare and peculiar symptoms
8. Generalities
9. Modalities
10. Clinical symptoms/pathology
11. Etiology
12. Local symptoms
13. Organ and system affinities
14. Keynote and confirmatory symptoms
15. Concomitant symptoms
16. Remedy relationships
    a. Relationships within the *materia medica*
    b. Relationships of substances (e.g., botanicals, mammals, spiders)
    c. Periodic table relationships
    d. Antidotes, affinities, inimicals, complementaries, remedies that follow well
17. Acute/first aid uses
18. Comparative and differential study
19. Progressive stages of pathology of remedies
20. Chemistry of the substance
D. The differences among polychrests, so-called "small remedies," nosodes, sarcodes, isopathics, tautopathics and imponderables
E. The use of case studies (live, paper and video)
F. The use of journals and electronic sources in the study of *materia medica*
G. The use of repertory comparisons

V. Repertory

A. History and organization of repertories
1. Boenninghausen and Kent through modern repertories
2. Organization and limitations of various repertories
   a) Grading of symptoms/rubrics in each
   b) Organization Kent's through newer organizing techniques
   c) Strengths and limitations of older repertories, especially Kent's
   3. The purpose of rubrics and sub-rubrics and how they are developed and organized
B. Terminology and abbreviations used in the repertories, including contemporary and anachronistic medical terminology
C. Converting symptoms into repertory language
D. Various tabulation tools—their strengths, limitations and uses
1. Paper graphs
2. Computers, and their use in modern practice
E. The different roles of repertorization in selecting a remedy

VI. Case Taking

A. Evaluating whether a case is suitable for homeopathic treatment based on initial information. Includes knowing when to refer to a different modality or a different homeopathic practitioner
B. Communicating with the client about the nature of the homeopathic interview and the nature of homeopathic treatment, including its limitations. This should take place prior to formal case taking
C. Conducting a comprehensive homeopathic interview
1. Individualizing the case: the ability to vary techniques for eliciting information according to the client
2. The need for freedom from bias, for healthy senses and astute observation
3. Guidelines for recording the case
4. Special considerations for epidemic diseases
D. Consideration of previous and current therapeutic history/treatment, including homeopathy, allopathy and other therapeutic modalities
E. Conducting the interview with sensitivity to the client's needs, privacy, dignity and psychological safety
F. Accurate and systematic recording of the case according to the prevailing medical model

G. Understanding the value, limitations and use of medical reports in homeopathic case taking

H. After case taking, re-evaluating the suitability of a case to homeopathic treatment: when to treat and when and how to refer elsewhere

I. After case taking, ongoing communication with the client about the nature of homeopathic treatment, including its limitations, if any, in this particular case

J. The value and limitations of client forms in homeopathy (e.g., medical history, informed consent)

VII. Case Analysis

The practitioner must be able to synthesize disparate information into meaningful totality and treatment strategy based on sound classical homeopathic principles.

A. Analyzing what needs to be cured—determining the central disturbance and themes of the case based on distinguishing symptoms in the mental, emotional and physical spheres. Includes understanding of:
   1. Sensations and function of the organism
   2. Vitality and health of the person
   3. Totality of the disease
   4. Hierarchy of symptoms—mental, emotional and physical
   5. Characteristic/strange, rare, peculiar symptoms
   6. Family and miasmatic history
   7. Modalities
   8. Affinities and systemic effects
   9. Pathology, including knowledge of common symptoms of allopathic disease and being able to distinguish them from characteristic symptoms
   10. Obstacles: e.g., antidoting, environmental, iatrogenic influences
   11. Etiology/exciting and maintaining causes
   12. Susceptibility
   13. Onset, duration, and intensity/severity of symptoms
   14. Prognostic evaluation

B. Converting symptoms into repertory language

C. Repertorizing in a manner appropriate to the case presented

D. Researching remedies in the materia medica and applying this research to the case

E. Posology/Potency
　　1. Assessing strength of the vital force
　　2. The relative benefits of various homeopathic potencies and their relevance to the case
　　3. Choosing the right method of administering remedies (e.g., dry, in water, olfaction)

VIII. Case Management

The practitioner must be able to evaluate and supervise the entire course of homeopathic treatment as an ongoing and cumulative process, an extended cycle of reflection and response. The process must encompass knowledge of a hierarchy of change within the curative process. It requires

A. Appropriate communication with clients both during and between follow-ups
B. Appropriate scheduling of follow-ups based on strategy of treatment, anticipated remedy action, prognosis and the client's needs
C. Assessment of remedy action
　　1. Recording the individual's experience in treatment, while being able to assess the accuracy of this reporting
　　2. Evaluating the extent to which treatment has achieved the client's aims and goals
　　3. Evaluating results according to the homeopathic definition of cure versus palliation and suppression
　　4. The application of models of remedy actions by Kent and others
　　5. The homeopathic aggravation: how to recognize it and how to handle it
　　6. Obstacles to cure
　　　　a) Environmental considerations
　　　　b) Iatrogenic factors
　　　　c) Antidoting
　　　　d) Progress of pathology
　　7. Knowing when to wait, when to repeat and when to change remedies and potencies
　　8. Knowing when to retake the case
　　9. Knowing when to refer the case to another modality or another homeopath
　　10. Recognizing proving symptoms
D. Concepts of simillimum, similar, layers, zigzagging
E. The individual's motivation and commitment to treatment
F. Acute diseases during chronic treatment
G. Intercurrent prescribing
H. The value, limitations and uses of medical reports in homeopathic case management

Council for Homeopathic Education January 2000 Summit

Part III: Statement of Medical Standards and Competencies

Part A: General Principles

Medical competence in the practice of homeopathy is viewed in this document from the perspective of the minimal set of knowledge, skills and attitudes necessary to prescribe homeopathic therapy in a fashion that is effective and safe for the client. These standards recognize the interdependence of homeopathy with other fields of health care, the need for effective communication among health-care professionals, and the need for consultation in clinical medicine.

These subjects have purposely been expressed in terms of competency, not in terms of course hours.

These recommendations are made with a recognition that homeopathy is based in a vitalist paradigm (vitalism-the science or doctrine that all functions of the living organism are due to an unseen vital principle distinct from all chemical and physical forces)*, which views health-related events from a perspective that may differ significantly from that of the prevailing medical paradigm.

At a minimum, a homeopathic practitioner:

1. Must demonstrate through examination knowledge of the natural world and the human body sufficient to understand homeopathic philosophy and homeopathic therapeutics. These areas of knowledge include relevant aspects of chemistry, biology, botany, physics, human anatomy and physiology

2. Must demonstrate through examination knowledge of medical terminology, clinical pathophysiology and therapeutics. The level of competence must be sufficient
   a) for accurate homeopathic prescribing;
   b) to interface appropriately with members of the complementary and allopathic medical communities;
   c) to recognize the signs and symptoms of conditions that may pose immediate or long-term risk to the client;
   d) to distinguish between disease-specific signs and symptoms, iatrogenic signs and symptoms and those signs and symptoms that are characteristic of the client's individuality;

e) to assess the appropriate role of homeopathy in a specific case, and discuss this and other therapeutic options with the client;

f) to obtain and assess informed advice and research on unfamiliar conditions;

g) to know one's limits of competency, including when and how to make appropriate referrals

3. Must demonstrate through examination knowledge of allopathic and herbal pharmacology. The level of competence must be sufficient;

a) to recognize the effects, side-effects and interactions of drugs and substances;

b) to understand the influence of these substances on the natural history of the client's illness and how to differentiate between characteristic and iatrogenic signs, symptoms and modalities;

c) to know the dangers or consequences of an individual's withdrawing from drugs and substances, both prescribed and self-administered (for example, adrenal crisis on sudden withdrawal of steroids);

d) to recognize the danger of interfering with regimes of prescribed medications

4. Must demonstrate through examination knowledge of the psychological and emotional functioning of individuals and how this may affect their health and well-being. Specifically, the practitioner must demonstrate;

a) a familiarity with the normal stages of child and adult development;

b) a familiarity with the normal stages of response to stressful life events (e.g., death and dying, child and adult responses to trauma);

c) an appreciation of the dynamics of family and other relationships and their impact on the client's life circumstances and mental and physical health;

d) an appreciation for the nature of disability, the social resources available to the disabled, and the effects of disability on the individual, health-care providers and members of the client's support system;

e) a sufficient knowledge of the terminology of mainstream psychiatry to enable the homeopathic practitioner to interface with mental health providers

5. Must demonstrate consultation skills. Specifically, the practitioner must show;

a) clarity of perception: homeopaths should have sufficient knowledge of health on the mental, emotional and physical levels, to be able to perceive what needs to be healed in others;

b) the ability to recognize obstacles to cure, including:

 I)   the relationship between the physical, social, emotional and economic contexts in which people live and their health and well-being;

 ii) the implications for health and disease of personal and family health history, life events and environmental factors;

 iii) the potential effect of lifestyle (for example, diet, smoking, alcohol consumption) on an individual's health and social well-being;

 iv) the resources available to individuals to make changes in their circumstances and lifestyles;

 v)   how personal beliefs and preferences affect individuals' lives and the choices they make, the context in which they live and their health and well-being;

 vi) drugging resulting in masking, suppressing, alteration of individualizing characteristic symptoms of the original disease symptoms.

c) facility in effective and sensitive interviewing attitudes and techniques that will enable individuals to reveal and talk through relevant issues in their physical, mental and emotional health;

d) the ability to recognize and interpret significant aspects of a client's appearance, body language, speech and behavior;

e) the ability to explain to clients the nature and depth of homeopathic case taking, and a sensitivity to concerns and difficulties that can arise during this process;

f) the ability to take clear and coherent notes according to the standards and conventions of the healing professions;

g) knowledge of when it may be necessary or useful to involve someone besides the client in consultation (for example, when treating children). This includes recognizing the potential for reticence, misrepresentation and misunderstanding when others are involved in these discussions, and being able to minimize those risks;

h) awareness of the dangers of imposing one's own beliefs, values and attitudes on individuals and of the importance of respect for the client's beliefs, values and attitudes, both personal and cultural

6. Must demonstrate knowledge of alternative medicine. Specifically the practitioner must a) have sufficient knowledge of acupuncture, osteopathic, and chiropractic care to recognized the appropriate time for referral to practitioners of these modalities b) have sufficient knowledge of alternative modalities to be conversant with practitioners who refer patients from these modalities

Part B: Major Categories of Illness

Practitioners of homeopathy should be able to recognize signs and symptoms of the following common medical conditions. They should be familiar enough with these signs and symptoms to know when to refer clients for other evaluation and treatment.

The disorders are presented by system, with distinction made between those conditions that are urgent—meaning that appropriate evaluation and treatment must be made acutely—and those that can be handled in a routine manner. These distinctions cannot be kept completely separate. There can be acute exacerbations of some of the routine conditions, causing them to become urgent. However, what is listed below represents where these conditions will most commonly be found. The scope of formal evaluation, diagnosis, and management of disease is defined by licensing statutes and the standards of practice of the various professionals who practice homeopathy.

In addition, homeopaths must be able to recognize the common symptoms of these diagnosed diseases and conditions in order to distinguish them from a client¹s individualized symptoms.

A. Rheumatological / Musculoskeletal / Connective Tissue Diseases

◎ **Urgent Conditions**: Fractures, acute rheumatic fever, septic arthritis (gonococcal, Lyme, etc.), temporal arteritis, acute gouty arthritis

◎ **Routine Conditions**: Strains, sprains, osteoarthritis, osteoporosis, rheumatoid arthritis, gout, costochondritis, Reiter's syndrome, scleroderma, systemic lupus erythematosus (SLE), polymyalgia rheumatica, polyarteritis nodosa, dermatomyositis/polymyositis, Sjogren's syndrome, ankylosing spondylitis, fibromyalgia, chronic Lyme disease, carpal tunnel syndrome

B. Malignancy

◎ **Urgent Conditions:** Fever in the immunosuppressed client, bleeding in the thrombocytopenic client, acute spinal cord compression, intestinal obstruction, evaluation of any client suspected of having a diagnosis of cancer

◎ **Routine Conditions:** Chronic management of all types of cancer, with emphasis on skin, breast, brain, ovarian, testicular, prostate, bladder, oral, esophageal, stomach, liver, pancreas, colon, uterine, cervical, lung, kidney, lymphoma (including Hodgkin's disease), leukemia

C. Hematological

◎ **Urgent Conditions:** Disseminated intravascular coagulation (DIC), immune thrombocytopenic purpura (ITP), thrombotic thrombocytopenic purpura (TTP)

◎ **Routine Conditions:** Anemia (nutritional, hereditary, associated with systemic disease), polycythemia, thrombocytopenia, leukopenia

D. Endocrine

◎ **Urgent Conditions:** Diabetic coma and ketosis, hyperthyroid crisis, acute hypoglycemia, thyroid nodule

◎ **Routine Conditions:** Hyperthyroidism, hypothyroidism, diabetes mellitus, diabetes insipidus, Cushing's syndrome, Addison's disease, chronic hypoglycemia, thyroid enlargement, acromegaly

E. Dermatology

◎ **Urgent Conditions:** Melanoma, third degree burn, second degree burns over large surface areas, drug rash, erythema multiforme, gangrene, abscesses, cellulitis, syphilis, petechiae

◎ **Routine Conditions:** Eczema, psoriasis, seborrhea, nevi, boils, impetigo, monilial dermatitis, tinea capitis, tinea corporis, tinea cruris, tinea pedis, tinea versicolor, vitiligo, syphilis, varicella, herpes zoster, molluscum, rubella, rubeola, warts, scabies, lice, first and second degree burns over small areas, first degree burns, urticaria, contact dermatitis (Rhus dermatitis), acne, rosacea, alopecia, aphthous stomatitis, lipoma, keloid, dermatofibroma, hemangioma, insect bites, basal cell carcinoma, squamous cell carcinoma, seborrheic keratosis, solar keratosis, herpes simplex

F. Respiratory/ENT

◎ **Urgent Conditions:** Peritonsillar abscess, epiglottitis, foreign bodies (eye, ear, nose throat), streptococcal pharyngitis, mastoiditis, acute asthma, status asthmaticus, pneumonia, pulmonary embolus, pneumothorax, tuberculosis

◎ **Routine Conditions:** Otitis media and otitis externa, mastoiditis (see above), hearing disorders, epistaxis, adenoid and tonsillar hypertrophy, pharyngitis, sinusitis, allergic rhinitis, croup, laryngitis, bronchitis, chronic asthma, chronic obstructive pulmonary disease, pleurisy, tuberculosis, sarcoidosis, bronchiectasis, Meniere's disease, obstructive sleep apnea

G. Cardiovascular

◎ **Urgent Conditions:** Acute myocardial infarction, cardiac and aortic aneurysm, hypertensive crisis, endocarditis, unstable angina, pericarditis, pericardial tamponade, congestive heart failure, acute arrhythmia, acute deep vein thrombosis, cerebral aneurysm

◎ **Routine Conditions:** Hypertension, stable angina, chronic arrhythmia, coronary artery disease, valvular heart disease, congenital heart disease, cardiomyopathy, chronic congestive heart failure, peripheral vascular disease, superficial thrombophlebitis, carotid artery stenosis, cerebral aneurysm, Raynaud's syndrome

H. Gastrointestinal

◎ **Urgent Conditions:** Acute appendicitis, volvulus, intussusception, incarcerated hernia, acute abdomen and other surgical emergencies, upper and lower gastrointestinal bleeding, acute hepatitis, acute pancreatitis, pyloric stenosis, acute cholecystitis, acute diarrhea, acute diverticulitis

◎ **Routine Conditions:** Gall stones, flatulence, encopresis, constipation, chronic diarrhea, malabsorption syndromes, celiac disease, lactose intolerance, parasite infestation, hernia, peptic and duodenal ulcer, esophageal motility disorders, gastro-esophageal reflux, cirrhosis, acute gastroenteritis, Crohn's disease, ulcerative colitis, irritable bowel syndrome, hemorrhoids, chronic hepatitis B, hepatitis C, chronic pancreatitis, diverticulosis

I. Diseases of the Mouth

- ◎ **Urgent Conditions**: Epiglottitis, acute parotitis

- ◎ **Routine Conditions**: Aphthous stomatitis, herpes simplex, dental abscess, periodontal disease, caries

J. Nutritional and Metabolic Diseases

- ◎ **Urgent Conditions**: Failure to thrive

- ◎ **Routine Conditions**: Obesity, anorexia, osteoporosis, B12 deficiency, protein deficiency, phenylketonuria and other congenital metabolic disorders

K. Infectious Diseases

- ◎ **Urgent Conditions**: HIV, sepsis, meningitis, peritonsillar abscess, cellulitis, gonorrhea, syphilis, pneumonia, rheumatic fever, encephalitis, septic arthritis, pyelonephritis, acute hepatitis, acute cholecystitis, acute appendicitis, acute diverticulitis, tuberculosis, mycoplasma infections, malaria, pneumonia, smallpox, anthrax

- ◎ **Routine Conditions**: Influenza, common cold, mononucleosis, varicella, scarlet fever, pertussis, Fifths disease, chlamydia infections, systemic candidiasis, moniliasis, trichomonas, amebiasis, giardiasis, hookworm, malaria, scabies, conjunctivitis, bronchitis, urinary tract infections, chronic prostatitis, chronic hepatitis, otitis media, sinusitis

L. Immunologic Diseases

- ◎ **Urgent Conditions**: AIDS, anaphylaxis

- ◎ **Routine Conditions**: Chronic fatigue immunodeficiency syndrome, environmental illness, systemic allergy, acquired and congenital immunodeficiency syndromes

M. Ophthalmology

- ◎ **Urgent Conditions**: Retinal detachment, iritis, uveitis, corneal abrasion, papilledema, acute red eye, foreign body

- ◎ **Routine Conditions**: Conjunctivitis, sty, blepharitis, meibomian cyst, lachrymal duct obstruction, subconjunctival hemorrhage, glaucoma, diabetic retinopathy, myopia, hyperopia, astigmatism, strabismus, cataract, ocular tumors, ocular migraine

N. Occupational Illnesses

◎ **Urgent Conditions**: Carbon monoxide poisoning

◎ **Routine Conditions**: Occupational lung diseases (asthma, asbestosis, etc.), sick building syndrome; repetitive stress syndrome (as carpal tunnel syndrome, shin splints, low back pain, etc.)

O. Neurological

◎ **Urgent Conditions**: Stroke, subarachnoid hemorrhage, subdural hematoma, space occupying lesion/pathology, meningitis, encephalitis, cerebral abscess, skull fracture, vertebral fracture

◎ **Routine Conditions**: Headaches, vertigo, epilepsy, traumatic brain injury, multiple sclerosis, amyotrophic lateral sclerosis, myasthenia gravis, musculodystrophy, peripheral neuropathy, polio, vertebral disc disease, spinal stenosis, dementia, Parkinson's disease, cranial synostosis, Tourette's syndrome

P. Psychiatric

◎ **Urgent Conditions**: Suicidal or homicidal ideation, acute mania, acute psychosis, child abuse, spousal abuse, elder abuse, delirium

◎ **Routine Conditions**: Post-traumatic stress syndrome, dissociative disorder, alcoholism, drug addiction, other substance abuse, bipolar disorders, psychosis, depression, grief reaction, obsessive-compulsive disorder, anxiety disorders, personality disorders, eating disorders, autism, Asperger's syndrome, verbal and non verbal learning disorders, mental retardation, attention deficit disorder, dementia, somatization disorder, communication disorders (e.g., stuttering), conduct disorder, tic disorders, encopresis, enuresis, sexual dysfunction, sleep disorders, impulse control disorders, adjustment disorders

Q. Obstetrics/Gynecology

◎ **Urgent Conditions**: Ectopic pregnancy, uterine hemorrhage, pelvic inflammatory disease, acute gonorrhea and syphilis, toxemia of pregnancy, miscarriage, puerperal fever

◎ **Routine Conditions**: Pregnancy, nausea of pregnancy, hyperemesis gravidarum, bacterial vaginosis, vaginitis, papilloma virus, cervical dysplasia, herpes simplex, vaginal atrophy, premenstrual syndrome, metrorrhagia, menopause, endometriosis, ovarian cyst, polycystic ovarian disease, amenorrhea, infertility, breast lump, mastitis, uterine prolapse

R. Genital-Urinary

⊚ **Urgent Conditions:** Pyelonephritis, kidney stones, testicular torsion, testicular cancer, acute renal failure, acute prostatitis, epididymitis

⊚ **Routine Conditions:** Urinary tract infection, impotence, enuresis, incontinence, inguinal hernia, femoral hernia, chronic renal failure, chronic prostatitis

S. Pediatric

⊚ **Urgent Conditions:** Congenital heart disorders, congenital gastrointestinal disease, newborn hyperbilirubinemia, fetal alcohol syndrome or drug withdrawal, child abuse, epiglottitis, failure to thrive, pyloric stenosis

⊚ **Routine Conditions:** Lachrymal duct obstruction, herpangina, accident prevention, immunization, mental retardation, pica, lead poisoning, esophageal reflux, worms, cerebral palsy, urinary tract infection, atopic disease, developmental delay, encopresis, enuresis, anticipatory guidance, congenital hip dislocation, club foot

Part C: Medical Diagnostic Testing

1. The practitioner should have a basic knowledge of the common forms of diagnostic testing, including X-ray, ultrasound, computerized tomography (CT), magnetic resonance imaging (MRI), radioisotope scanning, electroencephalography, electromyography, electrocardiography and echocardiography

2. The practitioner should have a basic knowledge of the common laboratory tests, including, papanicolaou (PAP) smear, bacteriologic and viral culture, urinalysis, complete blood counts (CBC), measurements of serum lipids, liver and kidney function, electrolytes, glucose, glycohemoglobin, hormonal function, including thyroid (T3, T4,TSH), HCG, LH, FSH, sedimentation rate and coagulation rates (PT, PTT).

Part D: Major Categories Of Allopathic Medicatons

Practitioners should be familiar with the therapeutic uses and usual adverse reactions of common classes of allopathic pharmaceuticals, including:

> Analgesics, Narcotics, Acetaminophen, NSAID's, Anti-anginals, Antiarrhythmics, Anticoagulants, Antidiabetics, Oral hypoglycemics, Insulins, Anti-infectives, Antibiotics, Antivirals, Antifungals, AIDS Chemotherapies, Antihypertensives, Calcium channel blockers, Beta-blockers, Diuretics, ACE Inhibitors, Anticonvulsants, Anti-inflammatories, Corticosteroids, NSAID's, Salicylates, Antihistamines, Anti-anxiety agents, Antidepressants, Antipsychotics, Anti-asthma agents, Bronchodilators, Mast cell stabilizers, Corticosteroids, Antacids, Histamine receptor antagonists, Hormones, Thyroid Hormonal replacement therapy, Contraceptives Devices, Hormonal contraceptives, Dermatological agents, Scabicides, Topical steroids, Anti-psoriatic agents, Acne preparations

Part E: Herbs And Dietary Supplements

Practitioners of homeopathy should have some knowledge of herbal and dietary supplements frequently utilized by clients, including:

> Acidophilus/bifidobacter, Aloe Vera, Antineoplastons, Astragalus, Bee Pollen, Bilberry, Black Cohosh, Blessed Thistle, Bromelain, Burdock, Calcium, Calendula, Cat's Claw, Chamomile, Chondroitin, Co-Enzyme Q10, Comfrey, Cranberry, Creatine, Dandelion, DHEA, Devil's Claw, Dong Quai, Echinacea, Elderberry, Ephedra, Essiac, Evening Primrose Oil, Feverfew, Fish Oil, Flax Seed Oil, Garlic, Ginger, Gingko, Ginseng (Asian and Siberian), Glucosamine Sulfate, Glutamine, Goldenseal and Barberry, Gotu Kola, Green Tea, Hawthorn, Hops, Horse Chestnut, Hoxsey Formula, Hydrazine Sulfate, Kava Kava, Lavender, Lemon Balm, Licorice, Magnesium, Melatonin, Milk Thistle, Mistletoe, Nettles, Passion Flower, Pennyroyal, Peppermint, Pine BarkExtract/Grape Seed Extract/Pycnogenol, Pygeum, Red Yeast (Cholestin), Rhubarb Root, SAM-e, St. John's Wort, Saw Palmetto, Selenium, Shark Cartilage, Skullcap, Slippery Elm, Sorrel, Soy, Tea Tree Oil, Uva Ursi, Valerian, Vitamins: B12, Folic Acid, B Complex, C, D, E; Vitex (Chasteberry), Wild Yam, Willow Bark, Zinc

Source: *The Longwood Herbal Task Force* (Lhtf)
www.Mcp.Edu/Herbal/Default.Htm#Herbs
www.Mcp.Edu/Herbal/Default.Htm#Herbs

Part F: Other Treatment Issues

Treatment requires competency in the safe administration of homeo-pathic remedies, including the safety of both the client and the homeopath. The practitioner must also have the ability to manage the clinical case using clinical skills. Necessary areas of knowledge include:

a. Appropriate use of referrals for emergency care, medical evalua-tion, acupuncture, osteopathic or chiropractic care and other types of evaluation and treatment

b. Appropriate use of supervision and homeopathic consultation

c. The ability to use feedback from others, including clients and colleagues

d. Maintaining effective collaborative relationships

e. The ability to engage in self-evaluation

f. The ability to access and integrate new information to assist in decision making

g. The ability to use research, including provings, audits and case studies, to plan implement and critically evaluate concepts and strategies leading to improvements in care

h. The ability to critically evaluate professional knowledge, legisla-tion, policy and research in order to refine clinical practice

i. The ability to predict the development and limit the effect of difficult situations in clinical practice

* *Webster's Dictionary*, 1902 Edition.

Appendix F
Class Exercise: Creating Fairy Tales

Break into small groups. Choose one of the remedies covered today and make a fairy tale incorporating the key elements. Have someone record the fairy tale and be prepared to present the fairy tale by the end of class. Use the following guidelines in constructing the fairy tale:

1. Begin with "Once upon a time…" and use the past tense in your narrative.

2. Give each element of the story a name and capitalize it.

3. Exaggerate. For example, make small things very small and large things very large. The man might be the most handsome man in the kingdom or the woman might be the one with the most wealth.

4. Embellish or invent all settings.

5. Describe what people look like and what they are wearing.

6. Add the words "always" and "never" whenever you can.

7. Make up dialogue.

8. Use descriptive adjectives and adverbs whenever possible.

9. Title your fairy tale.

10. Come up with a moral for your fairy tale.

11. Make your fairy tale personal; put something of yourself into it.

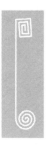

Appendix G
Interstate School Leaders Licensure Consortium Standards

Standard One:

A school administrator is an educational leader who promotes the success of all students by facilitating the development, articulation, implementation, and stewardship of a vision of learning that is shared and supported by the school community.

Knowledge:

The administrator has knowledge and understanding of:

◎ learning goals in a pluralistic society
◎ the principles of developing and implementing strategic plans
◎ systems theory
◎ information sources, data collection, and data analysis strategies
◎ effective communication
◎ effective consensus-building and negotiation skills

Dispositions:

The administrator believes in, values, and is committed to:

◎ the educability of all

◎ a school vision of high standards of learning

◎ continuous school improvement

◎ the inclusion of all members of the school community

◎ ensuring the students have the knowledge, skills, and values needed to become successful adults

- ◎ a willingness to continuously examine one's own assumptions, beliefs, and practices
- ◎ doing the work required for high levels of personal and organizational performance

Performances:

The administrator facilitates processes and engages in activities ensuring that:

- ◎ the vision and mission of the school are effectively communicated to staff, parents, students, and community members
- ◎ the vision and mission are communicated through the use of symbols, ceremonies, stories, and similar activities
- ◎ the core beliefs of the school vision are modeled for all stakeholders
- ◎ the vision is developed with and among stakeholders
- ◎ the contributions of school community members to the realization of the vision are recognized and celebrated
- ◎ progress toward the vision and mission is communicated to all stakeholders
- ◎ the school community is involved in school improvement efforts
- ◎ the vision shapes the educational programs, plans, and actions
- ◎ an implementation plan is developed in which objectives and strategies to achieve the vision and goals are clearly articulated
- ◎ assessment data related to student learning are used to develop school vision and goals
- ◎ relevant demographic data pertaining to students and their families are used in developing the school mission and goals
- ◎ barriers to achieving the vision are identified, clarified, and addressed
- ◎ needed resources are sought and obtained to support the implementation of the school mission and goals
- ◎ existing resources are used in support of the school vision and goals
- ◎ the vision, mission, and implementation plans are regularly monitored, evaluated, and revised

Standard Two

A school administrator is an education leader who promotes the success of all students by advocating, nurturing, and sustaining a school culture and instructional program conducive to student learning and staff professional growth.

Knowledge:

The administrator has knowledge and understanding of:

◎ student growth and development

◎ applied learning theories

◎ curriculum design, implementation, evaluation, and refinement

◎ principles of effective instruction

◎ measurement, evaluation, and assessment strategies

◎ diversity and its meaning for educational programs

◎ adult learning and professional development models

◎ the change process for systems, organizations, and individuals

◎ the role of technology in promoting student learning and professional growth

◎ school cultures

Dispositions:

The administrator believes in, values, and is committed to:

◎ student learning as the fundamental purpose of schooling
◎ the proposition that all students can learn
◎ the variety of ways in which students can learn
◎ life-long learning for self and others
◎ professional development as an integral part of school improvement
◎ the benefits that diversity brings to the school community
◎ a safe and supportive learning environment
◎ preparing students to be contributing members of society

Performances:

The administrator facilitates processes and engages in activities ensuring that:

- all individuals are treated with fairness, dignity, and respect

- professional development promotes a focus on student learning consistent with the school vision and goals

- students and staff feel valued and important

- the responsibilities and contributions of each individual are acknowledged

- barriers to student learning are identified, clarified, and addressed

- diversity is considered in developing learning experiences

- life-long learning is encouraged and modeled

- there is a culture of high expectations for self, student, and staff performance

- technologies are used in teaching and learning

- student and staff accomplishments are recognized and celebrated

- multiple opportunities to learn are available to all students

- the school is organized and aligned for success

- curricular, co-curricular, and extra-curricular programs are designed, implemented, evaluated, and refined

- curriculum decisions are based on research, expertise of teachers, and the recommendations of learned societies

- the school culture and climate are assessed on a regular basis

- a variety of sources of information is used to make decisions

- student learning is assessed using a variety of techniques

- multiple sources of information regarding performance are used to staff and patients

- a variety of supervisory and evaluation models is employed

- pupil personnel programs are developed to meet the needs of students and their families

Standard Three

A school administrator is an educational leader who promotes the success of all students by ensuring management of the organization, operations, and resources for a safe, efficient, and effective learning environment.

Knowledge:

The administrator has knowledge and understanding of:

◎ theories and models of organizations and the principles of organizational development

◎ operational procedures at the school and district level

◎ principles and issues relating to school safety and security

◎ human resources management and development

◎ principles and issues relating to fiscal operations of school management

◎ principles and issues relating to school facilities and use of space

◎ legal issues impacting school operations

◎ current technologies that support management functions

Dispositions:

The administrator believes in, values, and is committed to:
◎ making management decisions to enhance learning and teaching
◎ taking risks to improve schools
◎ trusting people and their judgments
◎ accepting responsibility
◎ high-quality standards, expectations, and performances
◎ involving stakeholders in management processes
◎ a safe environment

Performances:

The administrator facilitates processes and engages in activities ensuring that:

◎ knowledge of learning, teaching, and student development is used to inform management decisions

◎ operational procedures are designed and managed to maximize opportunities for successful learning

◎ emerging trends are recognized, studied, and applied as appropriate

◎ operational plans and procedures to achieve the vision and goals of the school are in place

◎ collective bargaining and other contractual agreements related to the school are effectively managed

◎ the school plant, equipment, and support systems operate safely, efficiently, and effectively

◎ time is managed to maximize attainment of organizational goals

◎ potential problems and opportunities are identified

◎ problems are confronted and resolved in a timely manner

◎ financial, human, and material resources are aligned to the goals of schools

◎ the school acts entrepreneurially to support continuous improvement

◎ organizational systems are regularly monitored and modified as needed

◎ stakeholders are involved in decisions affecting schools

◎ responsibility is shared to maximize ownership and accountability

◎ effective problem-framing and problem-solving skills are used

◎ effective conflict resolution skills are used

◎ effective group-process and consensus-building skills are used

◎ effective communication skills are used

◎ a safe, clean, and aesthetically pleasing school environment is created and maintained

◎ human resource functions support the attainment of school goals

◎ confidentiality and privacy of school records are maintained

Standard Four

A school administrator is an educational leader who promotes the success of all students by collaborating with families and community members, responding to diverse community interests and needs, and mobilizing community resources.

Knowledge:

The administrator has knowledge and understanding of:

◎ emerging issues and trends that potentially impact the school community

◎ the conditions and dynamics of the diverse school community

◎ community resources

◎ community relations and marketing strategies and processes

◎ successful models of school, family, business, community, government, and higher education partnerships

Dispositions:

The administrator believes in, values, and is committed to:

◎ schools operating as an integral part of the larger community

◎ collaboration and communication with families

◎ involvement of families and other stakeholders in school decision-making processes

◎ the proposition that diversity enriches the school

◎ families as partners in the education of their children

◎ the proposition that families have the best interests of their children in mind

◎ resources of the family and community needing to be brought to bear on the education of students

◎ an informed public

Performances:

The administrator facilitates processes and engages in activities ensuring that:

- high visibility, active involvement, and communication with the larger community is a priority

- relationships with community leaders are identifies and nurtured

- information about family and community concerns, expectations, and needs is used regularly

- there is outreach to different business, religious, political, and service agencies and organizations

- credence is give to individuals and groups whose values and opinions may conflict

- the school and community serve one another as resources

- available community resources are secured to help the school solve problems and achieve goals

- partnerships are established with area businesses, institutions of higher education, and community groups to strengthen programs and support school goals

- community youth family services are integrated with school programs

- community stakeholders are treated equitably

- diversity is recognized and valued

- effective media relations is developed and maintained

- a comprehensive program of community relations is established

- public resources and funds are used appropriately and wisely

- community collaboration is modeled for staff

- opportunities for staff to develop collaborative skills are provided

Standard Five

A school administrator is an educational leader who promotes the success of all students by acting with integrity fairness and in an ethical manner.

Knowledge:

The administrator has knowledge and understanding of:

◎ the purpose of education and the role of leadership in modern society

◎ various ethical frameworks and perspectives on ethics

◎ the values of the diverse school community

◎ professional codes of ethics

◎ the philosophy and history of education

Dispositions:

The administrator believes in, values, and is committed to:

◎ the ideal of the common good

◎ the principles in the Bill of Rights

◎ the right of every student to a free, quality education

◎ bringing ethical principles to the decision-making process

◎ subordinating one's own interest to the good of the school community

◎ accepting the consequences for upholding one's principles and actions

◎ using the influence of one's office constructively and productively in the service of all students and their families

◎ development of a caring school community

Performances:

The administrator facilitates processes and engages in activities ensuring:

◎ examination of personal and professional values

◎ demonstration of a personal and professional code of ethics

- demonstration of values, beliefs, and attitudes that inspire others to higher levels of performance

- service as a role model

- acceptance of responsibility for school operations

- consideration of the impact of one's administrative practices on others

- use of the influence of the office to enhance the educational program rather than for personal gain

- treatment of people fairly, equitable, and with dignity and respect

- protection of the rights and confidentiality of students and staff

- demonstrates appreciation for and sensitivity to the diversity in the school community

- recognition and respect for the legitimate authority of others

- examination and consideration of the prevailing values of the diverse school community

- expectation that others in the school community will demonstrate integrity and exercise ethical behavior

- the school is open to public scrutiny

- fulfillment of legal and contractual obligations

- application of laws and procedures fairly, wisely and considerately

Standard Six

A school administrator is an educational leader who promotes the success of all students by understanding, responding to, and influencing the larger political, social, economic, legal, and cultural context.

Knowledge:

The administrator has knowledge and understanding of:

◎ principles of representative governance that undergird the system of American schools

◎ the role of public education in developing and renewing a democratic society and an economically productive nation

◎ the law as related to education and schooling

◎ the political, social, cultural, and economic systems and processes that impact schools

◎ models and strategies of change and conflict resolution as applied to the larger political, social, cultural, and economic contexts of schooling

◎ global issues and forces affecting teaching and learning

◎ the dynamics of policy development and advocacy under our democratic political system

◎ the importance of diversity and equity in a democratic society

Dispositions:

The administrator believes in, values, and is committed to:

◎ education as a key to opportunity and social mobility

◎ recognizing a variety of ideas, values, and cultures

◎ importance of a continuing dialogue with other decision makers affecting education

◎ actively participating in the political and policy-making context in the service of education

◎ using legal systems to protect student rights and improve student opportunities

Performances:

The administrator facilitates processes and engages in activities ensuring that:

◎ the environment in which schools operate is influenced on behalf of students and their families

◎ communication occurs among the school community concerning trends, issues, and potential changes in the environment in which schools operate

◎ there is ongoing dialogue with representatives of diverse community groups

◎ the school community works within the framework of policies, laws, and regulations enacted by local, state, and federal authorities

◎ public policy is shaped to provide quality education for students

◎ lines of communication are developed with decision makers outside the school community

Appendix H
Excerpts from Abrahm Flexner's Report "Medical Education in the United States and Canada"

"None of the fifteen homeopathic schools require more than a high school education for entrance; only five require so much. The remaining eleven get less—how much less depending on their geographical locations rather than on the school's own definition. The Louisville, Kansas city, and Baltimore schools cannot be said to have admission standards in any strict sense of all...

On the laboratory side, though the homeopaths admit the soundness of the scientific position, they have taken no active part in its development. Nowhere in homeopathic institutions with the exception of one or two departments at Boston University, is there any evidence of progressive scientific work. Even "drug proving" is rarely witnessed. The fundamental assumption of the sect is sacred; and scientific activity cannot proceed where any such interdict is responsible for the spirit of the institution. The homeopathic departments at Iowa and Michigan are in this respect only half schools-clinical halves. For their students get their scientific instruction in pathology, anatomy etc., in the only laboratories which the university devotes to those subjects under men none of whom sympathizes with homeopathy...

Of complete homeopathic schools, Boston University, the New York Homeopathic College, and the Hahnemann of Philadelphia alone possess the equipment necessary to the effective routine teaching of the fundamental branches. None of them can employ full-time teachers to any considerable extent. But they possess fairly well equipped laboratories in anatomy, pathology, bacteriology, and physiology, a museum showing care and intelligence and a decent library. Boston University deserves special commendation for what it has accomplished with its small annual income.

Of the remaining homeopathic schools, four are weak and uneven; the Hahnemann of San Francisco and the Hahnemann of Chicago have small, but not altogether inadequate, equipment for the teaching of chemistry, elementary pathology and bacteriology; the Cleveland school offers an active course in experimental physiology. Beyond ordinary dissection and elementary chemistry, they offer little else. There is, for example, no experimental physiology in the San Francisco Hahnemann: 'the instructor doesn't believe in it; the Chicago Hahnemann contains a small outfit and a few animals for that subject; the Cleveland equipment for pathology and bacteriology is meager. The New York Homeopathic college for Women is well intentioned, but its means have permitted it to do but little in any direction.

Six schools remain-all utterly hopeless: Hering (Chicago), because it is without plant or resources; the other five (Kentucky, Pulte, Baltimore, Detroit, Kansas City), because in addition to having nothing, their condition indicates the total unfitness of their managers for any sort of educational responsibility. They buildings are filthy and neglected. At Louisville no branch is properly equipped; in one room, the outfit is limited to a dirty and tattered mannequin; in another a single guinea pig awaits his fate in a cage. At Detroit the dean and secretary 'have their offices downtown' the so called laboratories are in utter confusion...

In respect to hospital facilities, the University of Michigan, Boston University, and the New York Homeopathic alone command an adequate supply of material, under proper control, through modern teaching methods are not thoroughly utilized even by them. The Iowa's school controls a small, but inadequate, hospital. All the others are seriously handicapped by either lack of material or lack of control, and in most instances by both. The Hahnemann of San Franciso relies mainly on 80 beds supported by the city and county in a private hospital; the Detroit school is cordially welcome at the Grace Hospital, but less than 60 beds are available, and they are mostly surgical; the Woman's Homeopathic of New York controls a hospital of 35 available beds, mostly surgical; the Southwestern (Louisville) and the Cleveland school get one-fifth of the patients that enter the city hospitals of their respective towns, but these hospitals are not equipped or organized with a view to teaching. The Kansas city school holds clinics one day a week at the City Hospital; Pulte (Cincinnati) and the Atlantic (Baltimore) have, as nearly as one can gather, nothing definite at all. Several of the schools appear to be unnecessarily handicapped. The Chicago Hahnemann adjoins a hospital with 60 ward beds. But as the superintendent 'doesn't believe in admitting students to wards,' there is little or nothing beyond amphitheater teaching. A bridge connects Hering (Chicago) with a homeopathic hospital, but 'students are not admitted'. The Cleveland school is next door to a hospital with which it was once intimate; their relations have been ruptured. An excellent hospital is connected with the building occupied by the Philadelphia Hahnemann, but there is no ward work…

Financially the two state university departments and the New york Homeopathic school are the only homeopathic schools whose strength is greater than their fee income. All the others are dependent on tuition. Their outlook for higher entrance standards or improved teaching is, therefore, distinctly unpromising. Only a few of them command tuition fees enough to do anything at all: The Chicago Hahnemann, boston University, and the Philadelphia Hahnemann, with annual fees ranging between $12,000 and $18,000. Nine of them are hopelessly poor: The San Francisco Hahnemann, Hering Medical all operate on less than $4000 a year; the Southwestern (Louisville) and Pulte (Cincinnati) on less than $1500.

In the year 1900 there were twenty two homeopathic colleges in the United States; today there are fifteen; the total student enrollment has within the same period been cut almost in half, decreasing from 1909 to 1009; the graduating classes have fallen from 418 to 246. As the country is still poorly supplied with homeopathic physicians, these figures are ominous; for the rise of legal standard must inevitably affect homeopathic practitioners. In the financial weakness of their schools; the further shrinkage of the student body still inhibit first the expansion, then the keeping up of the sect.

Logically, no other outcome is possible. The ebbing vitality of homeopathic schools is a striking demonstration of the incompatibility of science and dogma. One may begin with science and work through the entire medical curriculum consistently, espousing everything to the same sort of test; or one may begin with a dogmatic assertion and resolutely refuse to entertain anything at variance with it. But one cannot do both. One cannot simultaneously assert science and dogma; one cannot travel half the road under the former banner, in the hope of taking up the latter, too, at the middle of the march. Science, once embraced, will conquer the whole. Homeopathy has two options: one to withdraw into the isolation in which alone any peculiar tenet can maintain itself; the other to put that tenet into the melting pot. Historically it undoubtedly played an important part in discrediting empirical allopathy…

It will be clear, then why, when outlining a system of schools for the training of physicians on scientific lines, no specific provision is made for homeopathy. For everything of proved value in homeopathy belong of right to scientific medicine and is at this moment incorporate in it; nothing else has any footing at all, whether it be of allopathic or homeopathic lineage."

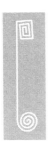

Appendix I
From AIH Convention on Education 1994

Question 1. What advice do you give concerning Materia Medica to a student beginning medicine by a year's preliminary study.

Answers:

Dr. R. E. DUDGEON, (Honorary Member, London.)—I have never had occasion to advise a student concerning the Materia Medica, and should think that, during his year's preliminary study, he had best give his whole attention to the subjects required for this preliminary study, and leave Materia Medica alone until he has mastered them.

Dr. RICHARD HUGHES, (Honorary Member, Brighton.)—On this point I should merge one thing, that the text book commended to such a learner shall not be one consisting of symptom lists. Of whatever use these may be to the practitioner, to a beginner they are uninteresting, confusing, disheartening. He wants an introduction which shall lead him by easy steps to the inner shrine. A literary work is required, one susceptible of continuous and not disagreeable reading; one that deals with outlines and generalities instead of burdening the memory with details. It was to supply such need mainly that I originally wrote my "Pharmacodynamics." Prepare your student to approach with zest his further studies in this sphere.

Dr. THOS. SKINNER, (Corresponding Member, London)—Let every candidate read and carefully study every sentence of the first volume of Hahnemann's Chronic Diseases and his Introduction to each medicine recorded in the Chronic Diseases and Materia Medica Pura; and if he has time and inclination let him not fail to peruse the pathogeneses of Hahnemann recorded in these two remarkable works. Lastly, let him do his best to comprehend the spirit and the letter of the Organon without a knowledge of which and a thorough belief in, no man can possibly practice the Homeopathy of Hahnemann.

Dr. E. T. BLAKE, (Corresponding Member, London.)—Though it may in some cases produce a stereotyped, inflexible physician, I would certainly not introduce Materia Medica nor Therapeutics till near the close of the curriculum. I take it that we are all agreed that students are taught too much, and that they remember too little.

Dr. J. W. HAYWARD, (Corresponding Member, Birkenhead, Eng.)—I would advise the student to spend most of his time and energies upon the Encyclopedia of Drug Pathogenesy, aided by Hughes', Dunham's and Farrington's and perhaps Hempel's Lectures; especially in passing the pathogenetic material through the "comparison" filter of Drs. Wesselhoeft and Sutherland, or (and ?) that of the Baltimore Club, and in the preparation of at least one of the drugs for the Materia Medica, Physiological and Applied.

Prof. MOHR, (Hahnemann of Phila.)—Should embrace a general description of the non metallic, vegetable and animal drug substances in their commercial or crude forms, and of the acids and special chemical products. The student should learn the methods required to convert these substances into the most active and least injurious medicinal forms, how these are administered, and what the maximum and minimum doses are. By carefully examining and handling specimens again and again he will become familiar with their characteristics.

Prot. HINSDALE, (Cleveland Univ. Med. and Surgery.)—Dunham says it requires seven years persistent study to measurably master our Materia Medica. I think he is right: the pursuit of this most important subject in point of time is co-extensive with a student's and physician's professional studies.

Prof. MCELWEE.—In the Homeopathic Medical College of Missouri it is customary to advise beginners to attend lectures, closely study the leading characteristics of the cardinal remedies, and endeavor to obtain only their "red-strings."

Prof. GILMAN, (Hahnemann of Chicago.)—First learn something of the rough work of the Materia Medica; the pharmacy and toxicological actions of the principal active poisons.

Prof. SNOW (Pulte of Cincinnati.)—Do not attempt too much in Materia Medica; select a few drugs; for instance the polychrests, and thoroughly master them. Each drug should be studied by itself and not left until it has become a part of the student. Advises particular attention to the physiological and pathological provings.

Prof. J. HEBER SMITH (Boston Univ. School of Med.)—Cause the student to become fairly proficient in human anatomy, physiology, biology and elementary microscopy, general and medical chemistry; elementary botany; the history of medicine leading up to Homeopathy; also pharmaceutics, Latin formulae and the Organon.

Prof. WESSELHOEFT, (same school as above.)—Devote much time to physics, (Natural Philosophy) chemistry, medical botany, and the brushing up of neglected Latin.

Prof. MACK, (Ann Arbor.)—Teach all the principles of medicine. When the field is once clearly mapped out, the student of Materia Medica and Therapeutics is prepared to intelligently accept all that is good in any system of medicine. I would show the student just what empiricism is; what rational practice is; and the same as to Homeopathic practice. If the student happens to be acquainted with the philosophy of Swedenborg and came as a private pupil, he would be given a direct and positive argument in favor of Homeopathy. Scrupulously avoid all dogmatism. Only in the fields of pathology and drug pathogenesy can a question of Homeopathicity be determined. Use the following books: Taylor's Treatise on Poisons; the volume on poisons in Wharton and Stille's Medical Jurisprudence; Reese's Medical Jurisprudence and Toxicology: also a number of old school authorities on Materia Medica. Then follow with Materia Medica Pura schematically arranged; so that if a question arises, whether it be pathogenesy or not, the most critical investigation of the question in the field of science (i. e. pathogenesy and never therapeutics) will always be in order.

Prof. COWPERTHWAITE, (Chicago Homeopathic)—Let them perfect themselves in botany and the chemistry of drugs, and follow with a study of the characteristic symptoms according to the Dr. Hering card plan. It is not wise to have students studying Materia Medica outside of these recommendations before they have listened to any lectures on the subject.

Prof. WOODWARD, (Chicago Homeopathic.)—They should obtain as distinct an idea of the toxical effects of drugs as they may from reading and comparing cases of poisoning. Also read Hughes's Pharmacodynamics, Taylor on Poisons, Woods or Bartholows Materia Medica, and U. S. Dispensatory.

Prof. ROYAL, (Iowa University.)—Give student Hughes' Pharmacodynamics, Dunham's Lectures and Farrington's Clinical Materia Medica. Look up all unfamiliar words and technical terms. Above all, do not let the student become disgusted with dry symptomatology.

Prof. DEWEY, (Hahnemann of San Francisco.)—Advises students to ground themselves well in the history of Homeopathy. Read Sharpe's Tracts, Dudgeon's Lectures, Ameke's History, and Fifty Reasons for being a Homeopath.

Prof. LEONARD, (Univ. of Minn.)—If he has not had preliminary college training, should learn something of botany, pharmacy and toxicology. If previously trained, should choose leading drugs in larger works on Toxicology, and Hughes' Pharmacodynamics. Also and better the Cyclopedia of Drug Pathogenesy.

Prof. EDGERTON, (Kansas City College.)—Select a work which gives general action of remedies and study them in groups and families, noting and memorizing the peculiar and characteristic symptoms.

Prof. PRICE, (Baltimore-Southern Hom. Coll.)—Pay no attention to details of symptomatology. Study botany and history of drugs. Occupy his attention with more preliminary studies.

Prof. CHEESEMAN, (National of Chicago.)—Study Hawkes' and Guernsey's Keynotes. Select from thirty to fifty polychrests, and endeavor to give him a good idea of these drugs.

Prof. NIELSEN, (Late of National of Chicago)—Acquire the physiological action of the principal drugs from Hughes' Pharmacodynamics, Shoemaker's or Bartholow's Materia Medica, Taylor on Poisons. Pay no attention to provings made from high potencies, but only such as have resulted from taking a tangible and reasonable dose.

Prof. HAWKES, (Herring College.)—Study the Organon. Read Farrington's Materia Medica, and Dunham's Homeopathy: The Science of Therapeutics. Give him an occasional case to look up. Also read carefully the Homeopathic Pharmacopeia and the Life of Hahnemann.

Prof. H. C. ALLEN, (Hering of Chicago.)—Don't let him study Materia Medica until he attends lectures.

Prof. MONROE, (Southwestern of Louisville.)—don't study Materia Medica in preparatory year. Ground the student in anatomy, physiology, chemistry, botany and pathology. Materia Medica is the pinnacle of the medical temple, the science toward which all other medical knowledge should ultimately converge.

Dr. GRAMM, (Ardmore, Pa.)— Familiarize the student with the nomenclature of his profession. Study the elementary steps of medicine. Be well grounded in botany, physiology and anatomy.

Dr. PECK, (Providence.)—Study Hughes' s Pharmacodynamics at the very beginning.

Dr. KRAFT, (Cleveland.)—Give him Dunham's books to read; talk, not read the Organon to him.

Question 2. When should the Organon be taught and how?

Dr. DUDGEON—The Organon being the best exposition of the homeopathic system, should be carefully studied by every one for himself and Its teachings accepted and endorsed by every teacher of Homeopathy when they are not inconsistent with the ascertained facts of modern science.

Dr. HUGHES—The teaching of the Organon does not seem to me to belong to the chair of Materia Medica, but rather to that of Theory and Practice of Medicine. From this I would have it at some time in every student's course, read and critically commented on. I recommend Dr Dudgeon's latest translation.

Dr. SKINNER—The Organon, in my estimation, should be studied from the very first. In fact, I do not believe it possible for any man to have any sound conception of what Homeopathy is until he thoroughly understands and can take into his comprehension the vast and important tenets and truths of the greatest work that ever was published in Medicine, theoretically, doctrinally or practically.

Dr. BLAKE—The Organon should be assimilated late in life probably.

Prof. MOHR—The Organon should be studied during the first year so effectually that its great or fundamental principles will be indelibly fixed on the mind of the student. In the class-room, in the clinic and at every opportunity its practical rules should be brought to the attention of the students, for they cannot be too often repeated.

Prof. DEWEY—The Organon should be taught during the second and third years of college course. And I believe in each homeopathic college a separate chair should be made for the Organon and Institutes of Homeopathy. Of course much of it can be taught in conjunction with lectures upon Materia Medica; but as it contains the philosophy of Homeopathy it seems to me that a separate chair for it is preferable, and it should be a chair insisted on by the American Institute, with two lectures a week at least.

Prof. HINSDALE—The principles of homeopathy should be taught to freshmen, well grounding them in the philosophy of the theory of homeopathy. The Organon can be taught by class-room readings, preferably by seniors. Comments can be made as the reading advances and papers prepared by the students upon topics suggested by the author. The teaching of this valuable book should be critical and impartial. Adoration for Hahnemann should give place to admiration for the truth to be taught.

Prof. McELWEE—The Organon should be taught when the student's mind is rested and fresh; consequently the first thing in the morning, one or two paragraphs only at a time, those paragraphs being read by the student, who gives his idea of it, and then later, under the supervision of the professor, discusses it before the class.

Prof. GILMAN—The Organon should be taught early and continually until it is mastered. It is the mother's milk to the medical student. It should be taught as the Bible is expounded— text by text, and explained and illustrated.

Prof. SNOW—The Organon should be systematically taught during the first year of college, as it is the foundation work of Homeopathy. Frequent reference should be made to it, however, during the whole three years as occasion may demand. It should be committed to memory as nearly as possible, so that its precepts may remain always engraved on the mind.

Prof. MACK—I do not use the Organon as a text-book. I think that one can better teach Homeopathy without the Organon as a text-book than with it.

Prof. COWPERTHWAITE—The Organon should be taught by a separate teacher. It has not fallen to my lot to teach the Organon to any extent and I do not consider myself a competent judge as to how it should be taught. My method is to take my old and much loved copy which I held in my hand when I attended the lectures by Dr. Hering, and which is profusely filled with annotations, comments and underlinings according to Dr. Hering's suggestions. From this book I talk to the class, giving them Hahnemann's ideas, Hering's comments and my own views on each particular section as we take it up.

Prof. WOODWARD—The Organon should be taught to beginners, not without judicious criticism.

Prof. ROYAL—The Organon should be studied and taught throughout the entire student's course.

Prof. LEONARD—For six years I have tried to teach the Organon in connection with Materia Medica and therapeutics; but whether from my own inability to do it well or from an incongruity of subjects, the results have not been satisfactory. A critical analysis of the Organon with an exposition of its essential parts before senior students, seems to me to be part of the work of the chair of Theory and Practice, and it is so taught in the University of Minnesota.

Prof. EDGERTON—The Organon should be taught to first course students. A text-book should be gotten up containing the essentials, and the student should commit the same to memory and recite in class.

Prof. PRICE—In my opinion the Organon should be taught from the chair of Institutes, first omitting the psoric theory, dynamization, primary and secondary drug action, alternating drug effects, etc. There is too much difference of opinion upon these subjects amongst the best minds in our profession to make a belief in them a point of vital necessity. Of course the chair of Materia Medica and Therapeutics should teach the fundamental principles of Homeopathy whether the Organon be quoted or not.

Prof. CHEESEMAN—The Organon should be taught by at least two lectures each week during the entire college course by a competent lecturer.

Prof. HAWKES—The Organon should be taught from the "cradle to the grave" of medicine. In my judgment it should be taught as the good preacher teaches his congregation: select a portion for a text (and each section of the Organon is a sermon in itself) and elaborate to the student and explain its philosophy. Then make him explain it to me.

Prof. ALLEN, H. C.—The Organon should be taught every year of the entire course and taught by one who practices what he preaches. It is the foundation of our system, and no student can ever practice Homeopathy who does not know, and know most thoroughly, its principles.

Prof. PEMBERTON DUDLEY—I hold to the view that every student should, first of all be made acquainted with the methods—perhaps in courtesy I should say "principles"-on which unhomeopathic treatment is applied to diseases and injuries by the various sects of physicians, and that his induction into the mysteries of Homeopathy should come later. I am quite sure that the uncompromising adhesion to the homeopathic law manifested by the "Homeopathic Fathers" was due to the fact that they knew from both study and experience all about allopathic methods and what these methods could and could not do for their patients; and holding this view it would naturally follow that the way to make staunch as well as intelligent homeopathists is to make them quite fully acquainted with the effects and defects of the other modes of medical practice first of all. Having accomplished this we proceed as follows: We endeavor to discover how the phenomenon known as "cure" is to be investigated. (The allopath never concerns himself on this matter save only as to the fact of its occurrence and the nature of the agencies by which it seems to be brought about. The phenomenon does not present itself to his mind as at all requiring investigation). This study forces us to the bedside as the only place where our curative studies can be pursued— the only "Laboratory" where principle of cure can be made known. Then having learned the reasonableness and practicability of this method of finding out how to find out cures for diseases, we turn to the Organon and there discover that the author of that book has been before us and has made the way plain for us. So we take up point after point in the development of curative science— first reasoning it out as well as we can and then turning to the book to find it all in Hahnemann's own words. One of the things that our students discover and often mention in this course is that the author of the Organon was anything but the dreaming visionary he has been so often represented to be. In these studies of Homeopathy both the student and the teacher are expected to have the open book before them. In last winter's class of about eighty first-year men I have counted over seventy copies of the Organon in the room at one time, and all of them in use. We call it our "Sunday School Class in the Organon."

Prof. MONROE—It is a question in my mind whether the Organon should be taught during the student years; that is systematically. It should be referred to by the professor frequently, and the student should be taught that he cannot regard himself as a well-rounded homeopathic physician until he is familiar with the Organon. To my mind, however, the book is not of such a character as will admit of its being properly digested during the rushing, cramming gallop that marks the career of a student during his last year; and previous to that time, he is not sufficiently far advanced to comprehend it.

Dr. GRAMM—Hahnemann's Organon should be read thoroughly by every student before entering a homeopathic college, and there it should be used by the regular professor of theory and practice as the foundation and guide for his teachings during all the four years. Every section should be properly read and carefully explained, and its teachings as much as possible illustrated by cases from actual practice from beginning to end.

Dr. PECK—The Organon should be the first book placed in the hands of a medical student. If he has not sufficient sense and knowledge to understand and to appreciate it he never can become a trustworthy physician. The youth should be told to read it slowly and deliberately, stopping at any (to him) obscure point, or at any utterance that does not commend itself to his sober judgment and refer it at once to his instructor for their joint investigation. Rarely will this happen a half dozen times. One or two more rapid re-readings will do no harm. Since many alleged homeopathic physicians do not provide their pupils this instruction it becomes necessary for the college to teach the Institutes of Medicine. These should be taught at the very beginning instead of at the close of a course of study, for it is as important that a doctor should know what he believes, and why, as for the preacher, or any other man; and the sooner he ascertains this the better. After a little talk on Hahnemann and his times, display on the blackboard or in other convenient manner singly and successively the various propositions. As each is exhibited ask the class if it accepts that assertion, then call for reasons pro and con.

Dr. NIELSEN—The Organon should be taught especially to the advanced student, but by a competent teacher and one able to read between the lines.

Dr. KRAFT—The Organon, like the bible, should be read through not less than once a year; its reading and study should not cease with the medical man's commencement exercises. During school-life it should be listened to from the chair of therapeutics at least once a week. Not read by the teacher but talked. The professor of therapeutics should have naught to do with Materia Medica; in him should be combined the present highly ornamental chair of Organon, and the rare chair of Institutes of Medicine.

To him should be given the duties of explaining the homeopathic law, the therapeutical application of Materia Medica, the Organon, and the potencies.

Dr. BOJANUS—According to my opinion I should think that the Organon should not be given before the end of the third year of study and must be explained and commented in a special course of lectures, and not before the students have visited the homeopathic and allopathic clinics and hospitals for at least two years. In the lectures upon the Organon, the whole homeopathic literature, with all its different tendencies, must be passed in review and particular attention must be paid that the youthful students should not prefer the literature which has given itself the task of clothing homeopathic therapeutics into a form more or less like allopathy.

Such compilations are a comfortable implement in the hands of those who wish to convert science into a milking cow; they are useful to establish a position and keep their disciple in the broad way of the beaten track, but this is preparing the ruin of homeopathy.

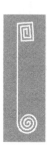

Appendix J
Homeopathic Board Certification Organizations

Author's Note: Please note that there is a distinction between licensure and certification. The homeopathic boards listed below only provide certification and not a license to practice.

Council for Homeopathic Certification

Description: This organization was founded in 1992, in response to a new vision for the future of homeopathy as a unified profession of highly trained and certified practitioners. To date, they have certified more practitioners than any other professional homeopathic organization. Their goals are to create a common standard to establish competence in classical homeopathy, define standards of homeopathic care and professional ethics, administer an exam process to certify homeopaths to this level of competence, assist the public to choose appropriately qualified homeopaths from all professional backgrounds with a national directory of certified practitioners, promote the inclusion of homeopathy within the recognized scope of practice of all health-care professions, and to cooperate with existing organizations to strengthen the homeopathic profession with an agreed credential and excellence in classical homeopathic training and practice.

Candidates for certification must fulfill educational and clinical experience prerequisites established by the CHC in order to undertake a challenging written exam. Those who pass the written exam subsequently take an oral examination. Successful candidates receive a certificate stating that they are "Certified in Classical Homeopathy" and are entitled to use the credential "CCH." This certification is not a license to practice, but is an important step toward defining a national identity for the homeopathic profession.

Certification by CHC is a public statement of recognition by a practitioner's peers of training, knowledge, skill, and competence in classical homeopathy. The certifying board includes homeopaths from major health-care professions, as well as the growing group of professional homeopaths. This certification also assists the general public in choosing appropriately qualified homeopaths from all professional backgrounds.

Designation: CCH
Contact:

1199 Sanchez St.
San Francisco, California 94114
Telephone: (415)789-7677
Fax: (415) 695-8220
chcmail@homeopathy-council.org

American Board of Homeotherapeutics

Description: The ABHt was founded in 1959 and incorporated (New York) in 1960 for the purpose of promoting the science of homeopathy, demonstrating its effectiveness to the medical profession, and insuring homeopathy's growth as a viable medical specialty in the U.S. The ABHt grants Diplomate (advanced specialty) status to those medical and osteopathic physicians applicants who meet the prerequisites and successfully pass a written and an oral examination. The ABHt in 1997 has also created a Homeopathic Primary Care Certification for the purpose of creating a minimum standard of competency in homeopathy. The ABHt grants Primary Care Certificate status to those licensed physicians, advanced practice nurses, or physicians assistants who meet the primary-care homeopathic education/training prerequisites and successfully pass the homeopathy primary certificate examination and who agree to practice within the bounds of their respective medical and homeopathic competence.

Designation: DHt
Contact:

801 N. Fairfax Street, Suite 306
Alexandria, VA 22314
#703-548-7790
Fax: 703-548-7792

Homeopathic Academy of Naturopathic Physicians

Description: The HANP is a certification organization for naturopaths only. Becoming a diplomate allows the individual to join a community of colleagues committed to the growth and development of classical homeopathy. The certified practitioner can contribute their skills and expertise through mentoring other homeopaths, participating as a member of the board of directors, writing cases for the naturopathic journal *Similimum*, or presenting cases at the Homeopathic Association for Naturopathic Physicians Annual Case Conference.

Designation: DHANP
Contact:

12132 SE Foster Place
Portland, Oregon 97266
503-761-3298
Fax: 503-762-1929
swolf@teleport.com

North American Society of Homeopaths

Description: The North American Society of Homeopaths was created in 1990. It is modeled after the Society of Homeopaths in the United Kingdom, the largest organization of competent yet non-medically licensed homeopaths in the world. The purpose of NASH is two-fold: the organization exists to set standards of competency and to certify individuals in the practice of classical homeopathy. This is an unusually effective way to inform and protect health-care consumers in search of homeopathic treatment. NASH exists to help non-medically licensed homeopaths to meet their needs as professionals in a variety of ways, including advocating for legality and licensure to practice, developing national recognition for the profession, and working to obtain malpractice insurance and coverage. NASH requires all applicants to pass the exam administered by the Council for Homeopathic Certification (see above).

Designation: RSHom
Contact:

1122 E. Pike Street, Suite 1122
Seattle, WA 98122
206-720-7000
Fax: 206-329-5684
www.homeopathy.org

National Board of Homeopathic Examiners

Description: The National Board of Homeopathic Examiners has been incorporated since 1987. The board evolved out of a vision of creating standardized interprofessional testing for the advancement of the homeopathic profession. The board administers an examination every six months that certifies the basic level of proficiency of homeopathic practitioners who successfully pass the exam. Applicants must have previously earned a PhD, DC, RPh, MD, DO, AP, ND, OMD, or equivalent degree and have received specialized training in a board-certified institution.

Designation: DNBHE

Contact:

PMB#832, P.O. Box 15749
Boise, Idaho 83715-5749
208-426-0847
Fax: 208-426-0848
msassodc@aol.com
www.nbhe.com

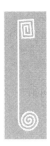

Bibliography

American Association of School Administrators. *America 2000: Where School Leaders Stand.* Arlington, VA: 1991.

——. *1994 Platforms and Resolutions.* Arlington, VA: 1993.

Armour, Robert A., and Fuhrmann, Barbara S. "Confirming the Centrality of Liberal Learning." In *Educating Professionals: Responding to New Expectations for Competence and Accountability,* edited by L. Curry and J. Wergin. San Francisco: Jossey-Bass Publishers, 1993.

Arredon, P., Toporek, R., Brown, S., Jones, L., Locke, D., Sanchex, J., and Stadler, H. "Operationalization of the Multicultural Counseling Competencies," *Journal of Multicultural Counseling and Development,* 24, 42-78.

Badaracco, J. L., and Ellsworth, R. *Leadership and the Quest for Integrity.* Boston, MA: Harvard Business School Press, 1989.

Banner, James, and Cannon, Harold. *The Elements of Learning.* New Haven, CT, and London: Yale University Press, 1999.

——. *The Elements of Teaching.* New Haven, CT, and London: Yale University Press, 1997.

Barker, J. A. *Paradigms: The Business of Discovering the Future.* New York: Harper Collins Publishers, Inc., 1992.

Baron, J. *Thinking and Deciding.* New York: Cambridge University Press, 1988.

Barrows, H. S., and Tamblyn, R. *Problem-Based Learning: An Approach to Medical Education.* New York: Springer, 1980.

Barrows, H. S. *How to Design a Problem-Based Curriculum for the Preclinical Years.* New York: Springer, 1985.

Bebeau, M. "Can Ethics Be Taught?" In *Journal of the American College of Dentists*, 58, 5-15, 1991.

Beck, L., and Murphy, J. *The Four Imperatives of a Successful School.* Thousand Oaks, CA: Corwin Press, 1996.

Belenky, M.F., Clinchy, B.M., Goldberger, N.R., and Tarule, J.M. *Women's Ways of Knowing: The Development of Self, Voice and Mind.* New York: Basic Books, 1986.

Bennis, Warren. *On Becoming a Leader.* Reading, MA: Addison Wesley, 1989.

Berends, Polly. *Coming to Life: Traveling the Spiritual Path in Everyday Life.* San Francisco, CA: Harper Publications, 1990.

Blake, R. R., and McCanse, A. A. *Leadership Dilemmas-Grid Solutions.* Houston, TX: Gulf Publishing, 1991.

Bland, C. J., Hitchcock, M. A., Anderson, W. A., and Stritter, F. T. "Faculty Development Fellowship Programs in Family Medicine." In *Journal of Medical Education*, 62 (8) (1987), 632-641.

Bligh, D. A. *What's the Use of Lectures?* Harmondsworth, England: Penguin Publishers, 1987.

Block, P. *Stewardship: Choosing Service Over Self-Interest.* San Francisco: Berrett-Koehler, 1993.

Bolman, Lee G. And Deal, Terrence E. *Leading with Soul, An Uncommon Journey of Spirit.* San Francisco: Jossey Bass Publishers, 1995.

Boud, D., Keogh, R., and Walker, D. (Eds). *Reflections: Turning Experience into Learning.* New York: Nichols Publications, 1985.

Boud, D., and Griffin, V. (Eds). *Appreciating Adults Learning: From the Learner's Perspective.* London: Kogan Page Publishers, 1987.

Boud, D., and Feletti ,G. *The Challenge of Problem Based Learning.* New York: St. Martin's Press, 1998.

Boyer, E. L. *Scholarship Reconsidered: Priorities of the Professoriate.* Princeton, NJ: Carnegie Foundation for the Advancement of Teaching, 1990.

Brandt, R. "On Building Learning Communities: A Conversation with Hank Levin", In *Educational Leadership*, 50(1) (Sept. 1992), 19-23.

Bratchell, F. F., and Heald, M. *The Aims and Organization of Liberal Studies,* Oxford, England: Pergamon Press, 1966.

Bridges E., and Hallinger, P. *Implementing Problem Based Learning in Leadership Development.* Eugene, OR: University of Oregon; ERIC Clearinghouse on Educational Management, 1995.

Brookfield, Stephen. *Understanding and Facilitating Adult Learning: A Comprehensive Analysis of Principles and Effective Practices.* San Francisco: Jossey-Bass Publishers, 1986.

Brookfield, Stephen. *The Skillful Teacher.* San Francisco: Jossey Bass Publishers, 1990.

Brown, G. A. *Lecturing and Explaining.* London: Methuen Publishers, 1980.

Brown, G. A., and Atkins, M. *Effective Teaching in Higher Education.* New York: Methuen Publishers, 1987.

Brown, J. H. U. "Medical Schools in Crisis." In *Evaluation and the Health Professions,* 11 (1988), 147-171.

Burke, Nancy. *Teachers are Special.* New York: Gramercy Books, 1996.

Butterwick, S. "Re-entry for Women: This Time It's Personal." In *Proceedings of the Adult Education Research Conference.* Calgary, Canada: Faculty of Continuing Education, University of Calgary, **#29, 1988**.

Buzan, Tony . *Use Both Sides of Your Brain.* New York: E. P. Dutton, Inc., 1984.

Buzan, Tony, and Buzan, Barry. (1996); *The Mind Map Book.* New York: Penguin Books, 1996.

Calderhead, J. *Teachers' Classroom Decision Making.* New York: Holt, Rinehart & Winston, 1984.

Candy, P. C. *Self Direction for Lifelong Learning: A Comprehensive Guide to Theory and Practice.* San Francisco: Jossey-Bass Publications, 1991.

Carter, G. LO. "A Perspective on Preparing Adult Educators." In *Strengthening Connections Between Education and Performance,* S. M. Grabowski (ed.). New Directions for Adult and Continuing Education, #18. San Francisco: Jossey-Bass Publishers, 1983.

Cervero R. M. "Professional Practice, Learning and Continuing Education: An Integrated Perspective." In *Professions Educator Research Notes*, 11 (1989), 10-13.

Chappell, Peter. "George Vithoulkas and the Supervision for Homeopaths." In *Homeopathic Links*, Summer 2000, Vol 13(2).

Cook, Daniel, and Naude, Alain, "The Ascendence and Decline of Homeopathy in America: How Great Was Its Fall?". In *Journal of the American Institute of Homeopathy*, Vol. 89, #3 (Autumn, 1996).

Cordeiro, P., and Loup, K. "Partnering Changes the Roles of School Leaders: Implications for Educational Leadership Preparation Programs." In *Border Crossings: Educational Partnerships and School Leadership,* P. Cordeiro (ed.). San Francisco: Jossey-Bass Publications, 1996.

Cordeiro, P., and Monroe-Kolek, M. "Connecting the School Communities Through the Development of Educational Partnerships." In *Border Crossings: Educational Partnerships and School Leadership,* P. Cordeiro (ed.). San Francisco: Jossey-Bass Publications, 1996.

Corey, M., and Corey, G. *Groups: Process and Practice.* Pacific Grove, CA: Brooks/Cole Publishers, 1997.

Covey, S. "Leading By Compass." In *A New Paradigm of Leadership,* K. Shelton (ed.). Provo, UT: Executive Excellence, 1997.

Coulter, Harris L. *Divided Legacy: Conflict Between Homeopathy and the American Medical Association.* Berkeley, CA: North Atlantic Books, 1973.

Craig, R. "Ethical Frameworks to Guide Action." In *The Principal as Leader,* L. Hughes, (ed.). Saddle River, NJ: Prentice Hall, 1999.

Cranton, P. *Understanding and Promoting Transformative Learning: A Guide for Educators of Adults.* San Francisco: Jossey-Bass Publications, 1994.

Cronin, Thomas E. *Chronicle of Higher Education,* Feb. 1, 1989.

Cunningham, William, and Cordeiro, Paula. *Educational Administration: A Problem Based Approach.* Boston: Allyn and Bacon, 2000.

Curry, Lynn, and Wergin, Jon. *Educating Professionals: Responding to New Expectations for Competence and Accountability.* San Francisco: Jossey-Bass Publishers, 1993.

Daloz, L. A. *Effective Teaching and Mentoring: Realizing the Transformational Power of Adult Learning Experiences.* San Francisco: Jossey-Bass Publishers, 1986.

Daloz, L. A. *Mentor, Guiding the Journey of Adult Learners.* San Francisco: Jossey-Bass Publications, 1999.

Davis, Madeleine, and Wallbridge, David. *Boundary and Space: An Introduction to the Work of D. W. Winnicott.* New York: Brunner/Mazel Publishers, 1987.

Deal, T., and Key, M. M. *Corporate Celebration: Play, Purpose and Profit at Work.* San Francisco: Berrett-Koehler, 1998.

Deal, T., and Peterson, K. *Shaping School Culture: The Heart of Leadership.* San Francisco: Jossey-Bass Publications, 1998.

Decker, Burt. *You Have to Be Believed, To Be Heard.* New York: St. Martin's Press, 1991.

Dennison, Paul, and Dennison, Gail. *Brain Gym.* Ventura, CA: Educational Kinesthetics, Inc, 1989.

Detterman, D. "The Case for the Prosecution: Transfer as an piphenomenon." In *Transfer on Trial: Intelligence Cognition and Instruction,* D. Detterman and R. Sternberg (eds.). Norwood, NJ: Ablex, 1993.

Devaney, K. *The Lead Teacher: Ways to Begin.* New York: Carnegie Forum on Education and the Economy, 1987.

Dillard, Annie. *Pilgrim at Tinker Creek.* New York: Harper and Row Publishers, 1980.

Dinham, S. M., and Stritter, F. T. "Research on Professional Education." In *Handbook of Research on Teaching* (M. C. Wittrock, ed., third edit.). New York: Macmillan, 1986.

Doll, R. *Curriculum Improvement, Decision Making and Process.* Boston: Allyn and Bacon,1986.

Drucker, P. F. *Managing for the Future: The 1990's and Beyond.* New York: Truman Tally Books, 1992.

Duke, D., and Grogan, M. "The Moral and Ethical Dimensions of Leadership." In *Ethics in Educational Leadership Programs,* L. Beck and J. Murphy (eds.). Columbia, MO: UCEA, 1997.

Eble, K. E. *The Craft of Teaching: A Guide to Mastering the Professor's Art* (second edition). San Francisco: Jossey-Bass Publications, 1988.

Eckstein, Rudolph, and Wallerstein, Robert. *The Teaching and Learning of Psychotherapy.* New York: International Universities Press, Inc., 1980.

Edwards, H. T. "The Role of Legal Education in Shaping the Profession." In *Journal of Legal Education,* 38(3) (1988), 285-293.

Eisner, E. W. *The Enlightened Eye: Qualitative Inquiry and the Enhancement of Educational Practice.* New York: Macmillan, 1991.

Elstein, A. S., Shulman, L. S., and Sprafka, S. A. *Medical Problem Solving: An Analysis of Clinical Reasoning.* Cambridge, MA: Harvard University Press, 1978.

Ennis, R. H. "A Taxonomy of Critical Thinking Dispositions and Abilities." In *Teaching Thinking Skills: Theory and Practice,* J.B. Baron and R. S. Sternberg (eds.). New York: W. H. Freeman Publishers, 1986.

Evans, R. *The Human Side of School Change.* San Francisco: Jossey-Bass Publications, 1996.

Fink, Dee. *The First Year of College Teaching.* San Francisco: Jossey-Bass Publications, 1984.

Fletcher, Leon. *How to Speak Like a Pro.* New York: Ballantine Books, 1983.

Flexner, Abraham *Medical Education in the United States and Canada.* New York: The Carnegie Foundation, 1910.

Freire, P. *Pedagogy of the Oppressed,* New York: Continuum Press, 1970.

Fullan, Michael. *Change Forces.* Bristol, PA: Falmer Press, 1993.

Fullan, Michael. *Educational Leadership.* San Francisco: Jossey Bass Publications, 2000.

Gaines, Wendy. Senior Research Project for Hahnemann College of Homeopathy, 1994.

Galbreaith, M. W. *Facilitating Adult Learning: A Transactional Process.* Malabar, FL: Kreiger Publishing Company, 1991.

Gardner, H. *Frames of Mind: The Theory of Multiple Intelligences.* New York: Basic Books, 1983.

Gardner, Howard. *Types of Intelligence: Reflections on Multiple Intelligences—Myths and Messages.* Phi delta Kappan (November, 1995).

Glazer, Steven (ed.) *The Heart of Learning: Spirituality in Education.* New York: Tarcher/Putnam, 1994.

Giroux, H. *Border Crossings: Cultural Workers and the Politics of Education.* New York: Routledge, 1992.

Glickman, C. D. *Renewing America's Schools.* San Francisco: Jossey-Bass Publications, 1998.

Goodlad, S., and Hirst, B. *Peer Tutoring: A Guide to Learning by Teaching.* New York: Nichols Publishers, 1980.

Grabowski, S. M. "How Educators and Trainers Can Ensure On-the-Job Performance." In *Strengthening Connections Between Education and Performance,* S. M. Grabowski (ed.). San Francisco: New Directions for Adult and Continuing Education, #18; Jossey Bass Publishers, 1983.

Gray, Bill. *Homeopathy Science or Myth.* Berkeley. CA: North Atlantic Books, 2000.

Greenblatt, C. S. *Designing Games and Simulations.* Newbury Park, CA: Sage Publications, 1988.

Greenleaf, R. K. *The Servant as Leader.* Indianapolis: Greenleaf Center for Servant Leadership, 1970.

Guggenbul-Craig, Walter. *Power in the Helping Professions.* Woodstock, CT: Spring Publications, Inc., 1971.

Hahnemann, Samuel. *Organon of the Medical Arts.* Wenda Brewster O'Reilly (ed.). Redmond, WA: Birdcage Books, 1996.

Halifax, Joan. "Learning as Initiation: Not-Knowing, Bearing Witness and Healing". In *The Heart of Learning: Spirituality in Education,* Steven Glazer (ed). New York: Jeremy P. Tarcher/Putnam, 1940.

Halpern, S. C. "On the Politics and Pathology of Legal Education." In *Journal of Legal Education*, 32(3) (1982), 383-394.

Harris, I. B. "An Exploration of the Role of Theories in Communication for Guiding Practitioners." In *Journal of Curriculum and Supervision*, **1**, (1986) 27-55.

Harris, I. B. "A Critique of Schon's View on Teacher Education: Contributions and Issues." In *Journal of Curriculum and Supervision*, 5 (1989), 13-18.

Harris, I. B. "Deliberative Inquiry: The Arts of Planning." In *Forms Curriculum Inquiry,* E. Short (ed.). Albany, NY: State University of New York Press, 1991.

Heaton, Jeanne Albronda. *Building Basic Therapeutic Skills.* San Francisco: Jossey-Bass Publications, 1998.

Heifetz, Ronald, and Sinder, Riley. "Political Leadership: Managing the Public's Problem Solving." In *The Power of Public Ideas,* Robert Reich (ed.). Cambridge, MA: Ballinger, 1987.

Hersey, P., and Blanchard, K. H. *Management of Organizational Behavior: Utilizing Human Resources.* Englewood Cliffs, NJ: Prentice-Hall Publishers, 1982. Hooks, Bell. "Embracing Freedom: Spirituality and Liberation." In *The Heart of Learning: Spirituality in Education,* S.Glazer (ed). New York: Jeremy Tarcher/Putnam, 1999.

Huang, C. A., and Lynch, J. *Mentoring: The Tao of Giving and Receiving Wisdom.* San Francisco: Harper Publications, 1995.

Hutchinson, E., and Hutchinson, E. *Women Returning to Learning.* Cambridge, England: National Extension College, 1988.

Jackson, P. *Life in Classrooms.* New York: Teachers College Press, 1986.

James, William. *The Writings of William James*, John J. McDermott (ed.). Chicago: University of Chicago Press, 1970.

Jehl, J., and Kirst, M. "Getting Ready to Provide School-Linked Services: What Schools Must Do." In *The Future of Children* (second edit.). Los Altos, CA: Center for the Future of Children, 1992.

Jencks, C., and Riesman, D. *The Academic Revolution.* Chicago: University of Chicago Press, 1977.

Jersild, A. *When Teachers Face Themselves.* New York: Teachers College Press, 1955.

Jolles, Robert. *How to Run Seminars and Workshops: Presentation Skills for Consultants, Trainers, and Teachers.* New York: John Wiley and Sons, Inc., 1993.

Jung, D. G. *Mysterium Coniunctionis.* R. F. C. Hull (trans). Princeton, NJ: Princeton University Press, 1977.

Kaplan, D. "Leader as Model and Mentor." In *A New Paradigm of Leadership,* K. Shelton (ed.). Provo, UT: Executive Excellence, 1997.

Kellogg Leadership Studies Project. *Leadership in the Twenty First Century.* College Park, MD: Center for Political Leadership and Participation, University of Maryland, 1997.

Kennedy, M. "Policy Issues in Teacher Education". In *Phi Delta Kappan*, May 1991: 661-666.

Kent, J. *Lectures on Homeopathic Philosophy.* Berkeley, CA: North Atlantic Books, 1979.

King. A. "Improving Lecture Comprehension: Effects of a Metacognitive Strategy". In *Applied Cognitive Psychology*, 5 (1991): 331-346.

King, A. "Comparison of Self-Questioning, Summarizing, and Notetaking-Review as Strategies for Learning from Lectures". In *American Educational Research Journal*, 29 (1992): 303-323.

King, A. "Making a Transition from 'Sage on the Stage' to 'Guide on the Side'. In *College Teaching*, 41 (1993): 30-35.

Kleinke, C. L. *Common Principles of Psychotherapy.* Pacific Grove, CA: Brooks/Cole, 1994.

Klopp, Sheldon. *If You Meet the Buddha On the Road, Kill Him!.* Ben Lomond, CA: Science and Behavior Books, Inc., 1972.

Kolb, D. A. "Future Directions for Learning Style Research." In *Learning Style in Continuing Medical Education,* L.Curry (ed). Ottawa: Canadian Medical Association, 1983.

Kolb, D. A. *Experiential Learning: Experience as the Source of Learning and Development.* Englewood Cliffs, NJ: Prentice Hall Publishers, 1984. Englewood Cliff, NJ.

Kotter, J. P. *The Leadership Factor.* New York: Free Press, 1988.

Krannich, Caryl Rae. *101 Secrets of Highly Effective Speakers.* Manassas Park, VA: Impact Publications, 1998.

Kreisberg, Joel. "Homeopathic Education: An Overview." In *Resonance* (March-April, 1996), 16-18.

Kreisberg, Joel, and Phelps, Molly. *Trends in Homeopathic Education: A Survey of Homeopathic Schools in North America,* Chatham, NY: Council for Homeopathic Education, 1998.

Kreisberg, Joel. "The Attitude of Homeopathic Education." In *Homeopathy Today* (Nov. 1999), 18-20.

Kreisberg, Joel. "Clinical Supervision." In *Journal of the American Institute of Homeopathy,* Vol 93, #3 (Fall 2000), 110-115.

Kridel, C., Bullough, R., and Shaker, P. *Teachers and Mentors: Profiles of Distinguished Twentieth Century Professors of Education.* New York: Garland Publishers, 1996.

Lambert, L., Walker, D., Zimmerman, D., Cooper, J., Lambert, M. D., Gardner, M., and Slack, P. J. *The Constructivist Leader.* New York: Teachers College Press, 1995.

Landis, M. C. "Mentoring as a Professional Development Tool." In *Continuing Higher Education*, Winter 1990.

Lewis, L. H. (Ed.). *Experiential and Simulation Techniques for Teaching Adults.* San Francisco: New Directions for Continuing Education, #30; Jossey-Bass Publications, 1986.

Lieberman, Ann, Ellen, Saxl R., and Miles, Matthew B. "Teacher Leadership: Ideology and Practice." In *Educational Leadership*. San Francisco: Jossey-Bass Publications, 2000.

Lillard, Joe. "The Past Present and Future of Homeopathic Study Groups in the United States." 1992.

Lindeman, E. C. *The Meaning of Adult Education.* Oklahoma City: University of Oklahoma, 1989.

Lombrozo, Tania. *The Language of Teaching.* Boulder, CO: Blue Mountain Press, Inc., 1999.

Lukinsky, J. "Reflective Withdrawal through Journal Writing." In *Fostering Critical Reflection in Adulthood: A Guide to Transformative and Emancipatory Learning,* J. Mezirow and Associates (eds.). San Francisco: Jossey-Bass Publications, 1990.

Maclaren, A. *Ambitions and Realizations: Women in Adult Education.* Washington, D.C.: Peter Owen Publications, 1986.

Mayburry, Richard. *Whatever Happened to Justice?* Placerville, CA: Bluestocking Press, 1993.

McGregor, D. *The Human Side of Enterprise.* New York: McGraw-Hill, 1960.

McKeachie, W. J. *Teaching Tips: A Guide for the Beginning College Teacher* (eighth edition). Lexington, MA: Heath Publishers, 1986.

Meno, L. R. "Sources of Alternative Revenue." In *Fifth Annual 1 (1984),* L. D. Webb and V. D. Mueller (eds.). Cambridge, MA: Ballinger.

Merriam, S. B., and Caffarella, R. S. *Learning in Adulthood.* San Francisco: Jossey-Bass Publications, 1993.

Mertz, N. "Knowing and Doing: Exploring the Ethical Life of Educational Leaders." In *Ethics in Educational Leadership in Programs,* L. Beck and J. Murphy (eds.). Columbia, MO: UCEA, 1997.

Meyers, C. *Teaching Students to Think Critically: A Guide for Faculty in All Disciplines.* San Francisco: Jossey-Bass Publications, 1986.

Mezirow, J. "Perspective Transformation". In *Studies in Adult Education,* 9(2) (1977), 153-164.

Mezirow, J., and Associates. *Fostering Critical Reflection in Adulthood: A Guide to Transformative and Emancipatory Learning.* San Francisco: Jossey-Bass Publications, 1990.

Miller, E. "Shared Decision Making By Itself Doesn't Make For Better Decisions." In *Harvard Education Letter,* XI(6) (November/December 1995), 1-4.

Milne, A. A. *The World of Pooh.* London: McClelland and Stewart Limited Publishers, 1957.

Milroy, E. *Role Play: A Practical Guide.* Aberdeen: Aberdeen University Press, 1982.

Modra, H. "Using Learning Journals to Encourage Critical Thinking at a Distance." In *Critical Reflection in Distance Education,* T. Evans and D. Nation (eds.). Philadelphia: Taylor and Francis Publishers, 1989.

Moffett, J. *The Universal Schoolhouse: Spiritual Awakening through Education.* San Francisco: Jossey-Bass Publications, 1994.

Moustakas, C. *The Authentic Teacher: Sensitivity and Awareness in the Classroom.* Cambridge, MA: Howard Doyle, 1997.

Murphy, J., and Lewis, K. *Handbook of Research in Educational Administration.* San Francisco: Jossey-Bass Publications, 1999.

NAESP. *Proficiencies for Principles.* Revised. Alexandria, VA: NASPP, 1991.

National Institute of Education. *Involvement in Learning: Realizing the Potential of American Higher Education.* Washington, D.C.: National Institute of Education, 1984.

Neuman, Erich. *The Origins and History of Consciousness.* Princeton, NJ: Princeton Universtiy Press, 1973.

Neuschel, Robert. *The Servant Leader: Unleashing the Power of Your People.* East Lansing, MI: Visions Sports Management Group, Inc., 1998.

Nichols, M. P. *The Lost Art of Listening.* New York: Guilford Press, 1995.

North, Vanda, and Buzan, Tony. *Get Ahead! Mind Map Your Way to Success.* Bournemouth, MA: Buzan Centre Books, 1991.

Oakeshott, M. *Rationalism in Politics: And Other Essays.* New York: Basic Books, 1962.

Ostrander, Sheila, and Schroeder, Lynn. *Superlearning.* New York: Laurel Confucian Press Books, 1979.

Ozar, D. "Building Awareness of Ethical Standards and Conduct". In *Educating Professionals: Responding to New Expectations for Competence and Accountability.* San Francisco: Jossey-Bass Publications, 1989.

Palmer, Parker. *The Courage To Teach.* San Francisco: Jossey-Bass Publications, 1998.

Palmer, Parker. "The Grace of Great Things: Reclaiming the Sacred in Knowing, Teaching and Learning." In *The Heart of Learning: Spirituality in Education,* S. Glazer (ed.). New York: Jeremy Tarcher/Putnam, 1999.

Parsons, T. "Professions." In *International Encyclopedia of the Social Sciences,* D. L. Sills (ed.), Vol 12 (1968). New York: Macmillan.

Paul, R. "Dialogical Thinking: Critical Thought Essential to the Acquisition of Relational Knowledge and Passions." In *Teaching Thinking Skills: Theory and Practice,* J. Baron and R. Sternberg (eds). New York: W. H. Freeman Publishers, 1986.

Pearson, S. Carol. *The Hero Within: Six Archetypes We Live By.* San Francisco: Harper and Row Publishers, 1989.

Perry, W. G., Jr. *Forms of Intellectual and Ethical Development in the College Years.* Troy, MO: Holt, Rinehart and Winston, 1970.

Peters, T. J., and Waterman, R. H. *In Search of Excellence: Lessons from America's Best-Run Companies.* New York: Harper and Row Publishers, 1982.

Phillips-Jones, L. *The New Mentors and Proteges: How to Succeed with the New Mentoring Partnerships.* Grass Valley, CA: Coalition of Counseling Centers, 1993.

Pratt, D. D. "Three Perspectives on Teacher Effectiveness". In *Proceedings of the Adult Education Research Conference.* Calgary, CAN: Faculty of Continuing Education, University of Calgary, 1988.

Rannells, Saul, J. "Women Speak about Their Learning Experiences in Higher Education." In *Proceedings of the Adult Education Research Conference, #30*. Madison, WI: Department of Continuing and Vocational Education, University of Wisconsin-Madison, 1989.

Resnick, L. *Education and Learning to Think*. Washington, D.C.: National Academy Press, 1987.

Rest, J. "A Psychologist Looks at the Teaching of Ethics." In *Hastings Center Report*, 12 (1982), 29-36.

Rest, J. "Morality." In *Manual of Child Psychology*, P. Mussed (ed.), *Vol 3 (1983)*. New York: Wiley.

Rice, Eugene, and Richlin, Laurie. "Broadening the Cencept of Scholarship in the Professions." In *Educating Professionals: Responding to New Expectations for Competence and Accountability*, L. Curry and J. Wergin (eds.). San Francisco: Jossey-Bass Publications, 2000.

Rilke, Rainer Maria. *Rodin and Other Prose Pieces*. London: Aquartet Books Limited, 1986.

Robbins, H., and Finley, M. *Why Teams Don't Work: What Went Wrong and How to Make It Work*. Princeton, NJ: Pacesetter Books, 1995.

Robinson, J., Saberton, S., and Griffin, V. (eds.). *Learning Partnerships: Interdependent Learning in Adult Education*. Toronto: Ontario Institute for Studies in Education, Department of Adult Education, 1985.

Rogers, Carl. *A Way of Being*. Boston: Houghton Mifflin Publishing, 1980.

Rogers, J. *Adults Learning* (third ed.). Philadelphia: Open University Press, 1989.

Rose, Colin, and Nicholl, Malcolm J. *Accelerated Learning for the 21st Century*. New York: Delacorte Press, 1997.

Rowe, Todd. *Homeopathic Methodology: Repertory, Case Taking and Case Analysis*. Berkeley, CA: North Atlantic Books, 1998.

Rowe, Todd, and Hesselmann, Lesley. *Building a Strong Homeopathic Community*. Copyright 2000; to be published.

Ruskin, K. B., and Achilles, C. M. *Grantwriting, Fundraising and Partnerships: Strategies That Work!*. Thousand Oaks, CA: Corwin, 1995.

Salzberger-Wittenberg, I., Henry, G, and Osborne, E. *The Emotional Experience of Teaching and Learning*. New York: Routledge, Chapman & Hall, 1983. Sankaran, P. *The Elements of Homeopathy: Volume Two*. Santa Cruz, CA: Homeopathic Medical Publishers, 1996.

Sankaran, R. *The Substance of Homeopathy*. Bombay: Homeopathic Medical Publishers, 1994. Bombay.

Scheele, Paul R. *Photoreading*. Wayzata, MN: Learning Strategies Corp, 1999.

Schein, E. *Organizational Culture and Leadership*. San Francisco: Jossey-Bass Publications, 1985 and 1991.

Schlossberg, W. K., Lynch, A. Q., and Chickering, A. W. *Improving Higher Education Environment for Adults*. San Francisco: Jossey-Bass Publications, 1989.

Schon, D. A. *The Reflective Practitioner: How Professionals Think in Action*. New York: Basic Books, 1983.

Schon, D. A. *Educating the Reflective Practitioner: Toward a New Design for Teaching and Learning in the Professions*. San Francisco: Jossey Bass Publications, 1987.

Schon, D. A. (ed.). *The Reflective Turn: Case Studies in and on Educational Practice*. New York: Teachers College Press, 1991.

Schwartz, W. *School Dropouts: New Information about an Old Problem*. Washington, D. C.: Office of Educational Research and Development, EDO-OD-96-5, 1995.

Senge, Peter. *The Fifth Discipline: The Art and Practice of the Learning Organization*. New York: Doubleday Currency, 1990.

Sergiovanni, T., and Starratt, R. J. *Supervision: Human Perspectives*. New York: McGraw-Hill, 1998.

Shakeshaft, C. S. *Women in Educational Administration*. Newbury Park, CA: Sage Publications, 1987.

Shapiro, J. P., and Stefkovich, H. "Preparing Ethical Leaders for Equitable Schools." In *Ethics in Educational Leadership Programs,* L. Beck and J. Murphy (eds.), Columbia, MO: UCEA, 1997.

Sherwin, Susan. *No Longer Patient: Feminist Ethics and Health Care*. Philadelphia: Temple University Press, 1992.

Shor, I. *Culture Wars: School and Society in the Conservative Restoration*. New Yrok: Routledge, Chapman and Hall, 1986.

Shor, I., and Freire, P. A. *Pedagogy for Liberation: Dialogues on Transforming Education*. Granby, MA: Bergin and Garvey Publishers, 1987.

Sizer, T. R. *Horaces' Hope: What Works for the American High School*. Boston: Houghton, Mifflin, 1996.

Slavin, R. *Cooperative Learning: Theory, Research and Practice*. Englewood Cliffs, NJ: Prentice-Hall, 1990.

Smith, M. L., and Glass, G. V. "Meta-analysis of Psychotherapy Outcome Studies". In *American Psychologist,* 32 (1977), 995-1008.

Smyth, W. J. *A Rationale for Teachers' Critical Pedagogy: A Handbook.* Victoria, Australia: Deakin University Press, 1986.

Snow, C. P. *The Corridors of Power.* New York: Macmillan Press, 1964.

Spear, G. "Beyond the Organizing Circumstance: A Search for Methodology for the Study of Self-Directed Learning." In *Self-Directed Learning: Application and Theory,* H. B. Long and Associates (eds.). Athens, GA: Department of Adult Education, University of Georgia, 1988.

Spear, G., and Mocker, D. "The Organizing Circumstance: Environmental Determinants in Self-Directed Learning." In *Adult Education Quarterly,* 35(1) (1984), 1-10.

"Standards and Competencies for the Professional Practice of Homeopathy in North America." Report of a Summit Meeting sponsored by the Council for Homeopathic Education, 2001.

Starr, P. *The Social Transformation of American Medicine.* New York: Basic Books, 1982.

Starratt, R. J. *Building an Ethical School: A Practical Response to the Moral Crisis in Schools.* London: Falmer Press, 1994.

Sternberg, R., and Frensch, P. "Mechanism of Tranfer." In D. Detterman and R. Sternberg (eds.), *Transfer on Trial: Intelligence, Cognition and Instruction.* Norwood, NJ: Ablex, 1993.

Stevens, R. and Slavin, R. E. "Effects of a Cooperative Learning Approach in Reading and Writing on Academically Handicapped and Nonhandicapped Students. In *Elementary School Journal,* 95(3) (1995), 241-262.

Stiles, W. B., Shapiro, D., and Elliot, R. "Are All Psychotherapies Equivalent?" In *American Psychologist,* 41 (1986), 165-180.

Tanner, D., and Tanner, L. N. *Curriculum Development: Theory Into Practice.* Englewood Cliffs, NJ: Prentice-Hall, 1995.

Tarule, J.M. "Voices of Returning Women: Ways of Knowing." In L. H. Lewis (ed.), *Addressing the Needs of Returning Women.* New Directors for Continuing Education, Jossey-Bass Publishers, San Francisco, 39 (1988).

Tennant, M., and Pogson, P. *Learning and Change in the Adult Years: A Developmental Perspective.* San Francisco: Jossey-Bass Publications, 1995.

Thompson, J. D. *Organizations in Action.* New York: McGraw-Hill, 1967.

Tomain, J. P., and Solimine, M. E. "Skills Skepticism in the Postclinic World." In *Journal of Legal Education,* 40(3) (1990) 307-320.

Topping, K. *The Peer Tutoring Handbook: Promoting Cooperative Learning.* Cambridge, MA: Brookline Books, 1988.

Van der Zee, Harry. *Miasms in Labour.* Haren, The Netherlands: Stichting Alonnisos Publications, 2000.

Van Ments, M. *The Effective Use of Role Play: A Handbook for Teachers and Trainers* (2nd ed.). New York: Nichols Publications, 1989.

Vargas, L. A., and Willis, D. J. "New Directions in the Treatment of Ethnic Minority Children and Adolescents." In *Journal of Clinical Child Psychology*, 23 (1994).

Vella, J. *Learning to Listen, Learning to Teach: The Power of Dialogue in Educating Aadultss.* Sand Francisco: Jossey-Bass Publications, 1994.

Wales, Chales E., Nardi, Anne H., and Stager, Robert A. "Emphasizing Critical Thinking and Problem Solving." In L. Curry and J. Wergin (eds.), *Educating Professionals: Responding to New Expectations for Competence and Accountability.* San Francisco: Jossey-Bass Publications, 1993.

Wallechinsky, David. *The Book of Lists.* New York: William Morrow Company, IInc., 1977.

Webb, L. D., and Norton, M. S. *Human Resource Administration.* New York: Merrill, 1999.

Wheatley, M. *Leadership and the New Science.* San Francisco: Berrett-Koehler, 1992.

Whitman, N. A. *Peer Teaching: To Teach Is to Learn Twice.* ASHE-ERIC Higher Education Report, #4 (1988). Washington, D.C.: Association for the Study of Higher Education.

Williams, G. *Western Reserve's Experiment in Medical Education and Its Outcomes.* New York: Oxford University Press, 1980.

Winston, Julian. *The Faces of Homeopathy: An Illustrated History of the First 200 Years.* Tawa, New Zealand: Great Auk Publishing, 1999.

Wurman, R. S. *Information Anxiety.* New York: Doubleday, 1989.

Yalom, Irvin D. *Love's Executioner and Other Tales of Psychotherapy.* New York: Harper Perennial Publishers, 1981.

Yukl, G. A. *Leadership in Organizations.* Englewood Cliffs, NJ: Prentice-Hall Publications, 1989.

Zachary, Lois. *The Mentor's Guide.* San Francisco: Jossey-Bass Publications, 2000.

Index

Bennis, Warren 204
Berends, Polly, 120
Blake, William, 11
Bolman, Lee, and Deal, Terrence, 201,
206, 211
Boundaries, 120, 124, 139, 150, 202
Bowen, Elizabeth, 75
Boyer, 90
Brecht, Bertolt, 241
Browning, Robert, 56
Buck, Pearl, 187
Buddha, 190, 194
Burn out, 71, 90-1
Buscaglia, Leo, 50

C

Campbell, Joseph, 16, 43
Camus, Albert, 44
Cantor, Nathaniel, 49
Carlson, Richard and Bailey, Joseph, 268
Carlyle, Thomas, 258
Carter, Forrest, 96
Carter, Jimmy, 266
Cases, failed, 12, 88, 134
Case taking (see teaching, clinical
training)
Case management (see teaching)
Celebrations, 26, 219-21, 231, 248, 257
initiation, 220
Certification, 13, 21, 23, 40, 105,
106, 127, 227, 235-6, 238-9,
247, 251, 336-9
Challenge, 5, 12, 13, 19, 22, 30, 34,
35, 37, 40, 48, 50, 55, 66, 75, 79,
80, 97, 103, 106, 106, 108, 109,
112, 114, 120, 121, 123-4, 128,
129, 131, 134, 135, 145, 146,
162, 169, 174, 186, 191, 194-5,
198, 200, 206, 211, 216, 231,
236, 237, 242, 244, 251, 252, 262
Chaos theory, 70
Charisma, 171
Cheney, Charles, 268
Chesterfield, Lord, 81
Chomsky, Noam, 93
Choosing a homeopathic program (see
training programs)
Churchill, Winston, 244
Cicero, Marcus Tullius, 68

Civility, 53
Class
discussion, 12, 76, 96-9, 100, 113,
115, 116, 119, 141, 185, 199
exercises, 12, 112, 135, 311
introductory, 174-181, 223, 225
power issues in, 87-88
Cleese, John, 262
Clinical training, 4,11,12,21, 22,
36-40, 112-18, 127-156, 226,
236, 247, 256-58, 282
acting as if, 37
apprenticeship, 36
attitudes, 131-7
billing, 139
business issues, 12, 139
case recording, 139
case taking, 37-8
certification, 40
clearing the energy, 37, 138
clinics, 147-8
communication skills, 62, 116,
117-18, 122, 132, 139
confidentiality, 140
consultation, 13
designing, 12
emergencies, 12
emotional expression, 133
ending sessions, 138
fear of the unknown, 38
greetings, 138
informed consent, 138
interpersonal skills, 37
knowledge, 12, 137-143
listening, 9, 37, 61, 128, 135
models, 12, 145-46
observation, 12, 146-47, 239
patients as teachers, 37
practice, importance of, 36-37
preparation for, 40
purpose, 129
renewal during, 37-38
schools of thought, 130
setting the tone, 138
skills, 12, 131-7
structure, 129